MW01641199

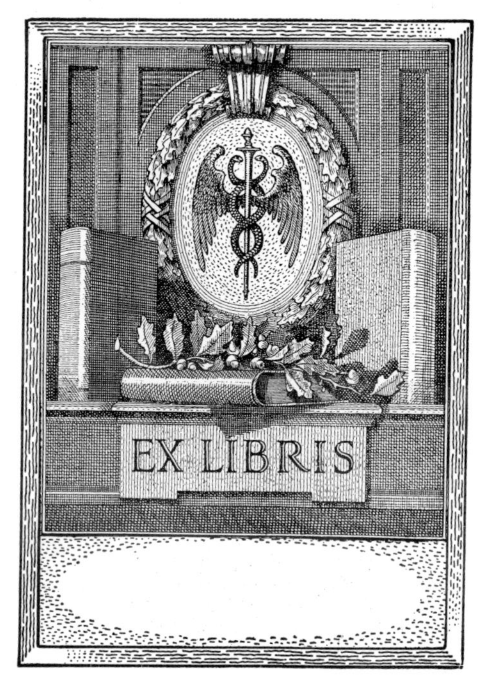
EX LIBRIS

Periodontal Disease
in Children and Adolescents

Periodontal Disease

in Children and Adolescents

PAUL N. BAER, D.D.S.

Diplomate, American Board of Periodontology, Professor and Chairman, Department of Periodontics, State University of New York at Stony Brook, School of Dental Medicine, Stony Brook, New York

SHELDON D. BENJAMIN, D.D.S.

Diplomate, American Board of Periodontology, Clinical Professor of Periodontics, University of Southern California in Los Angles, Consultant in Periodontics, Childrens' Hospital, Los Angeles

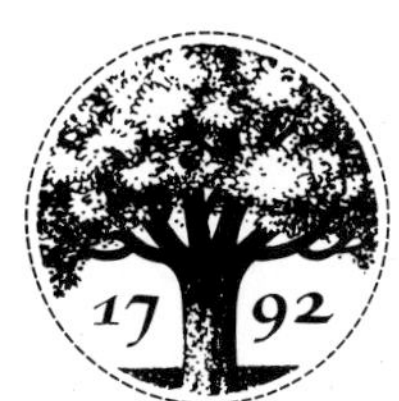

J. B. Lippincott Company

Philadelphia • Toronto

ISBN 0-397-50297-4
Library of Congress Catalog Card Number 73-15915
Printed in the United States of America

Library of Congress Cataloging in Publication Data

Baer, Paul N
Pediatric and Adolescent periodontology.

Includes bibliographies.
1. Pediatric periodontia. I. Benjamin, Sheldon D., joint author. II. Title. [DNLM: 1. Periodontal diseases—In adolescence. 2. Periodontal diseases—In infancy and childhood. WU240 B141p 1973]
RK306. C5B33 617.6′32 73-15915
ISBN 0-397-50297-4

To
Our Wives and Children
Without Whom It All
Might Still Have Been Possible
But Not Half as Much Fun

Contributors

Frank G. Everett D.M.D., M.D., M.S.
University of Oregon Dental School

Henry M. Goldman D.M.D.
Dean, Professor of Stomatology
Boston University
School of Graduate Dentistry

Corey H. Holmes D.D.S., M.SC.
Georgetown University
School of Dentistry

Hugh Kopel D.D.S.
University of Southern California
School of Dentistry

Gerald Lubin M.D.
Children's Hospital of Los Angeles and
University of Southern California School of Medicine

Maury Massler D.D.S., M.S.
Tufts University
School of Dental Medicine

Olaf Mickelsen Ph.D.
Michigan State University
College of Human Ecology

Morris P. Ruben D.D.S.
Assistant Dean, Professor of Stomatology
Boston University
School of Graduate Dentistry

Herbert L. Tanenbaum M.D.
Consultant, National Heart and Lung Institute;
Senior Attending, Cardiology, Washington Hospital
Center; Assistant Clinical Professor of Medicine,
Georgetown University,
School of Medicine

Preface

The idea for this book originated from a series of lectures first presented to graduate students in orthodontics and pedodontics. During this period of time, it became increasingly clear, that while textbooks on periodontology were generally in agreement that the onset of periodontal disease frequently originated during childhood or adolescence, minimal attention was given to the specific periodontal and oral problems which occurred during this most important period of life. It also became evident that systemic diseases which were reflected within the oral cavity in childhood and adolescence were frequently interrelated and many times confused with local diseases of the periodontium. Therefore, we felt it necessary to combine in a single textbook discussion of the diseases of the periodontium along with those systemic diseases which had oral manifestations.

Current knowledge on the etiology of the most common of all the destructive periodontal diseases, namely periodontitis, has established that it is largely preventible and arrestable. It is also a disease entity that is extremely well covered in all the recent textbooks on periodontology and there was little new that we could add. For these reasons juvenile periodontitis has been given minimal coverage in our book. Periodontosis or essential periodontitis, on the other hand, which is neither a common disease nor as amenable to treatment, is given extensive coverage, since this material is not as readily available.

Each chapter is a separate unit and may be randomly selected for study without adversely affecting the whole.

In brief, this book was written to fill a void. In doing this we have summarized our personal experiences and have reviewed the pertinent literature involving investigations on the etiology and treatment of the various periodontal diseases found in children and adolescents.

The bibliographies, rather than being all inclusive, have been carefully and selectively chosen. Furthermore, it is not the purpose of our book to describe basic "how-to-do-it" techniques, but rather to give to the practicing dentist and physician insight into the oral problems which they may encounter in treating patients in this age group. For these reasons we believe this book should prove to be useful to the student who desires extra "elective" knowledge, to the general dentist, the pedodontist, the periodontist and the pediatrician.

Paul N. Baer, D.D.S.
Sheldon D. Benjamin, D.D.S.

Acknowledgments

The chapters on the normal periodontium and the pathology of periodontal disease in children was largely the work of Dr. Henry M. Goldman and Dr. Morris P. Ruben. Dr. Frank G. Everett collaborated on the section on periodontosis. Dr. Herbert L. Tanenbaum was principally responsible for the patient with chronic heart disease. Dr. Hugh Kopel made major contributions to the treatment of the handicapped patient. Adolescent nutrition was the work of Dr. Olaf Mickelsen. Dr. Maury Massler and Dr. Corey H. Holmes contributed material to the chapter on prevention. Dr. Gerald Lubin was principally responsible for the chapter on the psychological management of the adolescent patient.

We are deeply indebted to our contributors and wish to express our appreciation for their contributions. However, in all instances, the final version of each chapter as to wording and ideas is our own responsibility.

Paul N. Baer, D.D.S.
Sheldon D. Benjamin, D.D.S.

Contents

1
The Normal Periodontium

GROWTH AND DEVELOPMENT

The periodontium during childhood and puberty is in a constant state of change owing to the exfoliation and eruption of the teeth. This makes a general description of the normal periodontium difficult because it varies with the age of the patient. Zappler,[18] however, has attempted a general description of the juvenile periodontium, listing its characteristics as follows:

Gingiva

1. *More reddish,* because of thinner and

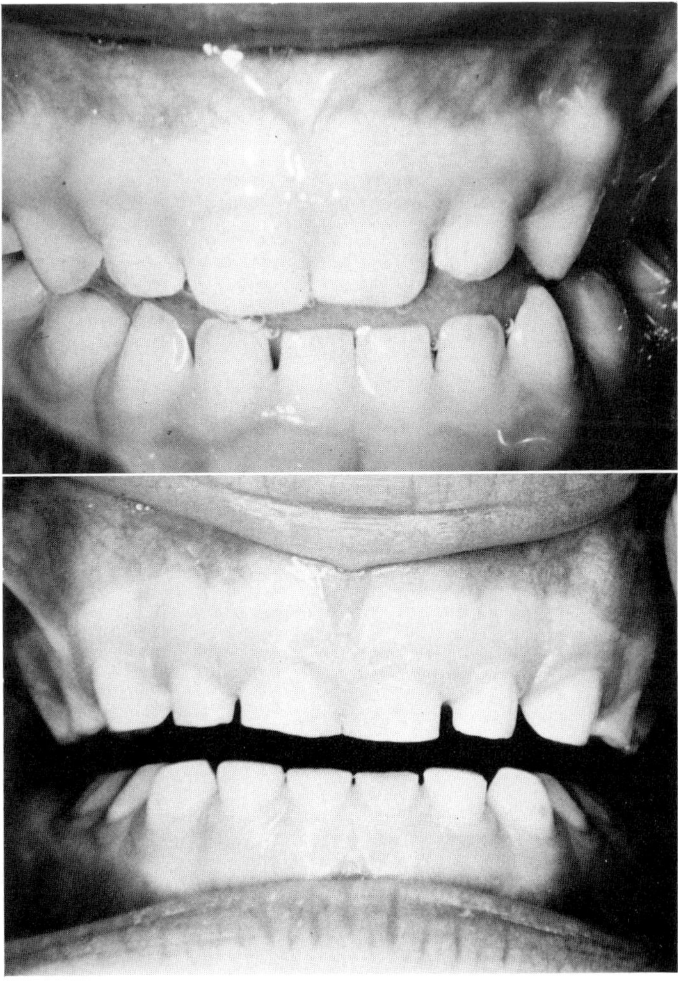

Fig. 1-1. *Top.* Normal gingiva in a 4-year-old child. The gingiva is firm and not readily retractable; there is usually a well-defined zone of attached gingiva present. *Bottom.* Normal gingiva in a 3-year-old child. Note wear facets (bruxism is common in young children).

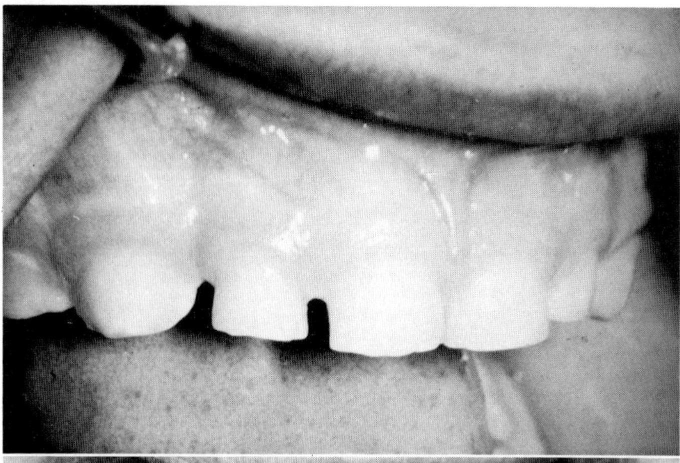

Fig. 1-2. Diastema formation is normal in the anterior region (6-year-old child).

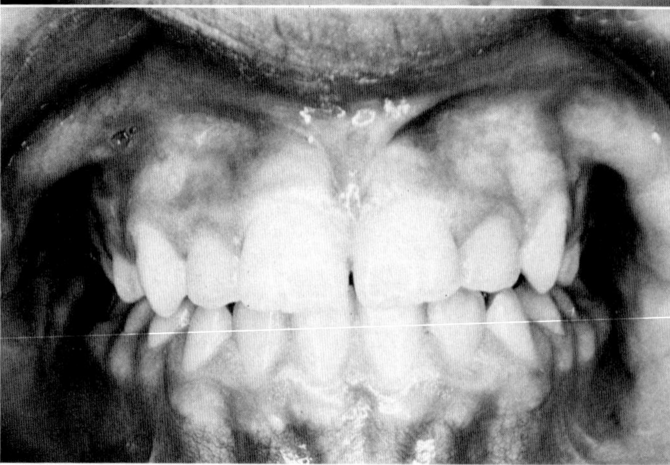

Fig. 1-3. Normal gingiva in a 10-year-old child. The gingiva margin is still not at its adult level. It is too high coronally. Passive eruption is generally not completed before the late teenage period.

less hornified epithelium and greater vascularity
2. *Lacks stippling,* because of the shorter and flatter connective papillae of the lamina propria
3. *Flabbier,* associated with decreased density of the connective tissue of the lamina propria
4. *Rounded and rolled margins,* related to hyperemia and edema that accompanies eruption
5. *Greater sulcular depth,* relative ease of gingival retraction

Cementum

1. Thinner
2. Less dense
3. Tendency to hyperplasia of cementoid apical to the epithelial attachment (quoting Gottlieb)

Periodontal membrane

1. Wider
2. Fiber bundles less dense with less fibers per unit area
3. Increased hydration, greater blood and lymph supply

Alveolar bone

1. Thinner lamina dura (radiologically)
2. Fewer trabeculae
3. Larger marrow spaces
4. Decreased degree of calcification
5. Greater blood and lymph supply

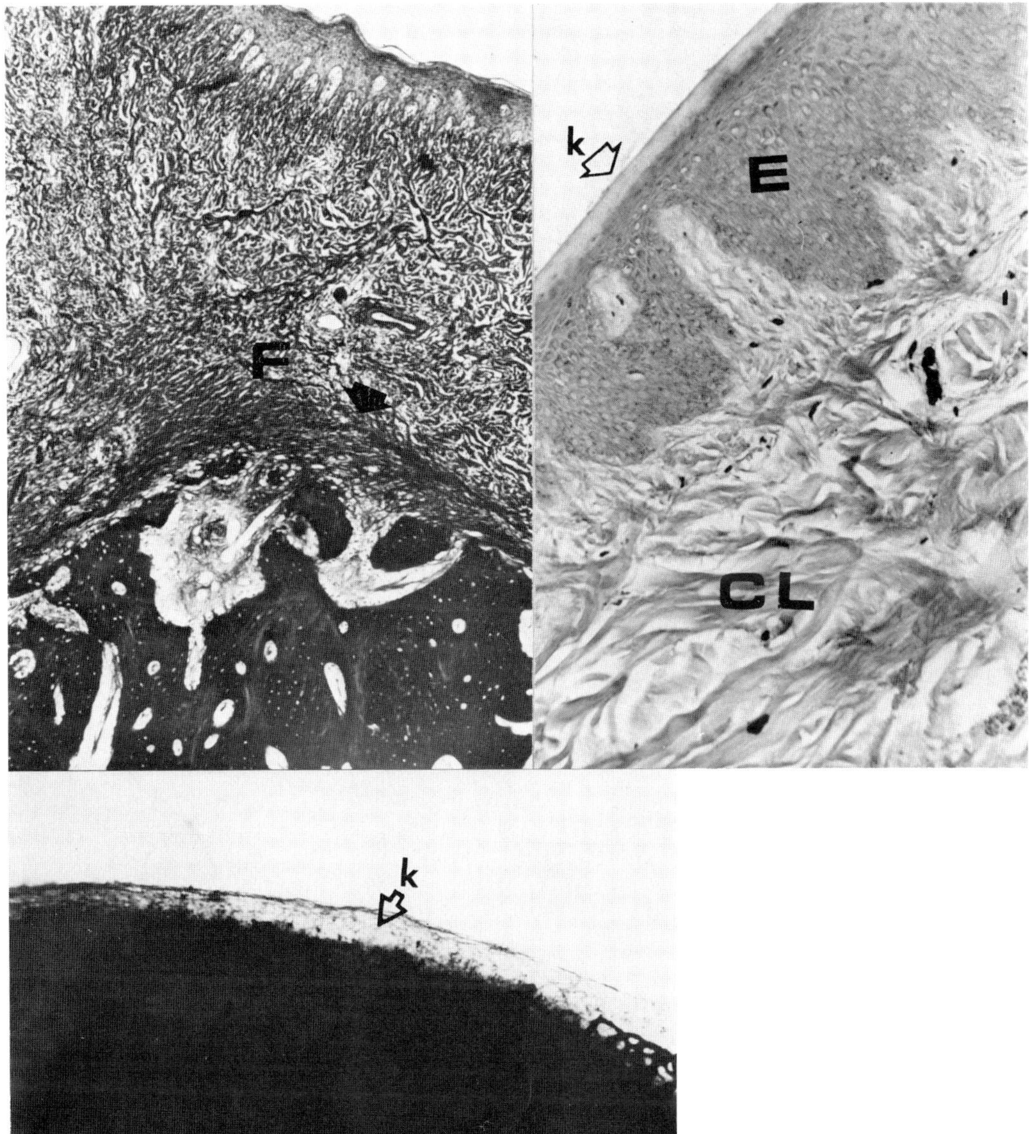

Fig. 1-4. *Top left.* Buccolingual section through interdental hard and soft tissues; an interdental diastema was present. Interdental gingiva is structured comparably to attached gingiva with dense collagenous corium and keratinizing epithelial cover. The soft tissue complex is usually tightly bound to crestal bone by means of anchoring fibers. *F* is the periosteal portion of the gingiva. *Top right.* This 100X photomicrograph reveals the quality of interdental epithelium (*E*) in the diastema zone. A definitive stratum corneum is indicated at *k*; it may be either para- or orthokeratotic. Both can be limiting to the penetration of exogenous irritants into the tissue (generally, only lipid-soluble substances may enter). The gingival corium (*CL*) is notable for stable and well-oriented collagen. *Bottom.* Perfusion specimen (dog perfused through carotid artery with patent blue violet and carbon suspension). The blue-dyed vascular transudate flows freely into the epithelium (*black band*) and is prevented from passing into the oral cavity by the stratum corneum (*k*).

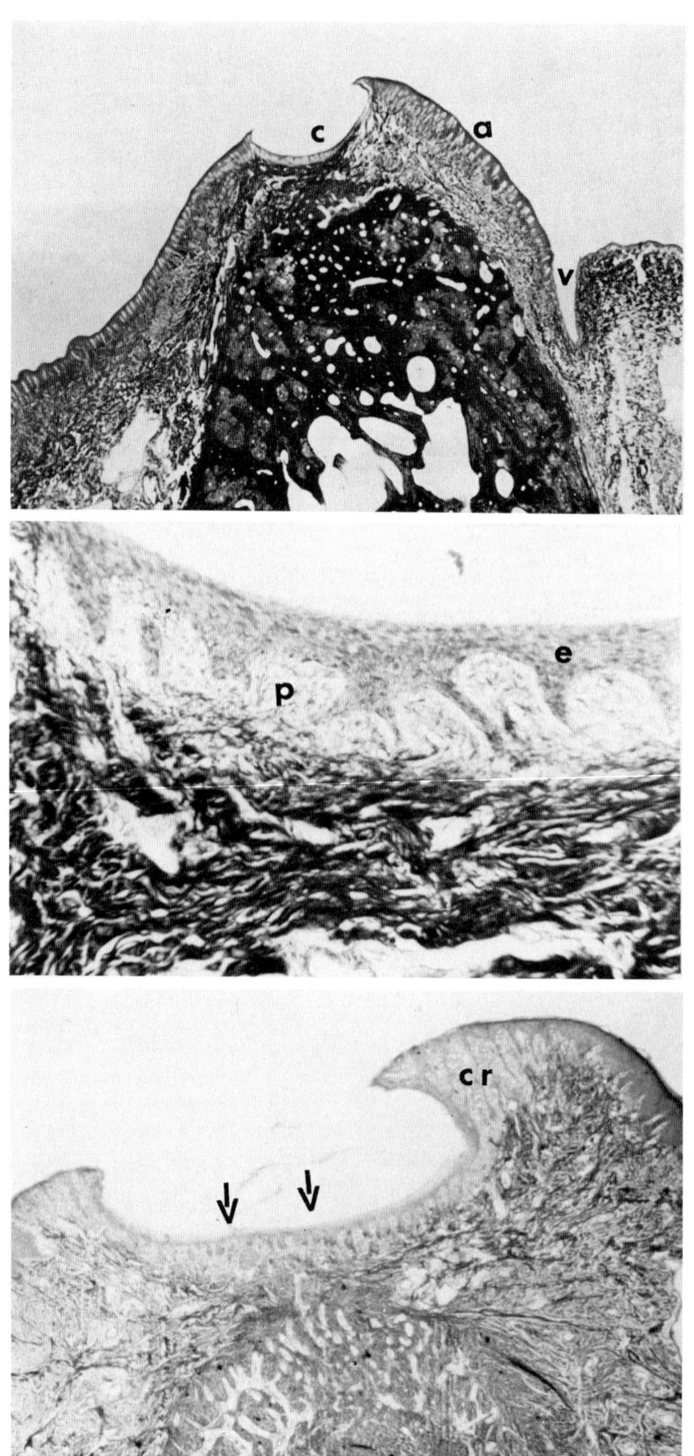

Fig. 1-5. *Top.* The bucco-lingual section (trichrome stain) through the interdental septum and contiguous soft tissues. The concavity (*c*) represents the col configuration of gingiva, the soft tissues conforming to the shape and dimensions of the proximal dental contact. It is lined by stratified squamous epithelium, thin and devoid of keratinization. *a* indicates the buccal zone of attached gingiva surmounted by keratinizing epithelium. *v* is the vestibular fornix. In this case the zone of attached gingiva is very broad apico-occlusally, while the dimension of alveolar mucosa is narrow. *Center.* In this 100X magnification of col epithelium and subjacent gingival corium note that the epithelium (*e*) is hyperplastic, an incipient response in inflammation. The area of ulceration is not evident; however, even the widening of the intercellular areas should be considered the equivalent of ulceration, since the deficiencies at the interface of epithelial cells allow bacteria and their toxins (exo- and/or endo-) to pass through the epithelial zone into the gingival lamina propria (*p*). There is reduction of collagen in the superficial aspect of the corium; resorption is mediated by enzyme activity. *Bottom.* In this more advanced interdental inflammation, the arrows point to inflammatory process at the col base. An inflammatory state has extended to involve both buccal (*cr*) and lingual walls of the col.

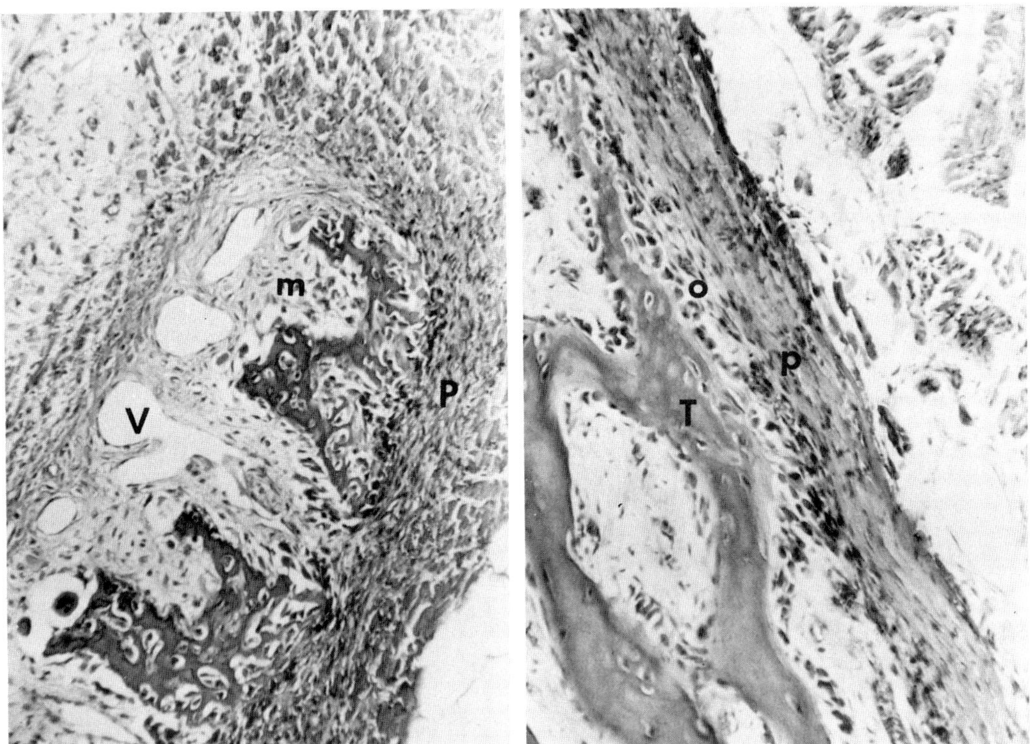

Fig. 1-6. *Left.* Developing alveolar process in fetus (about 6 months gestation). Highly cellular new bone adjacent to developing tooth. Trabecular pattern is evident without formation of buccal cortical plate. Cortices of a lamellated nature tend to be "completed" as the alveolar processes develop to their physiologic maximum in middle/late adolescence; osteogenesis becomes relatively quiescent on periosteal aspects of septa at this time. (*P*) periosteum; highly cellular adjacent to bone. *m* is the marrow area rich in osteoblasts contiguous to bone. *V* is the vascular channels. *Right.* Higher magnification of prenatal osteogenetic activity. *T* represents bony trabeculum with included osteocytes. Osteoblasts (*o*) as a part of the periosteum (*p*) engaged in elaboration of osteoid, seen here as a pale (eosinophilic) substance adjacent to osteoblasts.

6. Flatter alveolar crests associated with primary teeth

Similar comparisons are found in Finn's text and in publications by Cohen[4] and Bradley.[2]

In general, the authors agree with these descriptions, noting certain modifications: The gingiva in the young child with a totally deciduous dentition is generally pink and firm, with a well-defined zone of attached gingiva; it does not appear to be either reddish or flabby, as Zappler stated. The width of the attached gingiva varies between 1 and 6 mm. for the primary dentition and between 1 and 9 mm. for the adult dentition.[1A] The narrowest zone of the attached gingiva is found in the region of the maxillary and mandibular first premolars or first bicuspids. The widest area is found in the maxillary and mandibular incisor region (Fig. 1-1 *Top*). Present evidence suggests that there is an increase in the mean width of the attached gingiva from the primary to the adult dentition. After maturity, however, there is little additional change. During the period of the mixed dentition, Zappler's findings that the

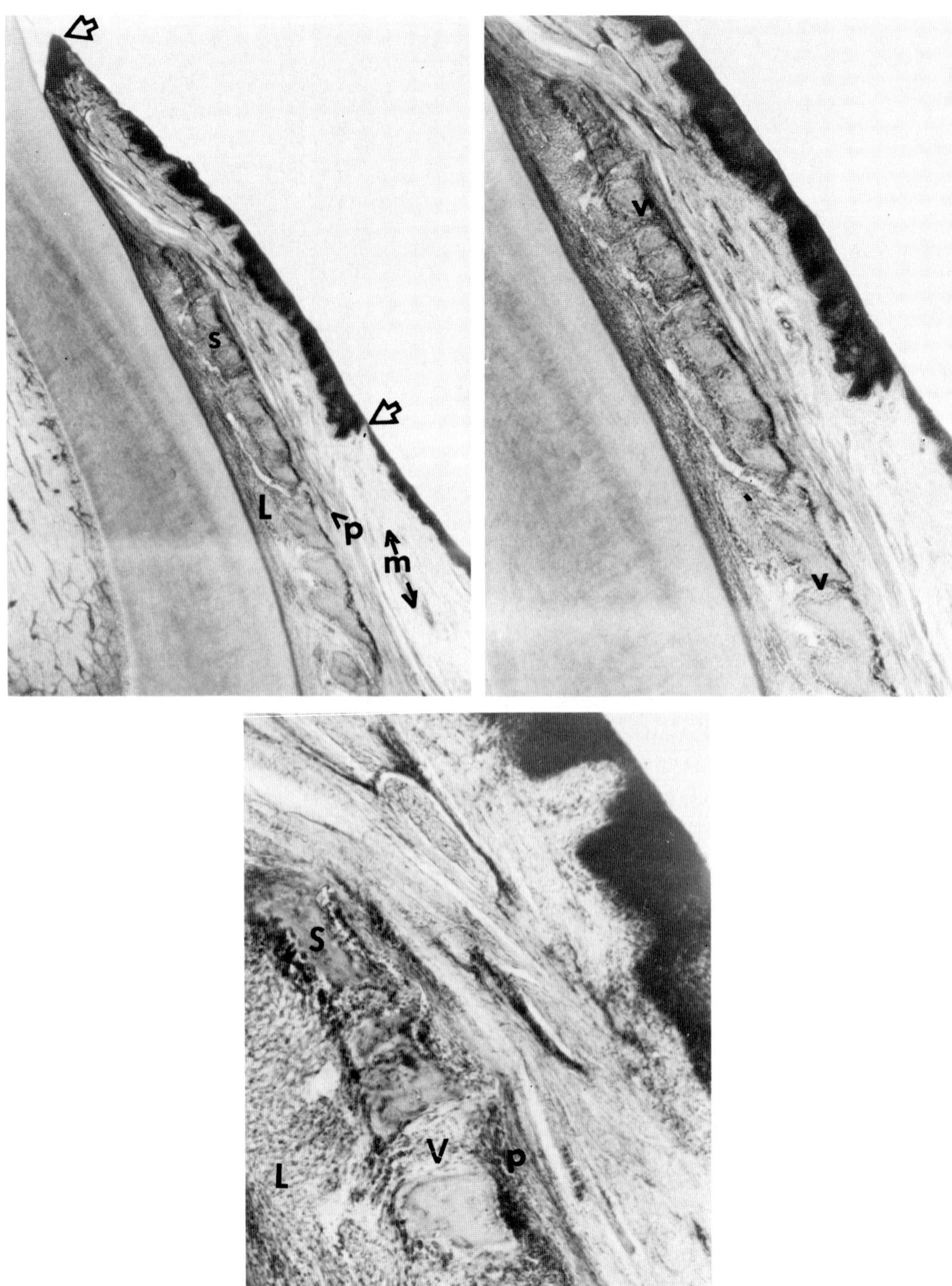

Fig. 1-7. *Top left.* The zone of attached gingiva (between *arrows*) in child tends to be inordinately wide in relationship to the width of the alveolar mucosa (←*m*→). Gingival connective tissue is usually denser and better organized than that of the alveolar mucosa. The epithelium of the attached gingiva is of the keratinizing type, while that of the alveolar mucosa lacks physiologic propensity for keratinization. The mucosa is resilient and pliable,

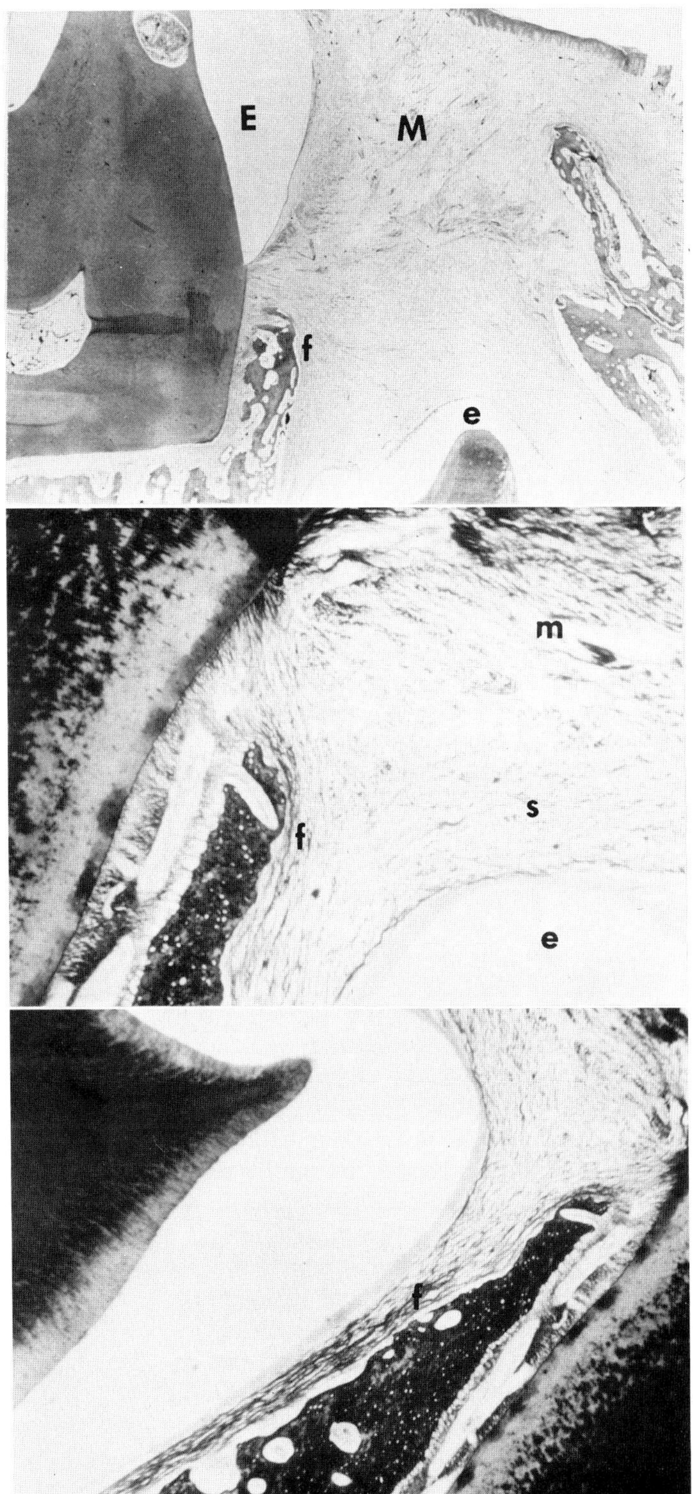

Fig. 1-10. *Top.* Tooth (*e*) is erupting from its bony crypt. A portion of the roof of the bone cavity has been resorbed and the dental sac of tooth is confluent with the connective tissue of the overlying retromolar mucosa (*M*). There is a paucity of collagen in such tissue, producing clinical flaccidity; adaptation to the crown of the tooth (at *E*) is long apico-occlusally and tends to be weakly apposed. The relationship favors plaque and debris accrual and initiation of inflammation, often of a clinically florid character. *F* shows the fibers of the dental sac. *Center.* Fibers of the dental sac (*f*) blend with supracrestal fibers and are the predecessors to the future transseptal fiber system. As the tooth erupts, there is shortening and remodeling of this fiber complex while the bone septum is apposed subjacently. Comparable processes take place at buccal and lingual aspects of teeth in the area of the Group C fiber system. *f* is the periosteal fibers; *m* is the mucosa; *s* is the dental sac; *e* is the enamel of the erupting tooth. *Bottom.* The developing transseptal fiber system at this time extends from the already erupted tooth *over* the bone crest alongside the septum (*f*) to insert into the cervical cementum of the forming and erupting tooth.

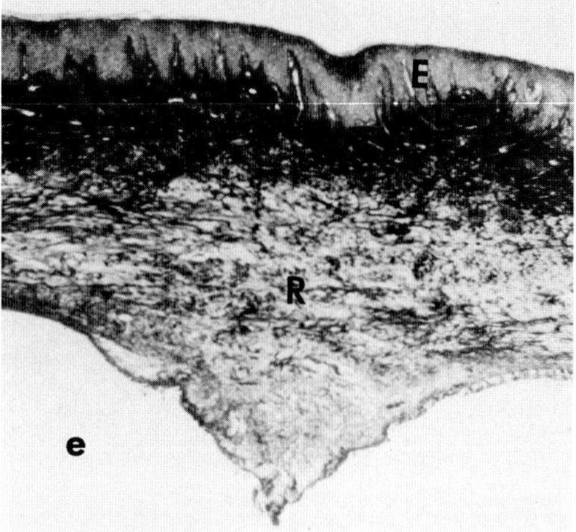

Fig. 1-11. Gingiva overlying erupting tooth (*e*). The dental sac has "blended" with the gingiva. The dense gingiva, cloaked in keratinizing epithelium (*E*), has a subjacent zone of tissue (*R*) manifesting collagen resorption. Collagen resorption leads to segmentation and disorientation of fibers, with their eventual dissolution and/or phagocytosis by tissue macrophages. Enzymatic dissolution possibly mediated by proteinases with collagenase potential, of fibroblastic origin. At this time the tooth crown is intimately covered by reduced enamel epithelium.

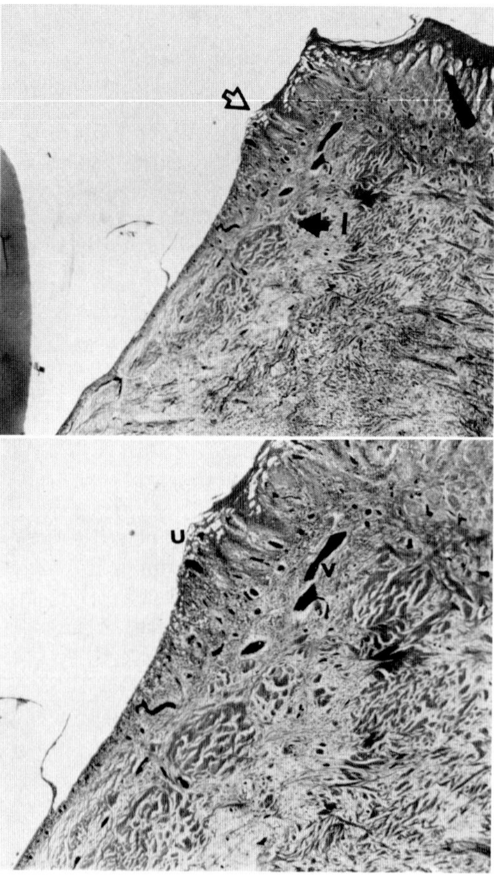

Fig. 1-12. *Top.* Retromolar mucosa. Note that the soft tissue's marginal level is nearly coincident with the disto-occlusal line angle of the tooth. Since this tissue is often weakly structured, with a deficit of organized and stable collagen, the approximation to the enamel of the distal surface may be tenuous. The deepened crevice favors plaque and debris lodgement. The resultant inflammatory lesion can be seen at arrows, the *open* arrow indicating the zone of epithelial ulceration and the *dark* arrow pointing grossly to the area of connective tissue resorption attending inflammatory process. Polychrome stain for connective tissue. *Bottom. u* is a closeup of the epithelial breach. Irregular black spots (*v*) represent perfused blood vessels (with Pelikan ink—Gunther Wagner), more numerous in inflammation as a consequence of augmented patency and blood vessel hyperplasia.

the eruption of the permanent teeth, is often characterized by incomplete passive eruption. One notes that there may be a long epithelial adherence to the enamel surface and that the gingival wall from the base of epithelial attachment to the gingival crest is relatively flaccid. The consequent retractability and diminished rigidity may be related to the large proportion of ground substance *to* collagen in the corium of the marginal gingiva. Melcher and Eastoe[12] have stated that young connective tissues are richer in protein-polysaccharide matrices, which are more markedly hydrated, than are older connective tissues. Sulfated protein-polysaccharides tend to increase with age. It is recognized that more "soluble" collagen is found in the young, with an increase in insolubility with aging.

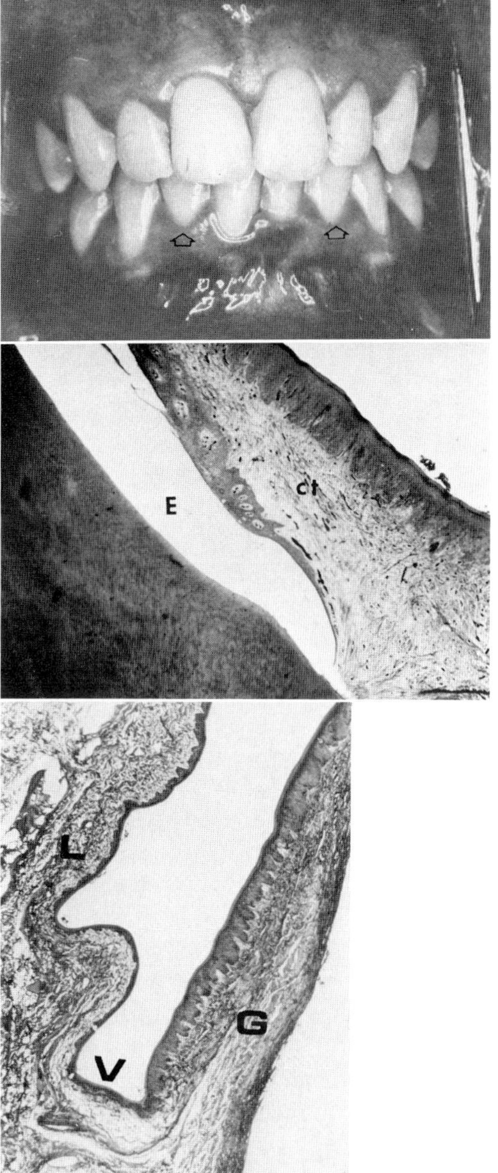

Fig. 1-13. *Top.* Teenage patient with multiple areas of gingivitis. Tissue distortion and color deepening are noticeable in papillary areas of maxillary anteriors. The mandibular gingival margin shows marked irregularity related to variability of the extent of passive eruption and to the edema and hyperplasia attending inflammation. The arrows point to two gingival zones of incomplete passive eruption. The distance from the gingival margin to the cemento-enamel junction is inordinately long; such gingiva may be weakly approximated to the enamel surface and clinically retractable and flaccid. *Center.* A histologic counterpart of the situation seen above. In this case fully one half of the distance from the cemento-enamel junction to the incisal edge of the tooth is covered by gingiva. The outer (surface) epithelium is of the keratinizing variety. The sulcular epithelium [next to enamel space (*E*)] is hyperplastic—an epithelial response to inflammation. The connective tissue (*ct*) has indifferent fiber organization along with collagenous deficit; abundance of tissue matrix connotes a myxomatous type of tissue. *Bottom.* Gingiva (*G*) abutting enamel (blank area at *right*) of erupting tooth. The cemento-enamel junction of the tooth is not in the photograph but is situated about 3 mm. below the observable base of soft tissue. The gingival wall is thin and retractable. The vestibular fornix is at *V* and is coronal to the cemento-enamel junction. *L* is mucosa on the inner aspect of the lip. This anomalous situation provides an environmental setting for accumulation of plaque, impairment of oral hygiene practices, and resultant "eruptive gingivitis."

As collagen "matures," its polypeptide chains become progressively more tightly cross-linked, with hydrogen and covalent bonding, while the fibers acquire greater tensile strength.

Histologically (Figs. 1-6 to 1-16) it is possible that the marginal gingiva of the young does not have the dense, well-oriented and organized collagen fiber systems seen in adult gingiva, but rather consists of numerous, more delicate collagen and reticulum fibers, deficient in the "bundle" arrangement evident in the adult. Thus it may be hypothesized that the strength of approximation of gingiva to the enamel is "weakened" because of incompletely differentiated circular and Groups A and B fiber complexes. The trans-septal and Group C fibers are excluded from this since they appear denser, well-aligned and with formed

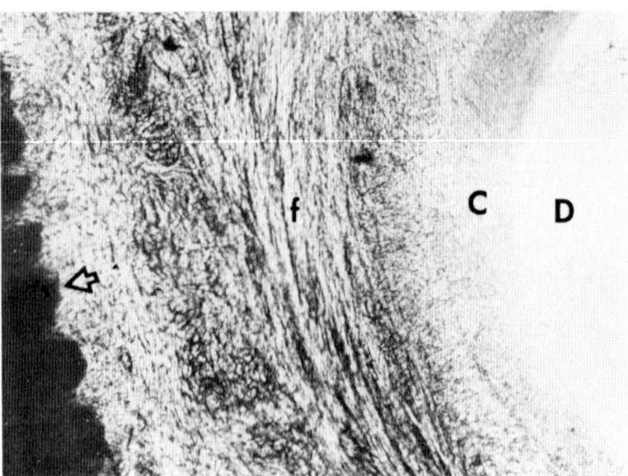

Fig. 1-14. Horizontal (x section) of tooth and supracrestal phase of gingiva. Unstained section cleared in methyl salicylate. *D* is dentin of the tooth. *C* is the cervical cementum. The arrow is in the area of subepithelial lamina propria and points to the gingival epithelium. The white semilunar and vertically directed striae (*f*) are the circular fibers of the gingival corium. These fibers are considered largely responsible for giving rigidity to the gingival wall (apico-occlusally from cemento-enamel junction to gingival margin) and for maintaining the soft tissue in tight approximation to the crown of the tooth. Their resorption (as in gingival inflammation) or their incomplete formation (as in incomplete passive eruption) lend to the retractability of tissue from the tooth.

attachments to cervical cementum and underlying bony septa. The Group C system also forms a continuum with periosteum. Although there is no information on the extent of development of the circular fiber complex in children, Arnim and Hagerman[1] postulate that their arrangement and quality contributed to tonus (i.e., support of the free gingiva and its adherence to the tooth surface). Loe[10] has added that since the fibers constitute the greater portion of the free gingiva, it is reasonable to assume that they are integral to the formation and continuance of the dentogingival relationship. This consideration of the characteristics of the marginal corium does not exclude the participation of any other factors in the preservation of the relationship, such as the ionic bonding of cells to the dental surface, the secretion of glycoprotein modalities from epithelial cells, the presence of a plasma filtrate or the effect of hemidesmosomes. One should note that the barrier of gingival attachment to tooth and bone appears to be well-developed at the time of tooth eruption and thereafter. In the child—even the edentulous infant—the zone of attached gingiva is firm, stippled, well bound to bone, and appears inordinately wide. The tooth erupts through the crestal aspect of this tissue with fibers of its dental sac merging with pre-existing gingival (periosteal aspect) collagen to form the trans-septal and Group III fiber complexes. This tooth emergence from the crypt and the blending of the dental sac with gingival collagen begins prior to the dental entry into the oral cavity and may continue, along with further development of the osseous phase, until the tooth reaches a functional occlusion. The collagenation of the basal aspect of the gingiva, its maturity and insolubility, and the tenacity of gingival attachment to bone and cementum may serve to limit the inroads of inflammatory disease into these areas (see chap. 2).

The gingiva of the young may also demonstrate a more extensive and patent vascularization at the marginal zone, made possible by reduction in containment of vascular patency, the extent of which is inversely proportionate to the degree of collagenation and matrical maturation of a tissue. This prominent vascularization may account for much transudation into the connective tissue proper, promoting its hydration, a looser constitution, and increase in turgidity. Furthermore, one would expect augmented passage of the transudate either into the sulcular area or into a more active venular and lymphatic drain. This fluid mediated "softening" of the connective tissue as well as the increased fluid transfer from the corium into the sulcus and the dentogingival interface may be responsible for the diminished adherence of the gingival wall to the tooth surface and may

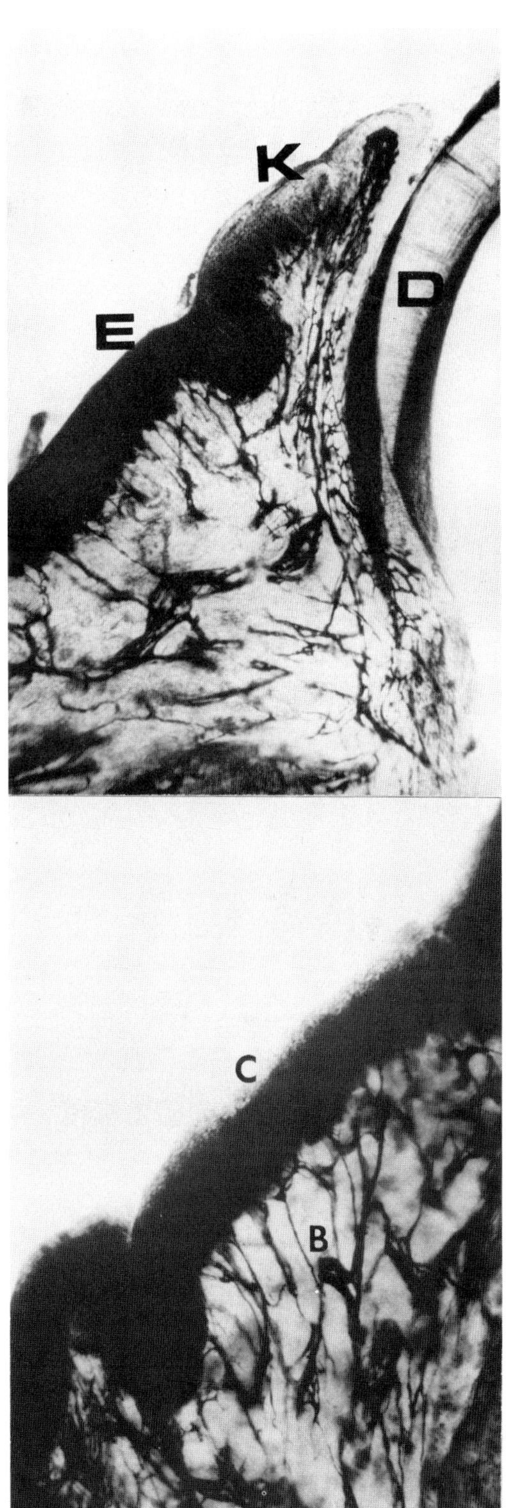

Fig. 1-15. *Top.* Cleared, perfused specimen of tooth (*D*) and associated gingiva. The gingival cuff at its buccal/labial/lingual phases is variably vascularized; centrally the number of patent vessels is decreased, conforming inversely to collagen density in the area. In the lamina propriae adjacent to the sulcular epithelium and to the outer epithelium (*E*) there are fairly elaborate networks of fine blood vessels. It is possible that much of the gingival fluid is derived from the subsulcular vascular arcade as a transudate or an exudate (in inflammation). *K* is the keratinized epithelium. *Bottom.* The keratinizing zone of the gingival epithelium (*C*) is seen as a pale linear area. The remainder of the epithelium is saturated with a perfusate of a diffusible dye (patent blue violet) which has entered the epithelium as a transudate derived from the subepithelial blood vessels (*B*). The surface keratinizing quality is one of the factors responsible for containing nutritive and hydrating fluids within the tissues. The nonkeratinizing epithelium of the sulcus and interdental col area allows freer passage of fluid through the epithelium into the sulcus/col areas. Keratinizing epithelia are also considered protective physically to the underlying tissues.

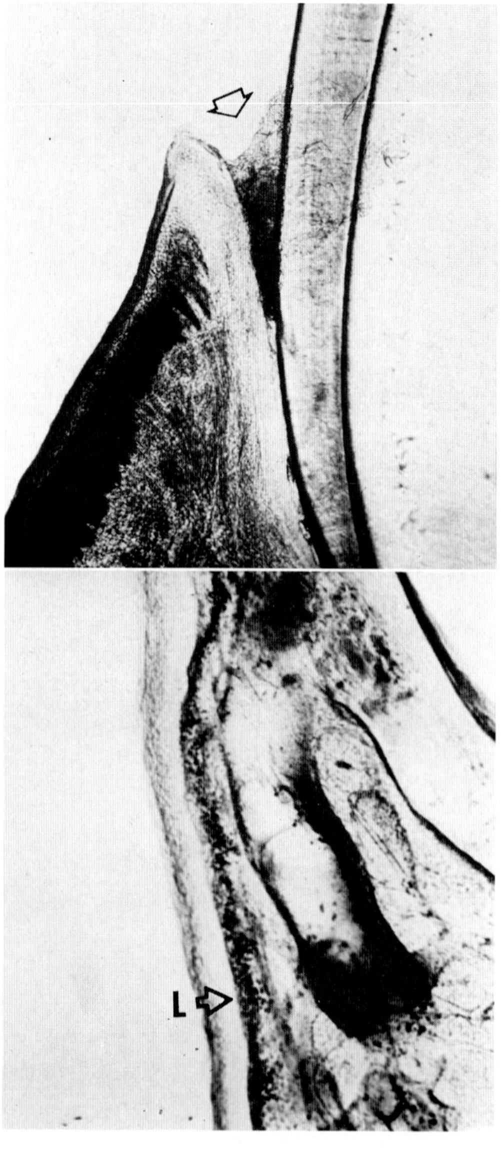

Fig. 1-16. *Top.* In this low magnification photomicrograph the gingival margin has been retracted from its adaptation to enamel by gingival fluid under a pressure of 30cm/ H_2O. A perfusate of carbon suspension and patent blue violet has been placed into the cervical lymphatic duct of a dog, inducing retrograde lymph flow into the gingiva and thence into the sulcus. Thin, incompletely formed or inflammation-altered gingival cuffs are particularly susceptible to retraction and colonization by bacterial flora. Generally, the shallower the crevice the more aerobic and coccal the bacterial genera. Deeper detachments favor multiplication of gram-positive organisms and the presence and activity of gram-negative strains. *Bottom.* Buccal septum of bone covered (*left*) by gingiva (seen as vertically oriented pallid area). *L* indicates the inner or periosteal aspect of gingiva carrying the major vascular supply to, and lymphatic drainage from, gingiva.

explain partially why Waerhaug[15,16] was able to pass delicate blades (0.005 mm. thick x 1.0 mm. wide) and cellulose strips to the cemento-enamel junctions of newly erupting teeth of dogs and the gingival crevices of children. Other investigators[13,17] using more adult tissue-tooth interfaces, found the adherence more tenacious.

The degree of adherence of the gingival wall to the tooth, then, is controlled or mediated by the following:

1. Tissue composition, particularly the ratio of collagen to ground substance and the viscosity of the matrical gel.[8,11]
2. The degree of structural rigidity afforded by the organization and arrangement of the gingival fiber system
3. The length of the "unattached" or adherent gingival wall, thus, the state of passive eruption. In this regard, it should be noted that gingival wall collagenation lessens as one proceeds from the base of the epithelial attachment toward the gingival margin

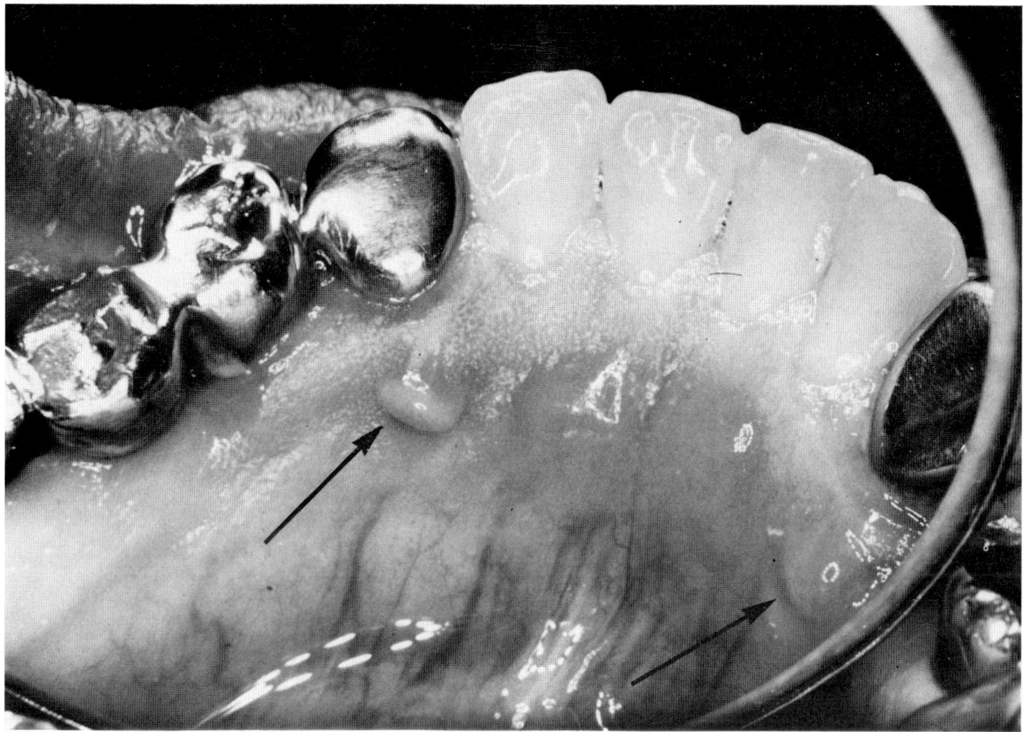

Fig. 1-17. Bilateral retrocuspid papillae. (From Everett, Hall, and Bennett.)[6]

4. The vascularity of the gingiva and concomitantly the amount of vascular transudate, tissue hydration, and sulcular fluid, with its possible effect on gingiva-to-tooth adherence

In the next chapter we will extrapolate from these anatomic findings to explain the nature and localization of the periodontal inflammatory lesion in the child.

RETROCUSPID PAPILLAE

This is a normal anatomical structure which most often occurs bilaterally and appears as a circumscribed, soft prominence between the free marginal gingiva and the mucogingival junction on the lingual aspect of the mandibular cuspid area (Figs. 1-17 and 1-18).

The retrocuspid papillae is composed primarily of thin-walled vessels and appears to represent a form of hamartomatous development. In many instances the vessels appear to be lymphatic.[6]

Prevalence. It is extremely common in children over 4 years of age and in teen-

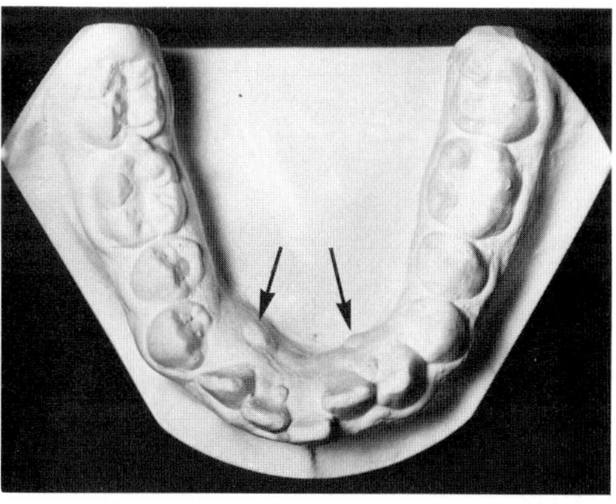

Fig. 1-18. Plaster cast of the mandibular arch of a 14-year-old boy displaying prominent bilateral retrocuspid papillae. (From Everett, Hall, and Bennett.)[6]

agers. The infrequent incidence of the retrocuspid papillae in persons over 40 years of age suggests that this clinical structure regresses with age.

Hirschfeld[7] reported it to be present in 99 percent of children 8 to 16 years old. Everett, Hale and Bennett[6] found it in 60 percent of individuals aged 2 to 21 years old, and Easley and Weiss[5] reported its occurrence in 85.2 percent of 331 individuals examined from birth to 25 years of age.

Significance. The main significance of this structure is that it can be confused with a periodontal abscess.

REFERENCES

1. Arnim, S. S., and Hagerman, D.: Connective tissue fibers of the marginal gingiva. J.A.D.A., *47:*271, 1953.

1*A*. Bowers, G. M.: A study of the width of attached gingiva. J. Periodont., *34:*201, 1963.

2. Bradley, R. E.: Periodontal lesions in children: their recognition and treatment. Dent. Clin. North Am., 671, 1961.
3. Cohen, B.: Morphological factors in the pathogenesis of periodontal disease. Br. Dent. J., *107:*31, 1959.
4. Cohen, M. M.: Periodontal disturbances in childhood. Dent. Radiogr. Photogr., *30:*41, 1957.
5. Easley, J. R., and Weiss, R. W.: Incidence of the retrocuspid papilla. J. Dent. Child., *37:*523, 1970.
6. Everett, F. G., Hall, W. B., and Bennett, J. S.: Retrocuspid papillae. Periodontics, *3:*81, 1965.
7. Hirschfeld, I.: The retrocuspid papillae. Am. J. Orthod., *33:*447, 1947.
8. Kent, P. W.: Mechanisms of Tooth Support. pp. 5–13. Bristol, England, John Wright, 1967.
9. Kohl, J. T., and Zander, H. A.: Morphology of interdental gingival tissues. Oral Surg., *14:*287, 1961.
10. Loe, H.: The dentogingival junction. In Miles, A. E. W.: Structural and Chemical Organization of the Teeth. vol. 2, 1964, p. 424. New York, Academic Press, 1964.
11. Melcher, A. L., and Eastoe, J. E.: Connective tissues. Melcher, A. H., and Bowens, W. H.: In Biology of the Periodontium. pp. 213–15, New York, Academic Press, 1969.
12. Ibid., p. 205.
13. Orban, B., Bathia, H., *et al.:* Epithelial attachment (the attached gingival cuff). J. Periodont., *27:*167, 1956.
14. Stallard, R. E.: Current concepts of periodontal disease. J. Dent. Child., *34:*204, 1967.
15. Waerhaug, J.: Current concepts concerning gingival anatomy. The dynamic epithelial cuff. Dent. Clin. North Am., pp. 715–22, 1960.
16. Waerhaug, J.: The gingival pocket. Odont. Tidsk. *60* (Supp. 1): 5, 1964.
17. Weinreb, M.: Epithelial attachment. J. Periodontal, *31:*186, 1960.
18. Zappler, S. E.: Peridontal disease in children. J.D.A., *37:*333, 1948.

2

Pathology of Periodontal Disease in Children: Development of the Gingival Inflammatory Lesion

In 1938, McCall[27] alerted the dental profession to the fact that the foundation of virtually all adult periodontal disease was laid in childhood. This warning was emphasized by Baer,[3] who stated that in many cases adult periodontitis must have had its inception at the time of puberty in order to be responsible for the severe destruction at times seen in 20- to 30-year-old patients. Parfitt[32] also felt that the early stages of periodontal disease were present before puberty and—if left untreated—would inevitably result in destructive manifestations in the adult. Recently, Stallard[44] expressed the belief that destructive periodontal disease often begins in childhood and is not recognized until the third decade, after irreversible changes have occurred. All agree that periodontal disease is a progressive, destructive lesion of the dental supporting apparatus that may have its origin in childhood or at puberty, the process then continuing into early adult life as an often unrecognized marginal periodontitis. Ramfjord, Emslie, *et al.*[33] indicate in their surveys that the transition between gingivitis and periodontitis begins at about 15 years of age.

If the above statements are valid, one would expect to find many instances of incipient marginal periodontitis in the younger population, since this disease process is the one most commonly observed in the periodontal patient. This, however, does not appear to be the case. If one discounts the reported instances of periodontosis, which may not necessarily begin primarily as an inflammatory lesion, the incidence of periodontitis in healthy children is rare. McIntosh,[29] Cohen, and Goldman[10] present histologic sections from cases of periodontitis involving children, and Butler[7] states that many vertical defects on the mesial aspect of the permanent first molars may be the result of periodontitis rather than periodontosis. No further documentation of periodontitis in the young was found except the notation that its occurrence in children was infrequent.

The periodontal disease entity most frequently observed in the young patient is gingivitis, a soft tissue lesion without affiliated bone destruction. This fact is confirmed in the epidemiological literature as well as in the clinical studies conducted by Zappler,[45] Bruckner,[6] and Massler.[30]

Massler further states that gingivitis is a biphasic phenomenon tending to be papillary, acute (implying overtness), and transient in the child, while it is marginal, chronic, and progressive in the adult. His findings are consistent with the clinical observations of Zappler, who noted that the child's gingival tissue reacts more quickly and more markedly than that of the adult, and with Cohen and Goldman who observed a marked tendency towards papillary hyperplasia.

TISSUE STRUCTURE AND THE ETIOLOGY OF GINGIVAL INFLAMMATORY LESIONS

The inflammatory lesion of the child is usually well confined to the more marginal

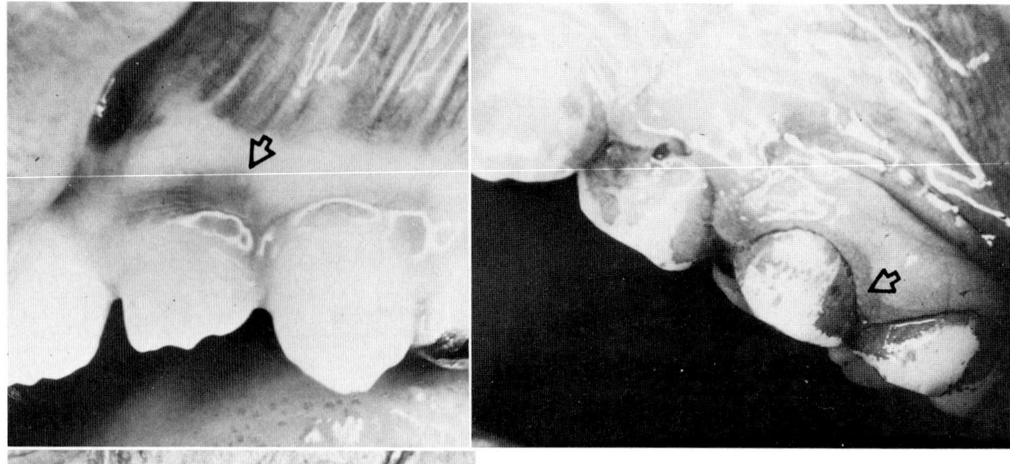

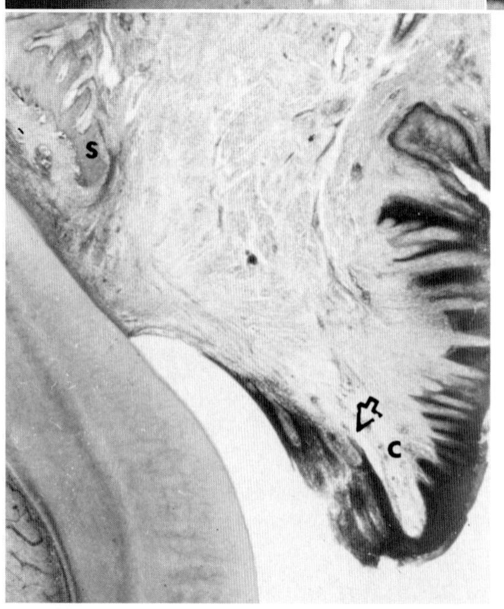

Fig. 2-1. *Top left.* Marginally restricted site of gingival inflammation. Note the shininess of the tissue as well as the absence of topical stippling. Coloration is deepened. Passive eruption is incomplete. *Top right.* Bacterial plaque deposits at cervical and interdental embrasure sites. The plaque is clinically stained with rosaniline dye. The arrow points to the area of gingival inflammation. *Bottom.* Comparable lesion seen histologically in 4½-year-old child. The arrow points to the affected sulcular epithelium. The adjacent connective tissue (at *c*) manifests collagen resorption and inflammatory cell infiltration. *s* is the crest of labial bone septum. (Specimen courtesy Dr. Walter Cohen, Philadelphia.)

aspects of the gingiva. It is of interest to note that little recognition or cognizance is given to the ubiquitous, contained marginal inflammatory state, or why clinically and histopathologically it exists and continues to exist, possibly for a protracted period. An exhaustive search of the pedodontic and periodontic literature reveals not a single, complete histologic analysis of the juvenile marginal lesion or any explanation of why such a lesion should be present, except on a temporal basis; that is, a mild lesion during youth slowly progressing with age into a more extensive and severe one. The literature does not contain a consideration of anatomic influences on the localization of the inflammatory state.

As presented in Chapter 1, there are structural attributes which may relate to the unique character of the juvenile lesion.

The anatomy of the interdental area in particular may influence the lesion. Observation has revealed that the inflammatory lesion is more often evidenced in these posterior segments and in anterior zones where proximal dental contacts are present; the character of the interdental tissues concomitantly changes. One cannot help but speculate that the fundamental structure helps to dictate the onset, presence, continuance and degree of inflammation.

Cohen's[9] description of the col area led him to speculate that the replacement of the reduced enamel epithelium by stratified squamous epithelium, which he felt essential to the health of the periodontium, would be interfered with by the chronic ulceration in this area.

Fish[16] noted that the col was susceptible to irritation, inflammation, and ulceration for the same reasons. Its increased susceptibility may be due, in fact, as stated by Cohen,[8] to the favorable morphologic location provided by the interdental region for bacterial growth. Recently, McHugh[28] challenged the role of col epithelial morphology in increasing its vulnerability to periodontal disease, and implicated the morphologic relationship of tooth to tooth and its association with the accrual of bacteria and debris.

In those areas where a diastema is present, a high degree of keratinization is also present, and protection against insult offered by the keratinization of the epithelium may be inferred. The permeability of these epithelia to labeled tissue fluids and intravascularly administered carbon suspensions suggests that the keratinizing effect limits transudation through such epithelium, containing hydrating and nutritive substances to the epithelium and by inference to the connective tissue. Other work by Brill,[5] Bader and Goldhaber[2] substantiates the inward-outward impermeability of such epithelium and the perviousness of sulcular epithelia. The surface keratinizing quality and an intra-epithelial zone of imperviousness (the barrier area at the junction between granular cells and the keratinizing layers) may also act to limit the action and penetration of exogenous irritants and thus protect the gingival corium.

In addition to the epithelial qualities, the observations that interdental connective tissues are structurally well organized, better endowed with collagen, and as a complex firmly bound to underlying bone and adjacent gingiva, may support a hypothesis that interdental tissues of a saddle nature are more resistant or less affected by inflammatory disease than interdental tissue topped by "col" configurations and the markedly different epithelial nature attending this morphology. Interdental saddle areas may also be shaped convexly, lending to the more effective self-cleansing by food abrasion and the detergency of liquids.

LOCALIZATION OF INFLAMMATORY LESIONS

It has previously been noted that the inflammatory lesion of the child is usually confined to the more marginal aspects of the gingiva—in the unattached, but adherent, gingival wall (cuff) (coronal to the CEJ) (Fig. 2-1). The process is more or less sharply separated from the rest of the gingiva by that part of its corium which is not only attached to the tooth by cementum but which comprises a well-oriented mat of connective tissue topping and attached to the rest of the bone interdentally and marginally. Since the marginal connective tissue is formed last, it may be conjectured that it is less defined until active and passive eruptions are completed. It is not possible to exclude, however, the consideration of *reactive fibroplasia,* as a response to inflammation, in the periosteal zone.

Clinically, normal childhood gingiva is often more flaccid marginally, probably more weakly attached to the tooth, with a tendency toward fullness and rounding of the gingival margin. When it is affected by the inflammatory process, there may be not only an accentuation of these features but also a sharply defined marginal erythema, induced by the vasodilatory phase of the disease. The free gingival groove which, even in inflammation may be difficult to define in the adult gingiva, may also be noticed in the incipient stages of inflammation.

This same localization of the inflammatory process, with rare extension into trans-septal or periosteal fiber areas and bone, can be seen in the young and adoles-

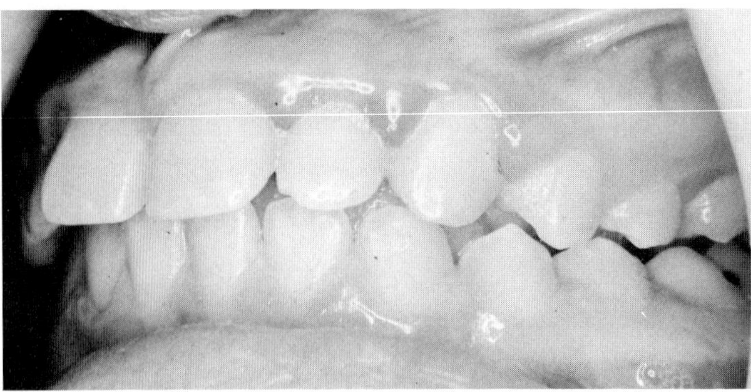

Fig. 2-2. Marginal gingivitis, in this 10-year-old child, is associated with plaque formation. Note the enlarged interdental papillae in the maxillary arch. This type of hyperplastic inflammatory response is common during puberty.

cents of other species, including nonhuman primates, rodents and dogs. In children and animals an expansion of a well-circumscribed marginal process into a state of more severe gingival and osseous involvement appears to depend on major local and/or systemic insult—as noted with vitamin deficiency in Italian children[37] as the grossly manifest necrotizing lesions in protein-deprived African children,[15] or the severe periodontitis in Down's syndrome.[20] The periodontal literature is replete with these documentations of severe manifestations in the young—human and animal. Recently, Sheiham,[41] in examining 15- to 19-year-old subjects, indicated that about 50 percent manifested periodontal disease with bony involvement.

From the material presented previously, it appears that the most logical hypothesis for the explanation of the well-defined marginal lesion in children involves structure. However, other hypotheses have been presented which, along with the structural concept, may have a modifying effect.

Robinson[34] has proposed that the strong periosteal activity found in children permits repair concurrent with or following disease and therefore offers resistance to the development of periodontitis. Kelsten[23] indicates that anabolism exceeds catabolism in young supporting bone, and this growth tendency favors healing following disease or injury. Hirsch[22] feels that the thinner epithelial lining and lesser degree of hornification are responsible for the overt nature of the gingival lesions and that the plasticity of young tissue accounts for both the rapid response to irritation and the expeditious healing that follows.

Bacterial and Pathologic Aspects

It is highly doubtful that gingival inflammation could exist without the presence of bacterial plaque[26] (Figs. 2-2 and 2-3).

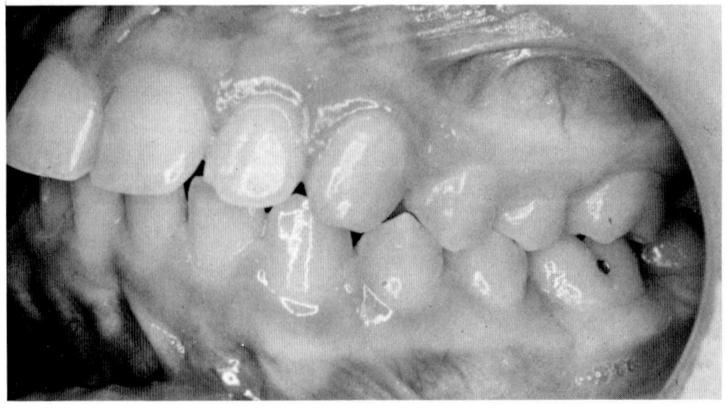

Fig. 2-3. The patient seen in Figure 2-2 shows return of normal gingival contour following plaque control. A gingivitis which occurs during puberty, the so-called "puberty gingivitis," does not regress spontaneously with age, but requires removal of plaque.

This extraneous material is evident not only in attachment to the surface of the tooth, with a predilection for roughened or irregular areas, but is also localized on gingival soft tissue and within the gingival sulcus; bacterial plaque may be discerned and localized clinically with disclosing dyes. In the latter instance, the retractability of incompletely developed gingival walls, associated with a deficiency of formed gingival fiber systems and a relative abundance and lowered viscosity of tissue matrical substances, may facilitate bacterial colonization within the crevice at the interface of epithelium and tooth. In areas of shallow detachment, usually associated with a short gingival cuff and concomitant improved collagenation, aerobic and gram-positive bacterial genera dominate, particularly nonhemolytic and alpha hemolytic streptococci. With deeper crevicular sites, and as inflammation supervenes, the bacterial population is increased and filamentous and gram-negative flora become ecologically significant.[4] Thus, the deepened sulcus/pocket may be noted for gram-positive bacterial forms at or near its orifice with a shift to a significant gram-negative population at its base; the latter include bacteroides, veillonella, spirochetes, vibrios, neisseria. The genus bacteroides (especially *B. Melanogenicus*)[20,31] is noted for its production of collagenase and for its release, upon lysis of the cell, of membrane lipoprotein-polysaccharides (endotoxin). The vibrios, veillonellas, and spirochetes may also liberate endotoxin. The aerobic types, especially the streptococcus, are able to polymerize sucrose and other sugars into highly viscous polysaccharides (i.e., dextrans, which adhere or attach to dental surface defects or acquired pellicle while forming much of the mucoid matrix of bacterial plaque). These and other gram-positive strains have the potential for release of exotoxins which may cause damage to the epithelial lining and in the adjacent connective tissue. Hyaluronidase, for example, has been shown[12,38] to attack the glycoproteins found at epithelial cell interfaces with consequent loss of cell approximation (an incipient ulcerative reaction). The enzyme may possibly enter the subepithelial zone and act upon the hyaluronate comprising much of the connective tissue matrix, with resultant liquefaction of this substrate. Other bacterial exotoxins may produce a direct proteolytic and polysaccharidolytic effect[39,40] with attendent damage to epithelial basement membranes, associated reticulum and subjacent collagen fibers. Bacterial complexes with immunoglobulins of the G and M series usually elicit complement fixation; their aggregation at tissue sites may also invoke damage. Complement inhibitors, such as cobra venom used experimentally, substantially reduce tissue destruction in inflammation.[19]

Inflammatory Cells. These cells are attracted to the site by the presence of bacteria and bacterial byproducts, and conjugates of antigen-complement-antibody, may not only act beneficially by phagocytizing these elements, with subsequent intracellular digestion, but may also liberate their cellular complements of acid hydrolases, as lysosomal membranes are dissolved. These enzymes are multiphasic in their effects and serve to invoke collagen resorption, matrix dissolution, cell disruption, vascular dilation and permeability—the destructive facets of the inflammatory state. The inflammatory cells with the greatest propensity for tissue destruction are the neutrophil,[1] and the monocyte. However, all altered or damaged cells[18] of the involved tissue, despite the fact that their complement of lysosomal enzymes is smaller and less varied qualitatively, could augment the destructive state. Both epithelium and connective tissue are involved. Lysosomal fractions may also act as antigens, precipitating immune responses.

Bacterial Endotoxins. These endotoxins have been demonstrated in plaque and in gingival exudates, along with the ubiquitous presence of their cellular sources.[14] In fact, it is possible to make a linear or parallel correlation between the amount of endotoxin recoverable from measured amounts of bacterial plaque/gingival exudate and the clinical and histologic severity of periodontal inflammation.[42,43] In other well-controlled human studies[26] in which the bacterial ecology of the pocket was correlated with plaque and debris accumulation, the more clinically overt manifestations of the inflammatory state coincided with quantitative flora increase and with the increased prevalence of the gram-negative bacterial strains.

Bacterial endotoxins and the agencies that they activate may have a number of pathologic potentials. Grossly, they invoke bleeding and necrotic manifestations by acting on blood vessel walls. Endothelium tends to be disrupted in continuity and may be destroyed. If the damage is slight, there may be sludging of blood flow through vascular lumina and the formation of mural thrombi; this leads to vascular obstruction and to ischemia related to loss of hydrating and nutritive transudates to the tissue. If the effect is more damaging to the vasculature, with endothelial necrosis and resorption of containing basement membranes and perivascular collagen/connective tissue, vasorupture will occur with a spilling of blood into the tissues (i.e., hemorrhage).

Recently, endotoxin has been allied to bone resorption[39]; it is conceivable that the resorption of bone in marginal periodontitis is associated with penetration of endotoxin to bone and periosteum as part of the spreading exudate seen in the conversion of gingivitis to periodontitis. It should be emphasized that this premise is unproved.

Endotoxin, per se, may not be the destructive factor. Endotoxin, alone or as a phase of endotoxin-antibody complexes, may join with complement (C'_3) at vascular basement membranes and accumulate at these sites, leading to nodular or diffuse thickening of the basement membrane.[13] In this way either enhanced vascular permeability or reduced perviousness may be produced, the latter leading to a relative local ischemic state.

Endotoxin-complement (C'_3) is also chemotactic for neutrophils attracting them to vascular (and possibly osseous) locales. The neutrophil may also phagocytize the antigen-complement *or* antigen-antibody-complement formations, at times negating their influences. In the majority of instances, however, the neutrophils undergo cytolysis as their lysosomal membranes rupture and release acid hydrolases into the cells. Cell membranes disintegrate and the hydrolases enter extracellular areas and invoke damage. A fraction of complement (C'_5) is also allied to mast cell disruption and histamine release, with concomitant vasodilation and permeability.

Endotoxins exert their detrimental effects by acting on cells, producing labilization of the limiting membranes of their cytoplasmic packets of lysosomal enzymes, allowing these substances to be *first,* endocytolytic and *second,* to leave the cells through ruptured cell-walls and express their lytic actions on other tissue components. These processes may take place in vasculature, connective tissue and epithelium. As a consequence, gingival exudates in periodontal inflammation contain measurable and increased quantities of hydrolytic enzymes in amounts comparable to the severity of inflammation. Among these enzymes are acid phosphatase, esterases, cathepsins, B-glucuronidase, aryl sulfatases, chondroitin sulfatases, lipases, ribonuclease, desoxyribonuclease.

Amino Acids. Such acids—for example, of collagenous origin, and released with fiber resorption—could also be expected to augment the exudate derived from the periodontal pocket. The hydroxyproline, hydroxylysine and hyroxyglycine content of gingival fluid should reflect and parallel the severity of collagen resorption attending inflammation. Studies of endotoxin, enzyme, and amino acid composition of exudates have been performed in relationship to adult lesions; study is required of these modalities in the young. It is not likely that gross discrepancies would be encountered in the comparison of similar lesions in the young and their elders.

Plaque, then, is undoubtedly of bacterial constitution being colonized by the indigenous flora of the individual. Bacteria certainly contribute (by polymerization phenomena) to the development of a sticky, viscous and thus adherent substrate, linking plaque tenaciously to the faulty/irregular surfaces of teeth and soft tissues.[17] Plaque harbors bacteria which release (the bacterial cell being preserved) enzymes capable of adversely affecting epithelium and adjacent connective tissue. Plaque furnishes a haven for other bacteria which lose their intact nature, liberating their cell wall constituents (endotoxin) which induce multiple tissue lesions.

Gingival Lesion Caused by Bacterial Agents. A most provocative hypothesis conceives of the possibility that once a gingival lesion is provoked by bacterial agencies, this lesion in turn can contribute to the continuance of the diseased state. With this concept, for example, immunologic processes engendered by bacteria and their products, while undoubtedly protective to the tissue complex by negating antigen directly or promoting phagocytosis, may also create tissue damage of a magnitude greater than the benefits derived from the immune processes. Endotoxins, especially with the addition of serum complement, and with or without additional antibody fixation, attract neutrophils by chemotaxis. The union often occurs in interendothelial sites or within the tissues immediately peripheral to the endothelium of blood vessels. Neutrophils phagocytize antigen-complement or antigen-complement-antibody complexes; at times, this leads to neutrophilic lysis or to neutrophilic release of acid hydrolases into these areas. Vascular or perivascular necrosis and resorption with associated hemorrhage and exudation may occur.

The exudates so liberated certainly become part of the exudative fluid found within the confines of the "pocket," with some of the material eventually escaping into the oral cavity at the pocket margin. At these areas, the exudate with all of its lytic potential could inflict additional epithelial damage and/or *may contribute to the formation of additional plaque,* being added to the plaque substrate as an additional structural component and augmenting the damaging capabilities of the plaque by virtue of its enzyme and cellular constitutents. In the latter context, neutrophilic emigration within exudative fluids into pocket zones and oral cavity can be directly related quantitatively to the severity of inflammation.[24] Tracer substances, placed into the living circulation, such as tetracyclines and Na fluorescein (fluorescent to UV irradiation), I^{131} labelled albumin, macromolecular substances such as carbon particles, have all been recovered from gingival exudates and have also been found to be localized in bacterial plaque, subgingival and supragingival calculus testifying as to the contribution of exudates to this potentially injurious material. It may be inferred that if macromolecular materials can leave the blood vasculature and finally emanate within the pocket, fibrinogen, albumin, and globulin-containing vascular exudates can likewise be carried to the pocket and gingival margin and participate in plaque formation; these are colloidal, viscous, hydrophilic and thus sticky substances which along with bacterial dextrans may constitute plaque matrices.

The hypothesis, extrapolated to clinical practice, indicates that if plaque removal and prevention by professionally and personally applied oral hygiene measures do not suffice to eliminate the clinical gingival inflammatory state, then it may be necessary to apply appropriate therapeutic regimens to the gingiva to eliminate the inflammatory locus within the tissues. Effective wound healing after efficient debridement and prevention of renewed eti-

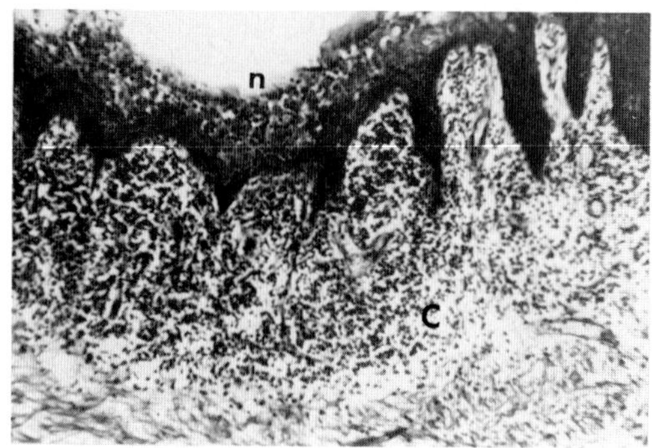

Fig. 2-4. 100X close-up of col lesion. There is dense subepithelial aggregation of the inflammatory cells (*C*) and concomitant paucity of collagen within the area, while at *n* there is epithelial cell desquamation and necrosis. Leukocytes have invaded the epithelium and are continuing through to the oral cavity as part of the exudate.

ology may then negate or inhibit the continuance of tissue destructive effects of inflammation[35] *and aid in the prevention of the redevelopment of bacterial plaque.*

Correlation of Histopathology to Clinical Lesion

Gingival inflammation in the young offers little to distinguish it clinically from that seen in late adolescence and adulthood. There appears to be a propensity for the lesions to develop initially in interdental zones, particularly where proximal dental contacts and allied tissue concavities (col form) coincide. When proximal tooth contacts are flattened or where carious lesions are present at contact areas, the square area of tooth-to-tooth approximation increases, often elongating its occluso-apical dimension as one or both of the teeth shift toward the contact area. Concomitantly the gingival embrasure may constrict in mesiodistal and occluso-apical directions, leading to a deepening of the col concavity. If the buccal and/or lingual peaks of tissue substantially retain their original heights, a situation is created in which there is a deep col with high, flaccid, and retractable buccal/lingual tissue boundaries. Such a deformity favors interdental plaque and debris lodgement,[28] the institution of inflammation, and the spread of exudates *laterally* into the poorly collagenated and supported tissue peaks (Fig. 2-4). Thus, the clinician can understand the contribution of dental and soft tissue form and relationships to the pathogenesis of many interdental lesions.

Tissue Enlargement. The indifferently collagenated, poorly structured, inflamed interdental gingiva becomes quickly enlarged because of edema and exudate accumulation in the tissue. As collagen and tissue matrix resorb under the influence of inflammation, much of the containing action of these constituents upon the patency and luminal diameters of blood vessels may be lost, allowing the vasculature to increase quantitatively and to dilate. The onrush of blood into this vasculature induces engorgement, manifested as clinical hyperemia, and permeability, reflected as tissue enlargement and exudation from the pocket margin (Fig 2-5).

Tissue enlargement is related also to hyperplasia of the elements of the gingival corium. In the characteristic low-grade, persistent gingival inflammatory state, the "destructive locus" is surrounded by a rim of retained and quantitatively expanded connective tissue (i.e., reactive hyperplasia). In this locale an increased fibroblastic population secretes additional collagen, reticulum, and the protein-polysaccharide constituents of matrix. Blood vessels increase in quantity and complexity of distribution by endothelial mitosis, leading to the extension of buds and cords of nonlumenized endothelium into the interfibrillar areas. As they connect with other cellular "shoots" or with already existing blood vessels, first, plasma, and then whole blood flow through interendothelial cell slits that expand to

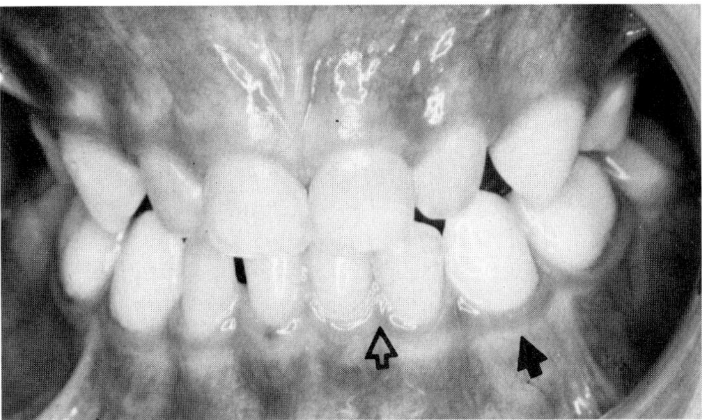

Fig. 2-5. Gingival inflammation in association with deciduous dentition. Clinically, there is a marginally restricted inflammatory state—characterized by redness (seen as deepening of coloration in black and white photograph), shine and tissue distortion—at the facial aspect of all the mandibular teeth. Probing elicited mild bleeding and limited gingival margin retractability. Evident was ballooning of the soft tissue margin at the buccal of the mandibular left first molar as well as at the gingival detachment apical to the cemento-enamel junction. The *dark* arrow indicates an area in which the zone of attached gingiva is inordinately narrow. The root of the cuspid is rounded and full while the entire tooth is tipped lingually; the buccal bone septum may be thin and cortical while the root is buccally prominent, lending to the presence of a broad area of alveolar mucosa and a concomitantly narrow band of attached gingiva. The *open* arrow points to inflamed interdental soft tissue.

become patent passages to connecting vessels. These new capillaries of the microcirculatory apparatus are easily damaged, and highly pervious to the passage of intravascular material. Hemorrhage and exudation are thus facilitated, particularly when the gingiva is subjected to mechanical irritation by probing, toothbrushing, or chewing of harsh food. While some of the blood accumulates in the tissue and eventually undergoes lysis and phagocytosis, another portion courses through the damaged (ulcerated) sulcular *or* col lining, eventuating in the "pocket" and in the oral cavity at the gingival crest. A final fraction may be taken from the scene by means of patent lymphatics.[36]

The Epithelium. This part of the attached gingiva and the marginal cuff (i.e., from mucogingival junction to gingival margin) is of the keratinizing variety in all but a limited number of instances. Keratinization implies either para- or orthokeratinization, the first with the retention of flattened, nucleated cells at the outer (oral) aspect of the epithelium, while the latter process connotes the aggregation of anucleate, flattened, nonfunctional epithelial cells external to the stratum granulosum. Both are physiologic at these sites and in areas where comparable masticatory mucosae are located (i.e., palatal gingiva, the mucosa of the hard palate, and the dorsum of the tongue). In the normal structure of gingiva,

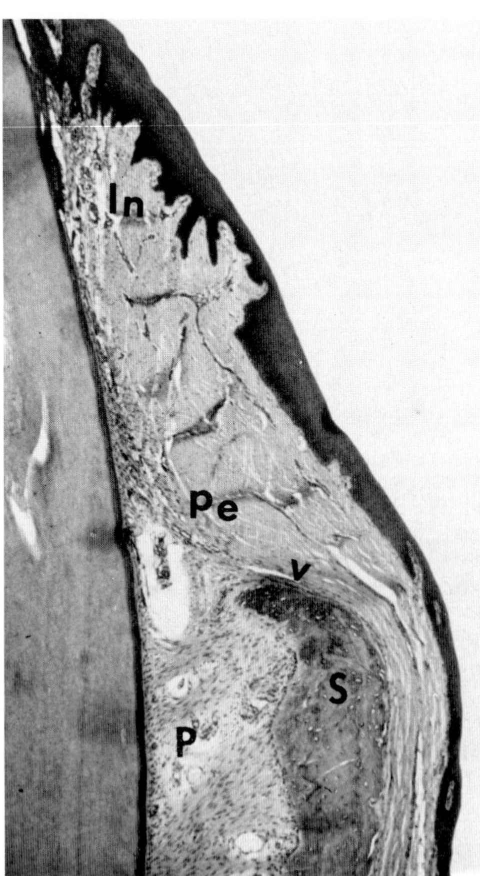

Fig. 2-6. A gingival inflammatory lesion in a child. The periosteal aspect of the gingiva is highly cellular (fibroblasts) suggesting reactive hyperplasia as a consequence of overlying inflammation. The apex of *v* points to the bone (*S*) crest where bone apposition is occurring; this appositional response may be related to inflammation in the gingiva (*In*) and/or to the physiologic development of the alveolar process. The periodontal ligament (*P*) is also highly cellular, not only intrinsically but also in relation to the cementum (cementoblasts) and bone (osteoblasts). The periosteal fiber complex extends from the periosteum to the cementum (*pe*). (Specimen courtesy of Dr. Walter Cohen, Philadelphia.)

the epithelial sheet is rippled or stippled on its external surface, while at its interface with the underlying connective tissue the rete pegs extend as a funnel into a gully, making blind, ending depressions in the connective tissue of the lamina propria. In the inflammatory response, when edema and hyperplasia invoke tissue enlargement and engorgement, the epithelium *may* lose its keratinizing phase and its rete projections into the tissue corium, the epithelium becoming thinner and "atrophic" in its configuration. In extreme instances, especially with topical gingival irritation, desquamative manifestations may lead to shedding of the entire thickness of epithelium with exposure of the subjacent connective tissue, the erosion characteristically topped with a thin fibrinomembrane of mixed epithelial and exudative origins; *clinical redness and tactile hypersensitivity are often present.* In therapy, as inflammation subsides and the tissues return toward their physiologic form, the epithelium regains keratinization, stature and durability, and its characteristic morphology.

In periodontal inflammation (Figs. 2-6 through 2-9) the epithelium of the sulcus/col, normally thinly stratified and nonkeratinizing, is converted to a hyperplastic and an ulcerative state. The epithelial breach ulcer serves as a pathway for the escape of exudate, leucocytes, blood, degraded connective tissue and epithelium into the "pocket" and thence toward its orifice. Exudative substance accrues between epithelial cells and at the dento-epithelial interface, "mechanically" detaching the epithelium (and thus the gingival cuff) from the tooth. Enzymatic processes of a degrading nature are also active at these sites and within the connective tissue of the gingiva, dissolving the interepithelial and dento-epithelial "cementing" agencies (glycoproteins) and resorbing the fibrillar components of the tissue. These changes are responsible for *gingival retractability* from the tooth.

Gingival Detachment. *Deepening of the gingival detachment* beyond the cemento-enamel junction is a consequence not only of connective tissue resorption apical to the pocket epithelium, but also of the chem-

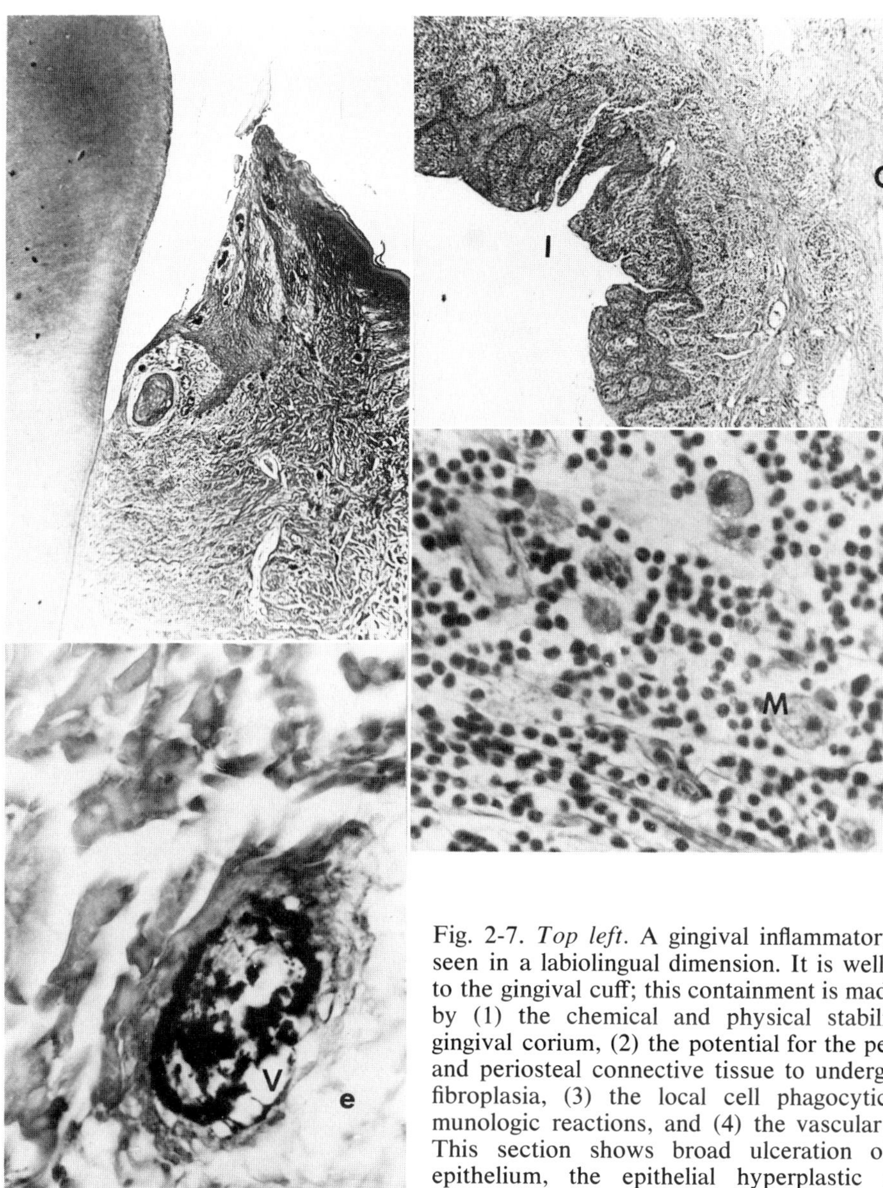

Fig. 2-7. *Top left.* A gingival inflammatory lesion is seen in a labiolingual dimension. It is well-restricted to the gingival cuff; this containment is made possible by (1) the chemical and physical stability of the gingival corium, (2) the potential for the perivascular and periosteal connective tissue to undergo reactive fibroplasia, (3) the local cell phagocytic and immunologic reactions, and (4) the vascular response. This section shows broad ulceration of sulcular epithelium, the epithelial hyperplastic state and numerous subepithelial blood vessels. *Top right.* The gingival biopsy specimen procured from the distobuccal aspect of the maxillary first deciduous molar. *I* is the epithelial breach in the pocket wall. *G* is the intact gingival corium. There is evidence of inflammatory cell infiltration adjacent to the epithelium. *Center.* 430X close-up of cellular reaction in inflammation. The small dark cells are largely lymphocytes and plasma cells; however, neutrophils and monocytes may pervade to a lesser extent. The large cells (as at *M*) with small nuclei and reticulated cytoplasm are mononuclear macrophages. *Bottom.* 430X view of perfused gingival blood vessel in inflammation. The carbon suspension is leaking from the venule (*V*) into the surrounding connective tissue, *e* is edema. Vasodamage is especially prevalent subjacent to the pocket's area of epithelial necrosis, accounting in part for the bleeding associated with gingivitis.

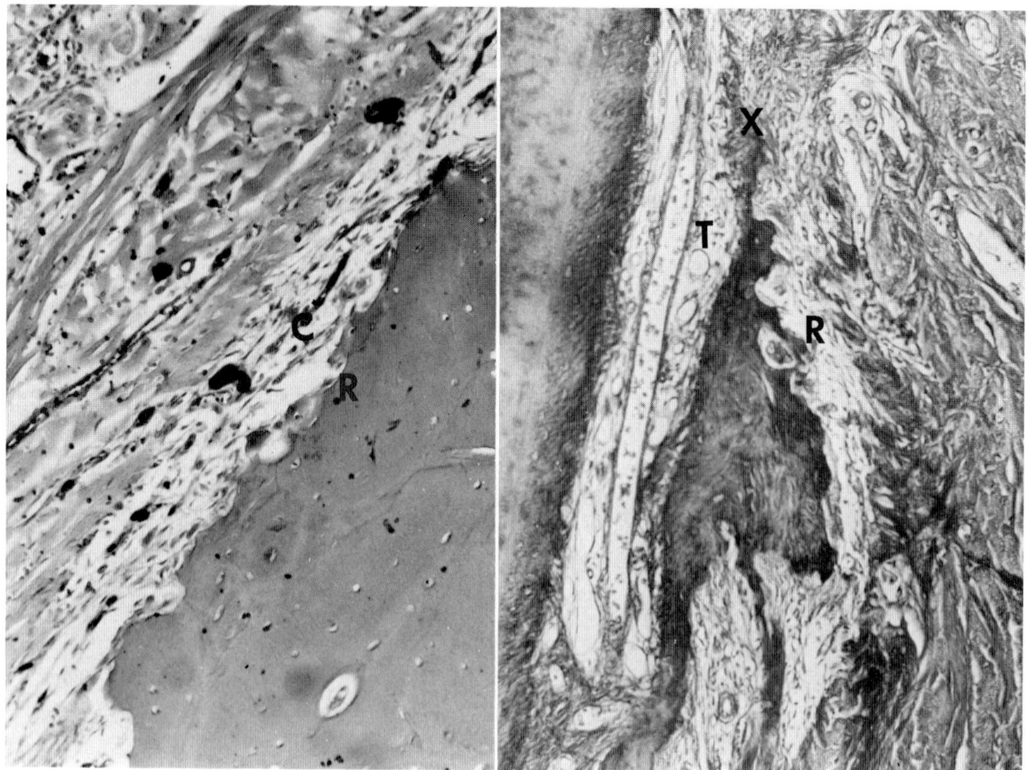

Fig. 2-8. *Left.* Resorption of the external face of the buccal septum in marginal periodontitis. Spread of exudate from the gingiva to the bone usually follows the course of periosteal blood vessels. lymphatics, and the planes of orientation of the fibers of the periosteum. *R* indicates the scalloped surface of the bone; the resorption is mediated by both osteoclasts and osteocytes. *C* are the connective tissue fibers undergoing collagenolysis. *Right.* Involvement of the labial septum by the inflammatory process. *R* denotes the irregular pattern of resorption. Osteoclasts can be seen in the resorptive lacunae in the bone. This very thin septum has been almost totally resorbed (*X*). An occlusal traumatic state also was present; manifestations of excessive pressure are evident in the coronal phase of the periodontal ligament. Notice the loss and segmentation of periodontal fibers and the vasodilatory reaction (*T*).

ical (enzymatic) severance of the gingival fiber insertion into cementum. The hyperplastic epithelium enters (a migratory phenomenon) the area of fiber detachment, with resulting epithelial approximation to the root. The process is repetitive, resulting in progressive or cyclic deepening of the pocket. The hydrolytic enzymes of the inflammatory state, cellular in derivation, act upon collagen fibers, dissolving the interfibrillar cementing substance (chondroitin sulfate) and inducing linear splaying of the fibrils. Fibrils in turn are segmented, and are seen as scattered and indifferently oriented bits and pieces. On ultrastructural and chemical[25] levels, collagen and reticulum may be subdivided into their polypeptide chains and amino acid components.

Cementum. This is attacked by enzymes which induce pitting and softening of its surface. Proteases and collagenases, for example, act on organic substrates—both fibrillar and ground substance—leading to their liquefaction/disruption. Demineralizing agencies, (i.e., lactic acid and citrates) found in the tissue exudate may be respon-

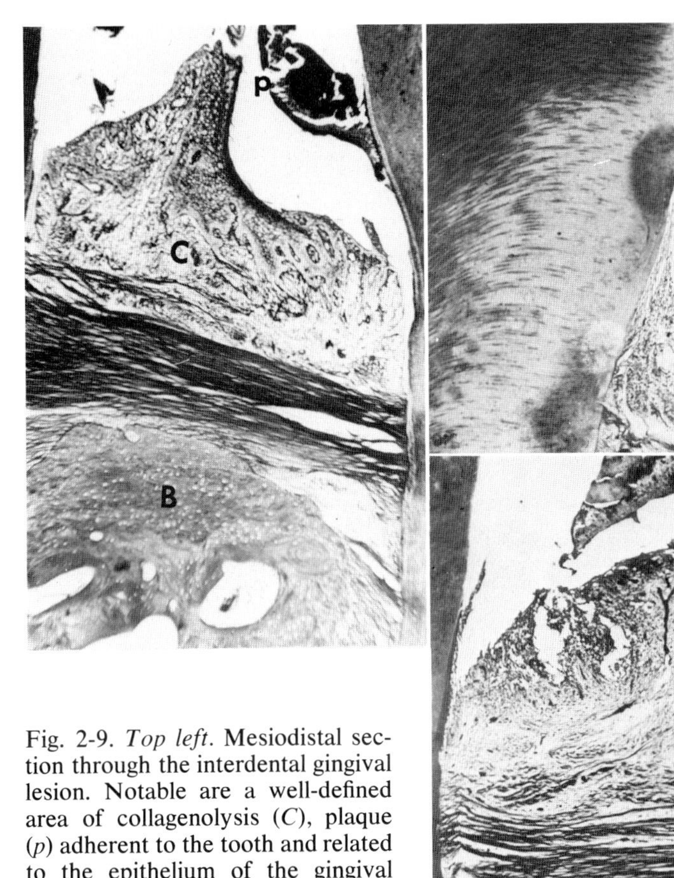

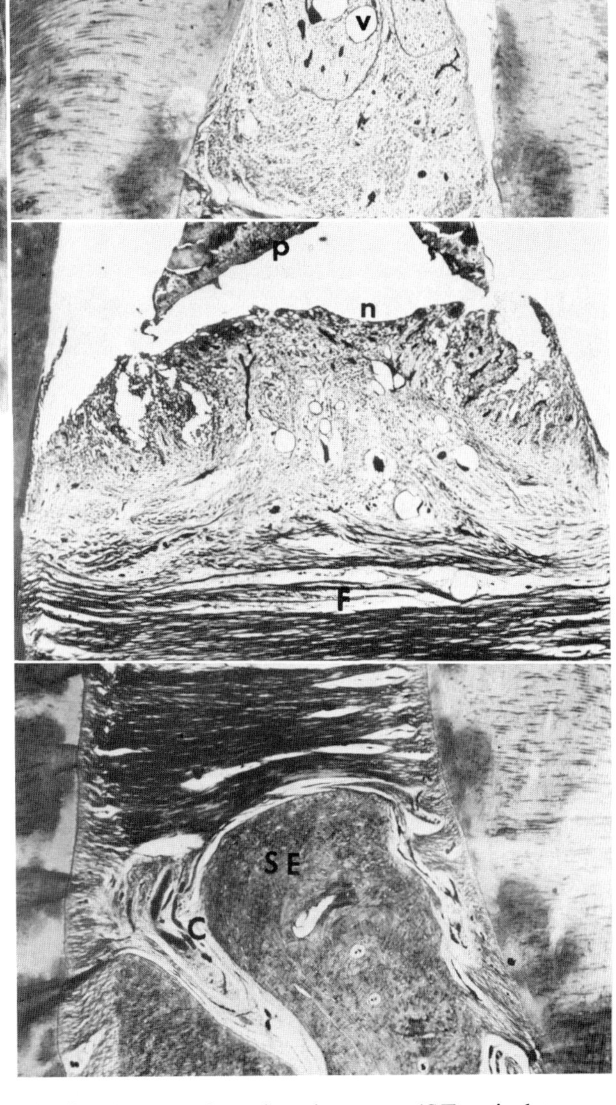

Fig. 2-9. *Top left.* Mesiodistal section through the interdental gingival lesion. Notable are a well-defined area of collagenolysis (*C*), plaque (*p*) adherent to the tooth and related to the epithelium of the gingival pocket, the uninvolved osseous septum (*B*), and the dense intervening band of transseptal fibers. *Top right.* Perfused gingival inflammatory lesion. The black blebs are dilated and patent vessels of the blood microcirculation. The variably shaped nonperfused vessels (as at *v*) are lymphatics. *Center.* In this interdental lesion there has been desquamation and necrosis of the entire epithelial cover (*n*) producing a broad ulceration/erosion. In the in vivo state, the soft tissue was undoubtedly in approximation to the bacterial plaque (*p*). The transseptal fibers (*F*) are intact despite the marked inflammatory involvement marginally. *Bottom.* Interdental septum (*SE*) apical to gingival lesion. The transseptal fibers are grossly unaffected. The vascular channel (*C*) may be portal for the extension of inflammatory exudate into the septum, resulting in periodontitis.

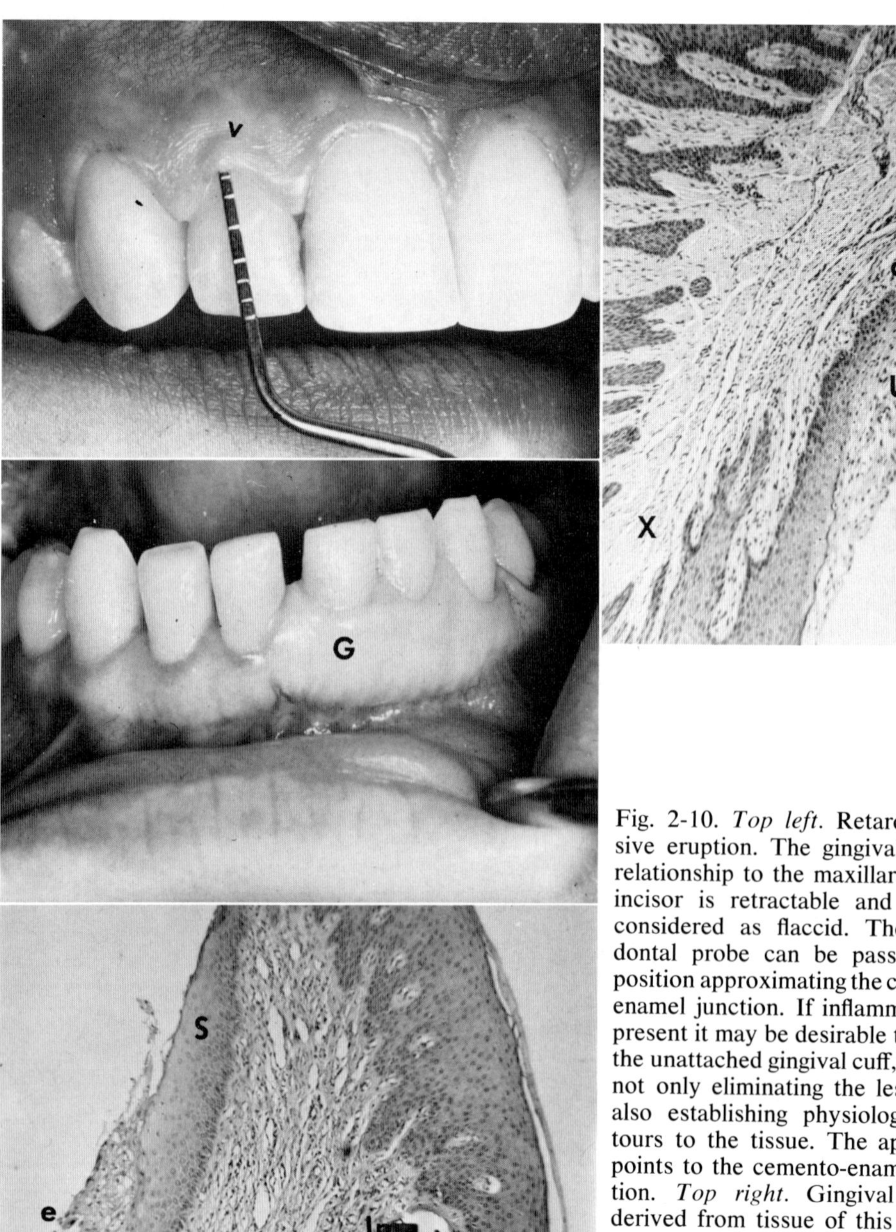

Fig. 2-10. *Top left.* Retarded passive eruption. The gingival cuff in relationship to the maxillary lateral incisor is retractable and can be considered as flaccid. The periodontal probe can be passed to a position approximating the cemento-enamel junction. If inflammation is present it may be desirable to resect the unattached gingival cuff, thereby not only eliminating the lesion but also establishing physiologic contours to the tissue. The apex of *v* points to the cemento-enamel junction. *Top right.* Gingival biopsy derived from tissue of this patient. The occlusal aspect of the gingival cuff (*X*) is thin and deficient in collagenation, accounting in part for the retractability of the tissue from the tooth. The micro-ulcer of the sulcular epithelium can be noted at *U* while a fairly well-localized inflammatory cell infiltrate can be discerned in the area of *c*. *Center.* In this instance of retarded passive eruption the lower incisors were ensheathed over approximately 50 percent of their labial surfaces by essentially thick, dense gingiva. The inflammatory lesion was well contained to the more marginal aspects of the tissue cuff. The tissue wall was rigid and well apposed to the enamel. The mandibular right reflects an area comparable to that at the mandibular left (*G*) which has been subjected to resection of the unattached gingiva (25 days postsurgery). *Bottom.* Photomicrograph of resected gingival cuff of above patient. The inner epithelium of the gingival wall can be seen

sible for the binding and withdrawal of cemental mineral. Scanning electron-microscopic views of the cemental surface reveal irregular pits and craters, projections of demineralized collagen, and spikes of cementum (like the ruins of Hiroshima). Exploration confirms these irregularities, as the surface is clinically roughened and etched, often discolored and softened. In areas where cementum has been in sustained exposure to oral fluids, or in the area of the "pocket" to exudative fluids, the previously marred cementum may be coated by a protein-polysaccharide film or "membrane" which undergoes mineralization by the binding of mineral from saliva and tissue fluid. In these areas, the surface of cementum may appear hypermineralized, thus glasslike and hardened clinically.

Treatment. Contrary to statements in the literature, we feel that although the gingivitis that occurs during pubescence is manifested as an exaggerated response to a local irritant, there is little justification for the term "puberty gingivitis." This latter term usually carries the connotation that a hormonal imbalance is responsible for the gingivitis and if left untreated the gingivitis will spontaneously regress with the approach of the late teens or early twenties. In our experience that is not the case. Meticulous plaque removal and oral hygiene are needed for both the prevention and cure of all forms of gingivitis, including the form that occurs during pubescence. Periodontal surgery is rarely indicated during pubescence because the gingiva is usually edematous rather than fibrous in nature. When tooth malalignment is severe, orthodontic treatment may be a necessary adjunctive procedure along with curettage and plaque control for complete case management.

RETARDED (ALTERED) PASSIVE ERUPTION

Concomitant with the active eruption of teeth and their movement toward the occlusal plane, there is a physiologic propensity for the enveloping gingival cuff to undergo contracture, thus shortening its apico-occlusal dimension. The apical base of the cuff is located at the coronal edge of the attachment of gingival fibers into cervical cementum, generally coincident with the cemento-enamel junction. Although there may be some remodeling of the gingival attachment to the tooth during the eruption of the tooth, the gingival fiber inclusion in forming and maturing cementum begins at the time of the commencement of root formation, continues during dental eruption, and is maintained spatially and structurally intact, barring agencies which provoke collagenolysis and fiber detachment, during the lifetime of the individual. There is no acceptable evidence that the progressive shift of sulcular epithelium and the base of the cuff onto the cementum, described by Gottlieb as phases three and four of passive eruption, constitutes a physiologic process. Rather they occur as a consequence of gingival inflammation and the associated severance of the gingival fiber insertion into cervical cementum.

The apically directed shift of the gingival margin clinically observable as gingival recession in relationship to the enamel surface, occurs physiologically and pro-

at *S*. The area of epithelial ulceration is deep within the cuff (*e*); epithelial cells are being shed into the pocket area. At *c* are cells of the inflammatory infiltrate. This is predominately a round cell aggregation of plasma cells and lymphocytes, but neutrophils are notable perivascularly and adjacent to the area of epithelial ulceration. At *I* is an inclusion of foreign material, neither precisely identifiable, directly relatable nor peculiar to the inflammatory lesion. It shows some fibrous encapsulation. The gingiva is essentially thick, fibrous and thus well supported clinically.

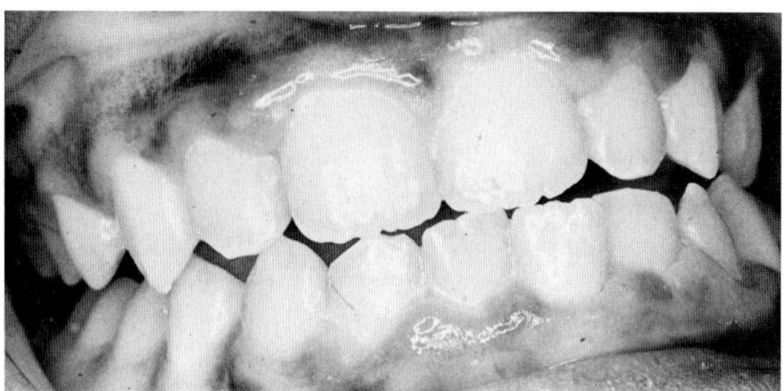

Fig. 2-11. In some adolescents, for reasons unknown, passive eruption is markedly delayed. This results in patients with "small" teeth and a deepened gingival sulcus which lends itself readily to bacterial invasion.

gressively until it reaches a linear position within the gingival one third to one fourth of the crown. The "ideal" structure configuration of the gingival cuff, once passive eruption has "terminated," is one in which the length of the inner sulcular aspect of the tissue pyramid is equivalent to the apico-occlusal dimension of its *outer* (oral) surface. The width of base of the pyramid is roughly equal to the individual lengths of the other two sides. The connective tissue corium of such an ideal cuff would consist of an organized, dense collagen fiber system encased by a matrix of maximal gelation viscosity.

In the condition of altered (retarded) passive eruption, the recession of the gingival margin is variably impaired leading to an elongated gingival cuff as seen in Figure 2-10. In some instances, the gingival wall is rigid and tightly adapted to the enamel surface; its structural stability is associated with dense collagenation (and bulkiness) of the gingival corium, and thick buccolingual dimensions of the tissue. When the gingival margin is thickened and positioned at or occlusal to the cervical convexity the altered dentogingival relationship (one which does not afford protection to the gingival crest) allows for plaque and debris accumulation with accompanying inflammation. The inflammatory process may be accompanied by hyperplasia and edema, augmenting the thickness and distortion of the tissue. In a majority of cases the faciolingual dimension of at least a portion of the tissue wall can be regarded as thin; it is therefore indifferently or incompletely collagenated, weakly supported, and in tenuous adherence to the enamel surface. While both (and intermediate) types of gingival cuffs may give clinical and histological evidence of inflammation, the disease process appears to be more dynamic and more overt where the tissue wall is thinned and poorly supported.

Treatment. Restoration of physiologic gingival form and sulcular depth by surgical resection of the excessive gingival tissue is the treatment of choice (Figs. 2-11 and 2-12). The morphology of the tissue postsurgically eventuates "physiologically" normal gingiva with a short, tightly adapted gingival cuff, a shallow sulcus, and a stoutly collagenated connective tissue corium. The gingival margin is now shielded from topical irritation by the deflecting contours of the cervical convexity of the crown. Physiologic dental and gingival contours are considered to be inhibitory to the accrual of debris and bacterial plaque and the renewal of inflammatory disease.

CONCLUSION

We must here recognize that microbiologic, traumatic, immunologic, inheritable, chemical and enzymatic, cellular, local and systemic influences are operative in periodontal disease and that their roles individually and in concert with each other may also be temporally variable. Cognizance must also be made of the variance of the

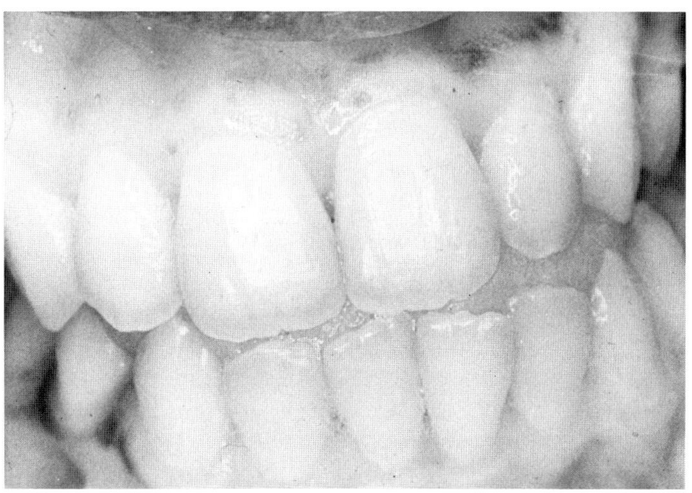

Fig. 2-12. The same patient in Figure 2-11 following surgical resection of excessive gingival tissue. The gingival margin is now shielded from topical irritation by the deflecting contours of the cervical convexity of the crown.

vague "resistance and reparative abilities" that exist at different periods of life and their mediation by the oral, systemic, atmospheric, psychologic, and social ecologies of the individual.

Fortunately, despite the complexity of influences on the individual and his periodontium, we find—on a near universal basis—that the young, when compared with his elders, manifests a well-defined, marginally restricted gingival inflammatory state which remains limited in severity and expanse, often cyclically, until he can no longer structurally, reparatively or immunologically contain the inflammatory process. At that point, the gingival inflammatory lesion progresses into a form of chronic destructive periodontal disease which, if left untreated, may result in the loss of teeth.

BIBLIOGRAPHY

1. Baer, P. N.: The case for periodontosis as a disease entity. J. Periodont., *42:*516, 1971.
2. Brill, N., and Krasse, B.: Passage of tissue fluid into clinically healthy gingival pocket. Acta Odontol. Scand., *16:*233, 1958.
3. Egelberg, J.: Gingival exudate measurements for evaluation of inflammatory changes in gingiva. Odont. Rev., *15:*381, 1964.
4. Friedman, L. A., and Klinkhamer, J. M.: Experimental human gingivitis. J. Periodont., *42:*702–705, 1971.
5. Glickman, I.: Occlusion—a factor in periodontal health and disease in the circumpubertal and adolescent periods. J. Periodont., *42:*513, 1971.
6. Goldman, H. M.: The variables in gingivitis and periodontitis during circumpubertal periods. J. Periodont., *42:*521, 1971.
7. Greene, J. C.: Oral hygiene and periodontal disease, Am. J. Public Health, *53:*913, 1963.
8. Kleinberg, I., Chatterjee, R., *et al.*: Plaque formation and the effect of age. J. Periodont., *42:*497, 1971
9. Klinkhamer, J. M.: Human oral leucocytes. Periodontology. *1:*109, 1963.
10. Larato, D. C.: Alveolar plate fenestrations and dehiscences of the human skull. Oral Surg., *29:*816, 1970.
11. Lindhe, J., and Mansson, V.: The bacteriology of the gingival crevices of erupting human incisors. J. Periodont. Res., *1:*14, 1966.
12. Loe, H., and Holm-Pedersen, P.: Absence and presence of fluid from normal and inflamed gingivae. Periodontology, *3:*171, 1965.
13. Ruben, M. P., Frankl, S. N., and Wallace, S.: Histopathology of periodontal disease in children. J. Periodont., *42:*473, 1971.
14. Sandalli, P., and Wade, A. B.: Crevicular fluid flow in young children. J. Periodont., *42:*713, 1971.

15. Socransky, S. S.: Relationship of bacteria to the etiology of periodontal disease. J. Dent. Res., *49:*203, 1970.
16. Socransky, S., and Manganiello, S. D.: The oral microbiota of man from birth to senility. J. Periodont., *42:*485, 1971.

REFERENCES

1. Attstrom, R.: Studies on the neutrophilic polymorphonuclear leucocyte at dento-gingival junction in gingival health and disease. J. Periodont. Res., (Suppl.), *8:* 1971.
2. Bader, H., and Goldhaber, E.: The passage of intravenously injected tetracycline in the gingival sulcus of dogs. J. Oral Ther. and Pharm., *2:*324, 1965.
3. Baer, P. N.: Periodontal disease in children and adolescents, a clinical study. J.A.D.A., *55:*629, 1957.
4. Bervell, S. F.: The bacteriology of physiological gingival pockets. Acta. Odontol. Scand., *22:*167, 1964.
5. Brill, N., and Krasse, B.: The passage of tissue fluid into the clinically healthy gingival pocket. Acta. Odontol. Scand., *16:*233, 1958.
6. Bruckner, M.: Gingivitis and Vincent's infection in children. J. Dent. Child., *23:*116, 1956.
7. Butler, J. H.: A familial pattern of juvenile periodontitis (periodontosis). J. Periodont., *40:*115, 1969.
8. Cohen, B.: An approach to the problem of parodontal disease. Parodontologie, *17:*13, 1963.
9. Cohen, B.: Morphological factors in the pathogenesis of periodontal disease. Br. Dent. J., *107:*31, 1959.
10. Cohen, D. W., and Goldman, H. M.: Periodontal disease in children. PDM, 1962: 1, Jul., 1962.
11. Cohen, M., and Winer, R.: Dental and facial characteristics of Down's syndrome. J. Dent. Res., *44:*197, 1965.
12. Dewar, M. R.: Bacterial enzymes and periodontal disease. J. Dent. Res., *37:*100, 1958.
13. Dixon, F. J.: Glomerulonephritis and immunopathology. In Good, R. A., and Fisher, D. W. (ed.): Immunobiology. Stamford (Conn.), Sinauer Associates, 1971.
14. Dwyer, D. M., and Socransky, S. S.: Predominant cultivatable microorganisms inhabiting periodontal pockets. Br. Dent. J., *124:*560, 1968.
15. Emslie, R. D.: Cancrum oris. Dent. Pract. Dent. Rec., *13:*481, 1963.
16. Fish, W.: Etiology and prevention of periodontal breakdown. D. Progress, *1:*234, 1961.
17. Fitzgerald, R. J., and Keyes, P. H., *et al.*: Effects of a dextranase preparation on plaque and caries in hamsters; a preliminary report. J.A.D.A., *76:*301, 1968.
18. Fullmer, H., Gibson, W. A., *et al.*: Origins of collagenase in periodontal tissues of man. J. Dent. Res., *48:*646, 1969.
19. Gewurz, H.: The Immunologic role of complement. *In* Good, R. A., and Fisher, D. W. (ed): Immunobiology, Stamford (Conn.), Sinauer Associates, 1971.
20. Gibbons, R. J., and McDonald, J. B.: Degradation of collagenous substrates by bacteroides melanogenicus. J. Bacteriol., *81:*614, 1961.
21. Hausman, E., *et al.*: Endotoxin: stimulation of bone resorption. Science, *168:*862, 1970.
22. Hirsch, J.: Periodontal disease in children. Study of etiological factors in childhood. D. Student's Mag., *34:*24, 1955.
23. Kelsten, L. B.: Periodontal and soft tissue diseases in children. J. Dent. Med., *10:*67, 1955.
24. Klinkhamer, J. M., and Zimmerman, S.: Function and reliability of the orgranulocytic migratory rate as a measure of oral health. J. Dent. Res., *48:*709, 1969.
25. Lapiere, G. M., and Gross, J.: Animal collagenase and collagen metabolism. *In* Sognnaes R. (ed.): Mechanisms of hard tissue destruction. Washington, D.C., American Association for the Advancement of Science, 1963.
26. Loe, H., Theilade E., and Jensen B. S.: Experimental gingivitis in man. J. Periodont., *36:*197, 1965.
27. McCall, J. O.: Gingival and periodontal disease in children. J. Periodont., *9:*7, 1938.
28. McHugh, W. D.: The interdental gingiva. J. Periodont. Res., *6:*227, 1971.
29. McIntosh, W. G.: Gingival and periodontal disease of children. J. Periodont., *25:*99, 1954.
30. Massler, M.: Co-report: periodontal disease in children. Int. Dent. J., *8:*323, 1958.

31. Mergenhagen, S. E., Hampp, E. G., and Scherp, H. W.: Preparation and biologic activities of endotoxin from oral bacteria. J. Infect. Dis., *108:*304, 1961.
32. Parfitt, G. J.: Periodontal disease in children. *In* Finn, S. B.: Clinical Pedodontics. Philadelphia, W. B. Saunders, 1963.
33. Ramfjord, S. Emslie, R., *et al.:* Epidemiological studies of periodontal disease. Am. J. Public Health, *58:*1713, 1968.
34. Robinson, H. G.: Periodontitis and periodontosis in children and young adolescents. J.A.D.A., *43:*709, 1951.
35. Ruben, M. P., Schulman, S., and Kon, S.: Healing of periodontal surgical wounds. *In* Goldman, H. M. and Cohen, D. W.: Periodontal Therapy ed. 5, St. Louis, C. V. Mosby, 1972.
36. Ruben, M. P., Prieto-Hernandez, J. R., Gott, F., Kramer, G. M., and Bloom, A. A.,: Visualization of lymphatic microcirculation of oral tissues. II. Vital retrograde lymphography. J. Periodont., *42:*774, 1971.
37. Schour, I., and Massler, M.: Gingival disease in postwar Italy. Gingivosis in hospitalized children in Naples. Am. J. Orthodont. Oral Surg., *33:*756, 1947.
38. Schultz-Haudt, S., Dewar, M. and Bibby, B.: Effects of hyalouronidase on human gingival epithelium. Science, *117:*653, 1963.
39. Schultz-Haudt, S., and Scherp, H. W.: Production of chondrosulfatase by microorganisms from human gingival crevices. J. Dent. Res., *35:*299, 1956.
40. Schultz-Haudt, S., and Scherp, H. W.: Production of hyalouronidase and B-glucoronidase by viridans streptococci isolated from gingival crevices. J. Dent. Res., *34:*924, 1955.
41. Sheiham, A.: Epidemiology of chronic periodontal disease in Western Nigerian school children. J. Periodont. Res., *3:*257-267, 1968
42. Simon, B., Ruben, M. P., and Goldman, H. M.: Role of endotoxin in periodontal disease. I. A reproducible, quantitative method for determining the amount of endotoxin in human gingival exudate. J. Periodontol., *40:*695, 1969.
43. Simon, B., Ruben, M. P., and Goldman, H. M.: Assessment of endotoxin in periodontal disease. II. Correlation with severity of inflammation. J. Periodont., *41:*81, 1970.
44. Stallard, R. E. Current concepts of periodontal disease. J. Dent. Children, *34:*204, 1967.
45. Zappler, S. E.: Periodontal disease in children. J.A.D.A., *37:*333, 1948.

3

Acute Lesions Affecting the Gingiva and Oral Mucosa

ERUPTION CYST

This type of dentigerous cyst is associated with erupting teeth, usually primary erupting teeth. It results from the accumulation of tissue fluid and/or blood in the dilated follicular space about the crown of the erupting tooth. The etiology is unknown.

Incidence. The cysts occur in children of all ages including the newborn. In the latter the cysts are most commonly associated with the partially formed crowns of the mandibular central incisors. In a study of 2,910 newborn infants, eruptive cysts were reported in 6 cases.[1]

Clinical Characteristics. The cyst generally appears as a bluish swelling over an erupting tooth (Fig. 3-1). The color depends upon the amount of blood present within the eruptive cavity and the thickness of the overlying mucosa.

Treatment. Treatment is usually unnecessary, since the tooth generally erupts without interference. However, in rare instances, in which the cyst apparently is responsible for undue delayed eruption of the affected tooth, surgical excision of the overlying tissue to expose the crown may be necessary.

ACUTE GINGIVAL PROBLEMS ASSOCIATED WITH EXFOLIATION OF A PRIMARY TOOTH

One root of a primary molar may resorb much more rapidly than another. Such uneven resorption can cause increased tooth mobility, thus encouraging food impaction, accumulation of bacterial plaque, and mechanical irritation of the underlying mucosa by the uneven, sharp, partially resorbed root end. Interproximal gingival

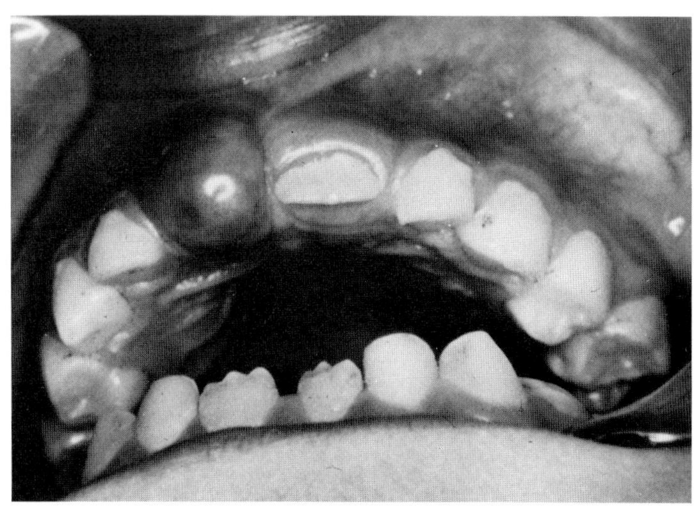

Fig. 3-1. An eruption cyst appears on the maxillary right central incisor.

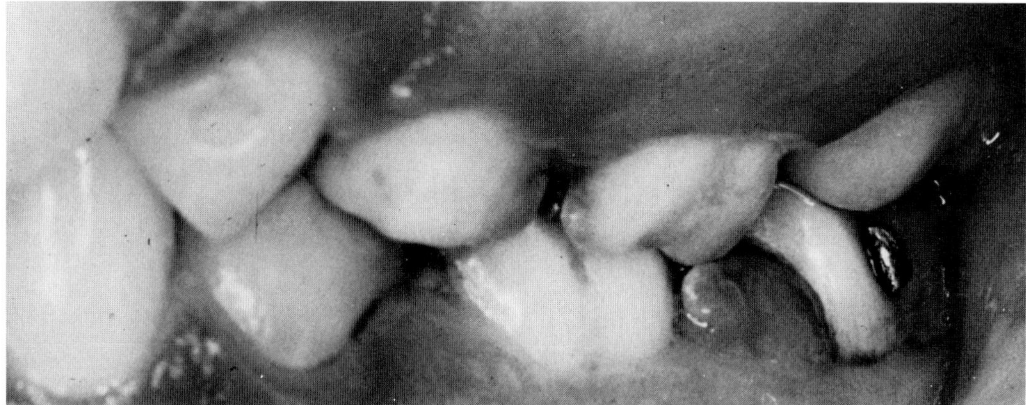

Fig. 3-2. *Top.* Note the interdental gingival enlargement between the mandibular primary molar and the first permanent molar.

enlargement (Fig. 3-2) associated with bleeding and discomfort may result.

Extraction of the primary tooth in such cases eliminates the pathologic condition and encourages the eruption of the underlying permanent tooth into good alignment.

ACUTE NECROTIZING ULCERATIVE GINGIVITIS (ANUG)

This disease has been known by many names throughout history, the most common of which are Vincent's infection and "trench mouth". In keeping with the modern trend towards nomenclature by clinical description, acute necrotizing ulcerative gingivitis (ANUG) has become the preferred term.

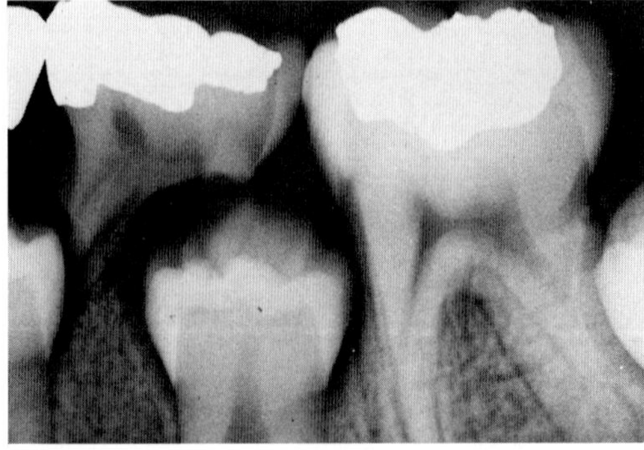

Fig. 3-2. *Bottom.* Roentgenograph of the above region shows that the primary molar is being exfoliated and the underlying permanent second bicuspid is erupting. This creates an environment that is favorable for the accumulation of plaque and the impaction and retention of food debris.

Cancrum Oris

In the United States and most other developed countries ANUG is primarily limited to adolescents. In less developed nations it also affects younger children. In malnourished children the intra-oral necrotic process may spread to the face, in which case it is termed cancrum oris (Figs. 3-3 through 3-6). Virtually all cases of noma occur in patients from low socio-economic groups who reveal a history of having had a debilitating disease prior to the onset of the oral symptoms. Usually the disease has been a viral infection such as measles or chicken pox.

Prevalence. Giddon, *et al.*[11] reported acute necrotizing ulcerative gingivitis present in 2.5 percent of entering college students; in United States military personnel Grupe and Wilder[14] found a frequency of 2.2 percent, and Goldhaber[13] a frequency of 3.4 percent. In Danish military personnel, Pindborg[30] reported a frequency of 4.4 percent, while Sillevius-Smith[40] found a frequency of 2.0 percent.

In Nigeria, Sheiham[39] found the disease present in 11.3 percent of children 2 to 6 years of age, while Emslie[7] found it occurring in 23 percent below the age of 10

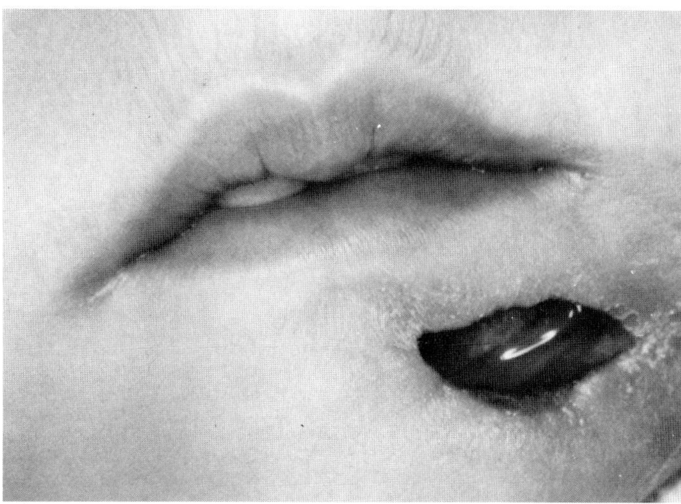

Fig. 3-3. At this early stage of cancrum oris or noma in a child the disease process is usually reversible with penicillin. (Courtesy of Dr. Mario Jimenez.)

years. In West Africa, Malberger[24] found ANUG present in 50 children aged 1 to 6 years, out of 7,650 patients who had the disease. In Bangalore, India, on the other hand, Pindborg[31] found only a prevalence rate of 2.36 percent, or 236 patients out of 10,000 examined who had the disease. It is interesting to note that 58 percent of these patients were below the age of 10.

The average age of the patients in the studies of Miller and Greenhut[26,27] was 15 to 30 years, whereas Stammer's[41] patients showed a range of 3 to 68 years of age, with the average being 19 to 30 years.

It is difficult to determine sex distribution, since most studies have been performed on military personnel. However, an analysis of the available studies indicates no sex differential.

Clinical Characteristics. The disease is characterized by rapid destruction of the interdental papilla with associated pain and bleeding. There is often a gray pseudomembrane found at the margin as a result of necrosis. Fetor exoris may be present, depending upon the severity of the disease, but is not found in all cases. Submaxillary gland enlargement and tenderness may occur in severe cases. Salivation may be excessive and the patient may complain of a metallic taste in the mouth.

The clinical picture may be quite varied (Fig. 3-7 through 3-10). One or many gingival papillae may be affected. The degree of destruction can be severe or mild. Those papillae exhibiting the disease most severely are usually subject to some local causative factor (e.g., overhanging restoration, calculus or rotated tooth). The lesions may remain limited to the interdental papilla or may extend onto the facial and lingual surfaces of the attached gingiva, but the alveolar mucosa is rarely involved. The disease is not self-limiting and will continue if untreated. However, there may be a spontaneous remission of the acute symptoms alternating with periods of exacerbation.

Systemic Findings. Systemic findings occasionally may accompany the disease. Anorexia and malaise may be present. While fever as high as 103° has been described, occurring in the acute phase, most authorities do not think that marked elevation of temperature is characteristic.[9,13,37]

Etiology. This disease has a multifaceted etiology.

Bacteria. The spirochete *Borrelia vincentii* and the *Bacillus fusiformis* have been implicated as causative agents because they appear in large numbers in this disease. These organisms, however, also exhibit a

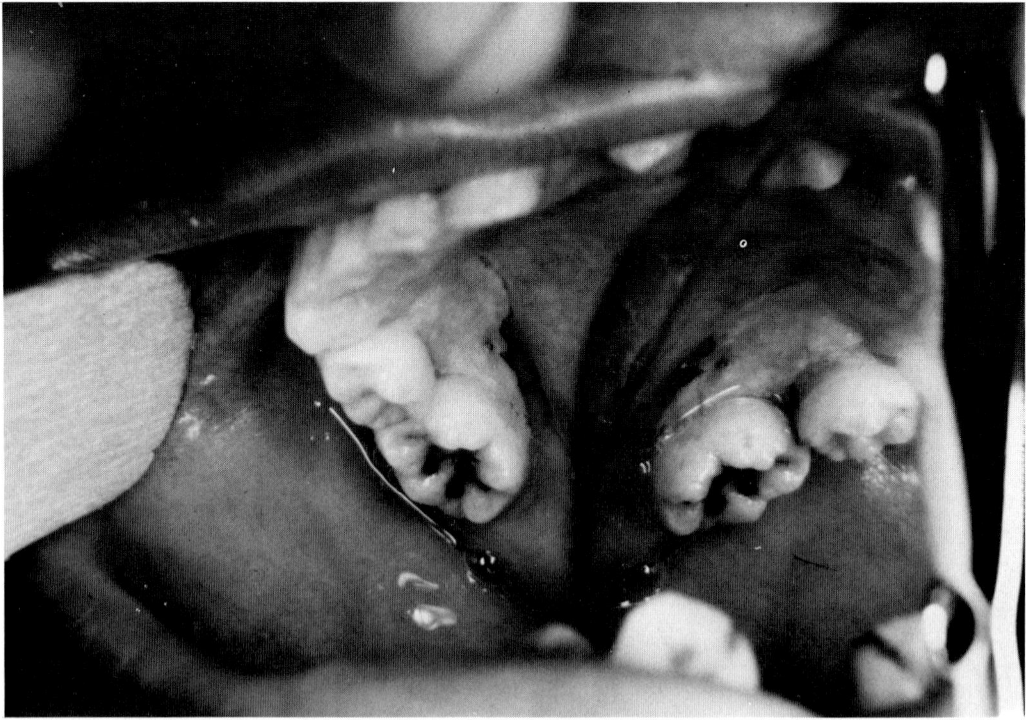

Fig. 3-4. In this case of cancrum oris with intra-oral lesions, necrotic bone is present about the palatal surface of the bicuspid-molar region. (Courtesy of Dr. Mario Jimenez.)

considerable increase in number in both chronic gingivitis and periodontitis, so that the mere presence of large numbers of organisms per se does not prove that they are responsible for the disease.[2,5,15,16,21,22,23,42] Spirochetes have long been considered to be secondary invaders in necrotic lesions. In acute necrotizing ulcerative gingivitis, for instance, spirochetes have not been found in the viable tissues underlying the areas of necrosis when examined by the ordinary light microscope. However, recent studies utilizing the electron microscope[17,20] have demonstrated spirochetes in the deep viable layer of tissue beneath the necrotic zones.

There is no question that bacteria play a role in the disease as evidenced by the dramatic response to antibiotic therapy.[3,34,35] However, the specific role of the oral microflora is still not understood.

Stress. Schluger,[36] in World War II, reported that stress rather than contagion was responsible for the outbreaks of acute necrotizing ulcerative gingivitis in bivouaced troops. Stammers,[41] in wartime England, thought there was an increased incidence of this disease during bombing raids. Goldhaber and Giddon[13] noted a higher incidence of necrotizing ulcerative gingivitis among college students who were dropouts, with 3 times those initially presenting having sought counseling over a random dental population. Davis and Baer[6] reported the onset of symptoms of ANUG in drug addicts during the period of drug withdrawal. Other investigators have also commented on the role of stress. Moulton,[28] for instance, demonstrated through psychiatric evaluations that patients with acute necrotizing ulcerative gingivitis were more unstable emotionally than a control group.

We have found similar results from our psychiatric examinations. The following is a case report taken from our files to illustrate this point.

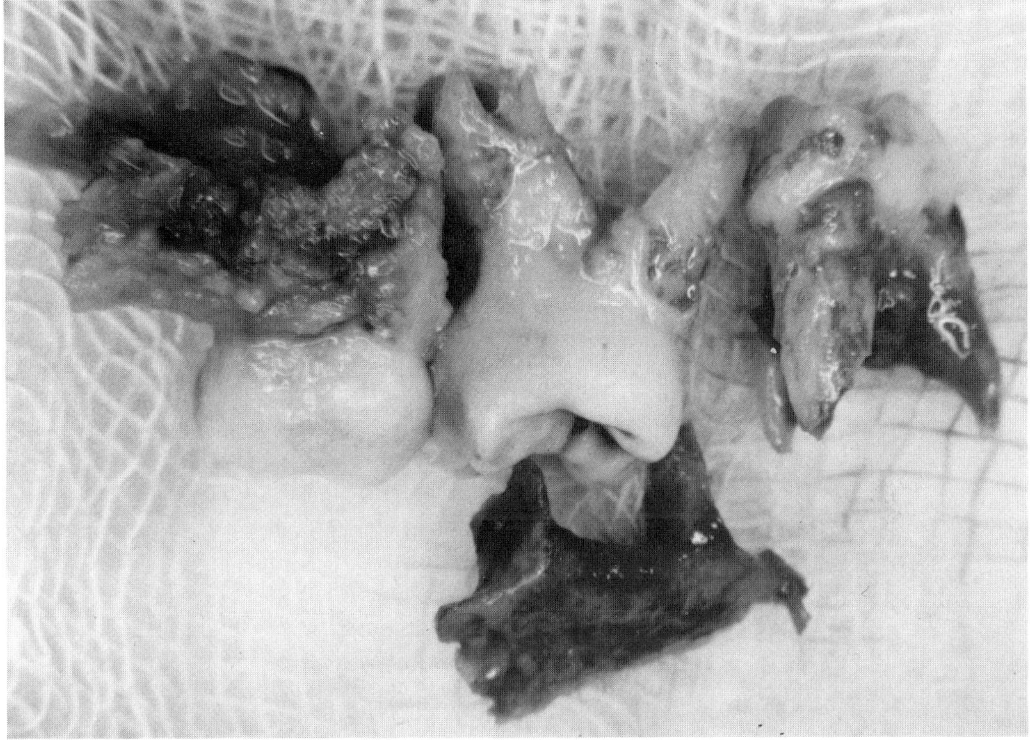

Fig. 3-5. The teeth and alveolar bone in the above case have sequestrated.

CASE HISTORY

A 20-year-old single male has complained of "trench mouth" of 3 years' duration, and has had feelings of inadequacy and pathological jealousy of at least that time. He is not aware of any relation between his oral and psychological symptoms but is convinced that he acquired the "infection" following a date with a girl who was similarly afflicted. Since leaving high school (for disciplinary reasons) he has felt inadequate at his jobs; he wants very much to succeed but is absentminded, does unaccountable "stupid" things and makes a fool of himself; in addition there is much absenteeism. At the same time, he feels very distrustful of his girl friend, whose fidelity he constantly and obsessively questions; he does not seem to realize that this feeling might be related to his own perfidy, which is quite flagrant. For the last 3 months he has been impotent, apparently in fear of impregnating his current girl friend, who wants to marry him. He also describes an obsession about being neatly dressed, which often prompts him to change his clothes up to 3 times a day.

His background is strikingly pathogenic. His father, now 56, has been tense, nervous, and markedly obsessive almost all his life and was hospitalized with a psychotic depression at the age of 40 when the patient was 4 years old. His mother is domineering, strict, and administered harsh physical discipline until the patient was 12 years old. The patient neither respects nor is close to either parent, his warmest feeling being one of pity for his father. There are 2 considerably older siblings who have left the family, and a younger sister who is involved with many of the girls the patient dates and who disapproves of his behavior.

During the interview the patient was outwardly cooperative, somewhat bland and compliant, and I did not think he was entirely reliable. He was dressed nattily in the style of the high school beat and the whole effect was quite effeminate (curly hair carefully coifed, ring with light blue stone, safety pin collar tie clip without tie). He seemed delighted to talk about himself and did so with a very transparent braggadocio through which his lack of confidence and his concern about himself were apparent. He was

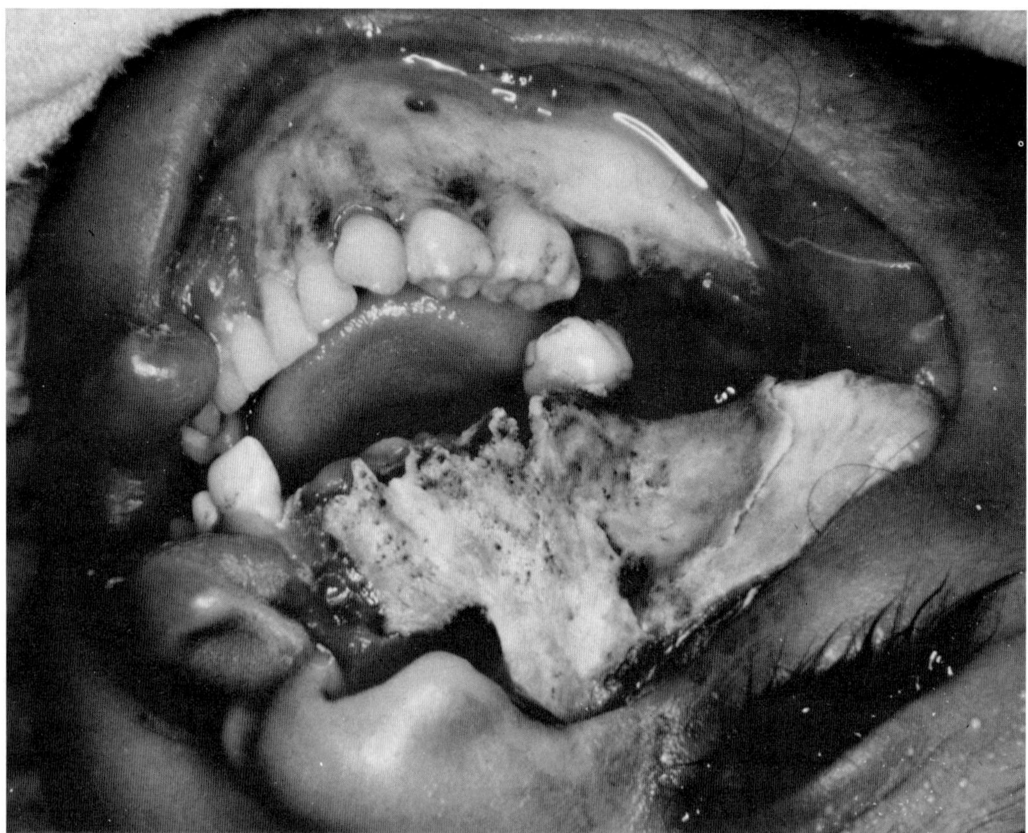

Fig. 3-6. Cancrum oris in the terminal stage. (Courtesy of Dr. Mario Jimenez.)

of average intelligence but without psychological insight. In addition to his blandness there was a flatness of effect and absence of feeling tone, but with no bizarre mental content and no secondary symptoms such as delusions or hallucinations. His defenses were chiefly denial, projection, and, to some extent, somatization. His obsessiveness was manifest in his dress. He denied depression, suicidal ideation or intent, and elation.

Impression. Schizoid personality with obsessive and psychopathic features. This was such a mixed picture that it was difficult to say what course it would take.

Recommendation. Appropriate dental management with further exploration of the patient's concept of disease (which is quite possibly venereal). I did not feel that this patient was likely to benefit from psychotherapy because of his limited capacity for insight.

Other Factors. Personality tests and physiologic tests which have been administered to patients with the disease have indicated that these patients display an abnormal peripheral vasomotor response during remission and tend to have dominant personality traits and a negative abasement trait.[4, 8, 10, 12, 38] This type of person when placed in a situation in which he could not be dominant and in which he had to humble himself would set into action the psychological factors which would contribute to the onset of necrotizing ulcerative gingivitis.

Smoking has been cited as another important etiologic factor.[29] However, it is difficult to separate the role of stress from that of smoking. Those people who smoke the most are also under the most stress. It is also possible that smoking exerts its deleterious effects through its influence on the vascularity of the gingival tissues. Vascular changes have been associated

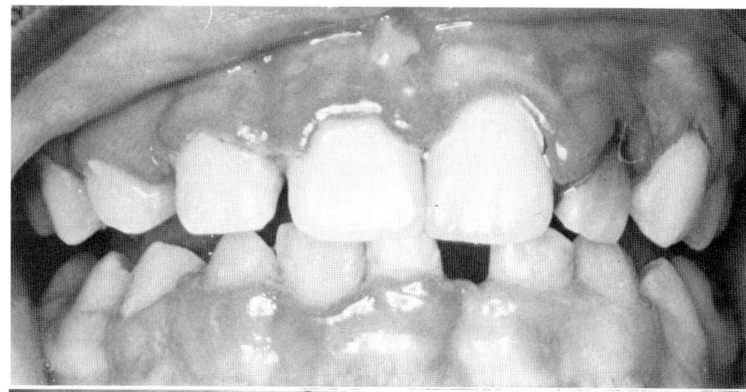

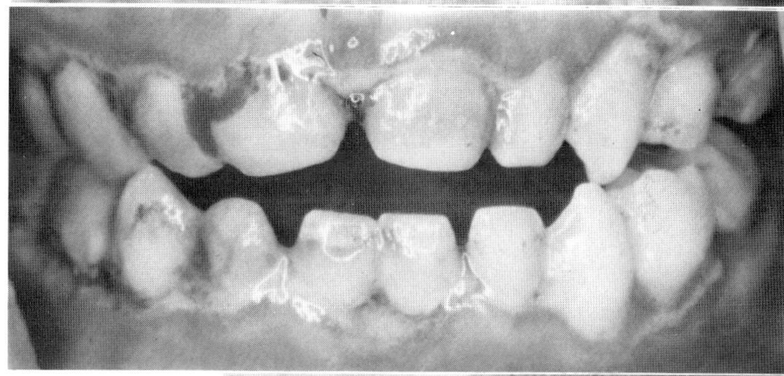

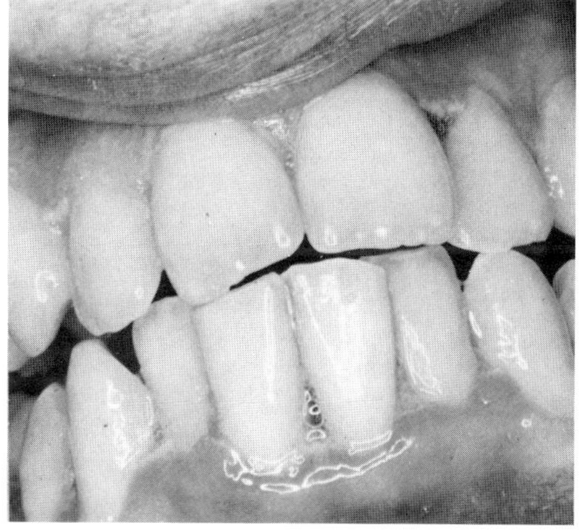

Fig. 3-7. *Top.* In this case of acute necrotizing ulcerative gingivitis, in a 14-year-old female, not only is necrosis of the tips of the interdental papillae present, but also the gingiva is hyperplastic and the papillae are enlarged and bleed spontaneously. In this case the acute necrotizing ulcerative gingivitis was probably superimposed upon a preexisting hyperplastic gingivitis.
Center. The necrosis may remain limited to the interdental papillae, or as in this case may extend onto the facial and lingual surfaces of the attached gingiva.
Bottom. In the young adult, as opposed to the adolescent, the lesions tend to be confined to the interdental papillae.

with the rapid production of certain types of necrosis. Both the Arthus and localized Schwartzman phenomena are immune reactions which produce alterations in the blood vessels, and the localized Schwartzman reaction has been produced in the oral cavity of hamsters.[33] Therefore, the possibility of an immunologic reaction in man must also be considered. Lehner[19] demonstrated that in acute necrotizing ulcerative gingivitis, and not in any other oral disease, there is a lowered IgG and elevated IgM immunoglobin concentrations within 1 to 4 days of the onset of symptoms.

The familial occurrence of ANUG has also been reported by several investigators.[6,18]

With the possible exception of protein deficiency,[32] there are no known nutritional deficiences that play an etiologic role.

In summary, the etiology of acute necrotizing ulcerative gingivitis appears to involve local traumatic factors coupled with an acute psychologic disturbance resulting in a lowered tissue resistance—which in turn permits the oral microbial flora to invade the gingival tissues.

CONTAGION

It is a noncontagious disease. Early reports classifying this disease as communicable were probably based on an incorrect diagnosis (i.e., the mistaken diagnosis of acute herpetic gingivostomatitis as acute necrotizing ulcerative gingivitis).

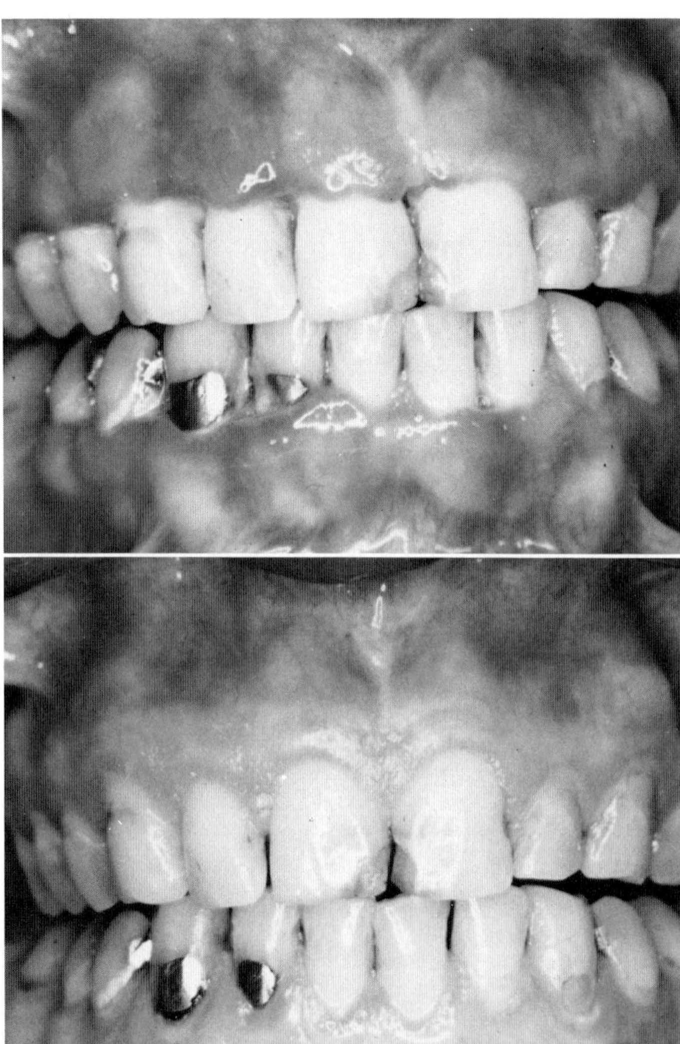

Fig. 3-8. *Top*. These gingival deformities are a result of necrotizing ulcerative gingivitis.
Bottom. Post-operative results in the above patient. Periodontal surgery was necessary to restore proper physiologic gingival contours.

Further confusion may exist when on occasion these diseases occur simultaneously.

Treatment. The treatment of choice is local therapy, consisting of the removal of local irritating factors and debridement of the necrotic portions of the wound. Systemic antibiotics are used only when massive necrosis has occurred or when there are systemic effects. Whether or not to use antibiotics systemically is a clinical judgment to be made by the therapist. The use of antibiotics usually does result in a rapid cessation of symptoms and a diminution in the amount of tissue lost from necrosis. Topical utilization of antibiotics by lozenge or troche is contraindicated because of the sensitization associated with topical antibiotic therapy. Several British publications have described the successful use of metronidazole (Flagyl) systemically; however, the potential side effects of this drug should mitigate against its routine use.

After relief of the acute symptoms, surgical treatment of the gingiva may be needed

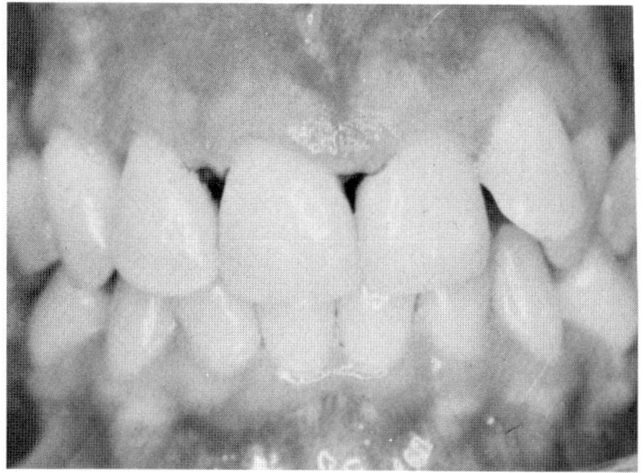

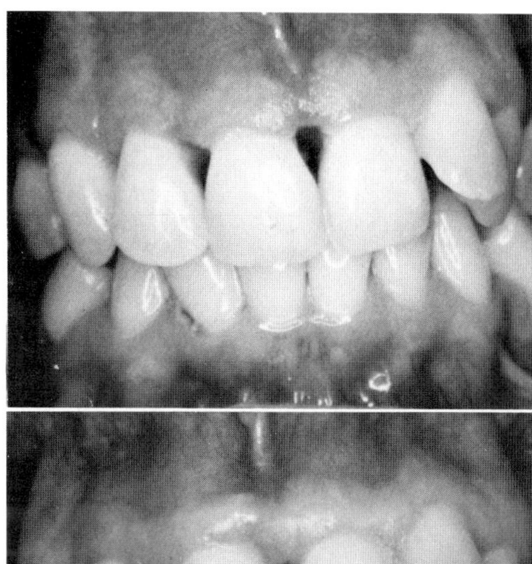

Fig. 3-9. *Top left.* This 16-year-old girl presented with necrotizing ulcerative gingivitis. *Top right.* Following treatment of the acute phase, interproximal craters developed. *Bottom.* Periodontal surgery was required to restore proper physiologic gingival contours.

to correct deformities created by the necrosis (Figs. 3-8, 3-9 and 3-10).

Recurrence. One of the difficulties in the treatment of this disease is the frequency of recurrence. Sillevius-Smitt[40] noted a 25 percent recurrence rate, while Manson and Rand[25] reported a 34.4 percent relapse rate in 6 months, 31.1 percent in one year and 24.7 percent after 2 years.

Lehner[43] has speculated that the recurrence may be the result of an immunologic phenomenon. Other investigators believe that recurrences are mainly due to persistent gingival deformity and the failure to eliminate local factors. Many times the fault lies with the patient, who is generally less stable than other dental patients and after cessation of the initial acute symptoms may not return for definitive therapy. Regardless of the causes the fact remains that there is a high rate of recurrence and the patient should be made aware of this fact. Because of this high recurrence rate, the patient should be kept under supervision after recovery for at least 6 months.

ACUTE HERPETIC GINGIVOSTOMATITIS

This acute inflammatory condition of the oral cavity is caused by the herpes simplex virus.[46] It was first identified as a clinical entity in 1938[45, 45] and has been held responsible for about one half of the sore mouths of childhood,[52] although the disease may occur at any age. It rarely affects children under the age of one year and reaches its peak at about 3 years of age. The incidence tends to be higher in the fall and winter months.[45, 52]

Etiology. The etiologic agent is the herpes simplex virus, which is usually spread by direct contact.[45, 46, 51] Exposure to the herpes simplex virus results in the formation of neutralizing antibodies.[49] The children affected, therefore, are those who do

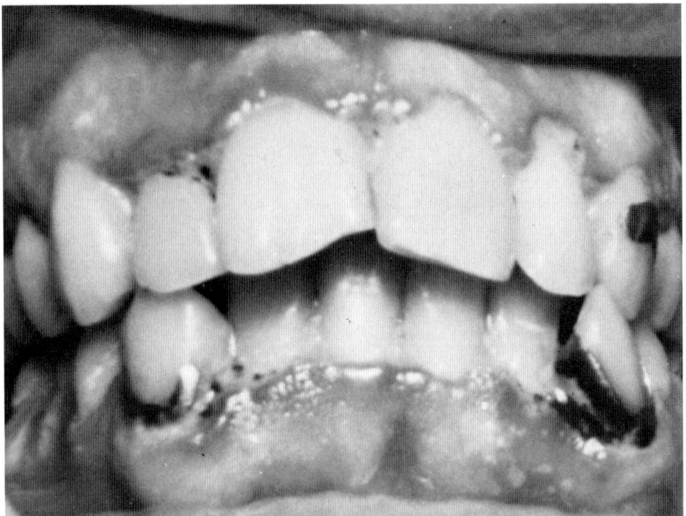

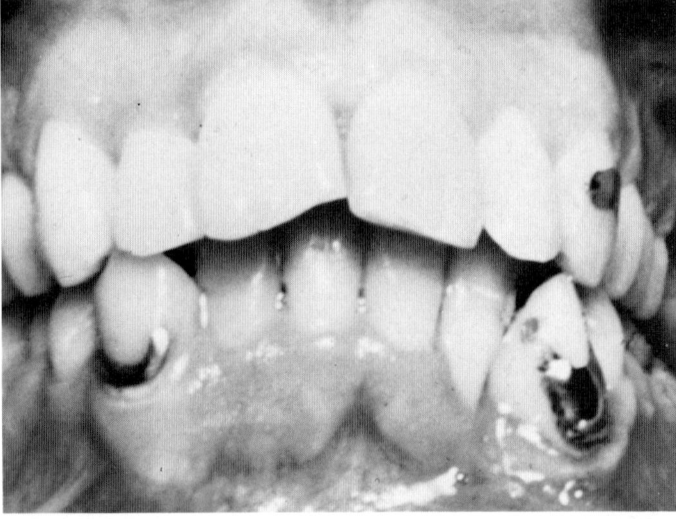

Fig. 3-10. *Top.* A 17-year-old male at the time of admission with ANUG. *Bottom.* Postoperative results in the above case. Periodontal surgery was needed to restore the proper physiologic gingival contour.

not possess these antibodies. After recovery from this disease the antibody titer drops to a low or nondetectable level in children, whereas in adults it usually remains at a detectable level.[47] Studies regarding the percentages of the population which have neutralizing antibodies vary from 40 to 90 percent.[50, 54] This large variation can probably be explained by the fact that the herpes simplex virus is transferred more readily among the lower socioeconomic groups.[48] Therefore, one would probably find a higher incidence of acute herpetic gingivostomatitis in young children of the lower socioeconomic groups and in adolescents and young adults of the middle and upper socioeconomic groups.[54]

Clinical Characteristics. The systemic findings appear first and are rather severe. They consist of a high fever (averaging between 101° to 103°), anorexia, malaise and submaxillary gland involvement.[44, 47, 53, 55]

The clinical appearance of the oral cavity is one of a fiery red diffuse inflammation throughout the gingiva (Fig. 3-11) and alveolar mucosa which often makes it difficult to distinguish the end of the attached gingiva and the beginning of the alveolar mucosa.[55] This is accompanied by the

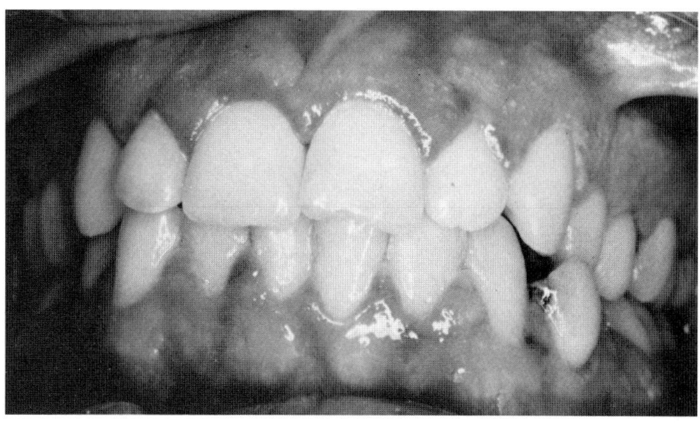

Fig. 3-11. The gingiva may show a diffuse and nonspecific type of inflammatory reaction in acute herpetic gingivostomatitis.

formation of multiple small vesicles over a 4- to 5-day period (Fig. 3-12), which burst, leaving shallow ulcers covered with a yellowish exudate. The borders of these ulcers are inflamed (Fig. 3-13). When the vesicles appear on the attached gingiva, they may be confused with acute necrotizing ulcerative gingivitis because of the presence of the exudate, which may be mistaken for the necrotic interdental papillae seen in that condition. Both of these diseases can occur together.

Treatment. Treatment is mainly supportive and palliative. The patient is usually dehydrated because of the high fever and the discomfort in ingesting fluids and food. He should be placed on a bland diet and the fluid intake increased. Analgesics should be given for relief of pain. An emollient, such as Orabase, or a demulcent, such as milk of magnesia, may be used locally to ease the discomfort in the oral cavity.

Prognosis. Good. The disease runs its course in 6 to 16 days, the average duration being 11 days. The oral lesions heal in 5 to 6 days without scar formation.[55] The disease is self-limiting and rarely causes secondary complications.

INFECTIOUS MONONUCLEOSIS

Infectious mononucleosis is usually an acute, benign, self-limiting disease characterized by irregular fever (ranging from 100° to 103°F), lymphadenopathy, pharyngitis, splenomegaly, extreme fatigability and an absolute lymphocytosis with many atypical lymphocytes. In addition, the patient's serum has an abnormally high concentration of heterophile antibodies against sheep erythrocytes (a positive Paul-Bunnell test)[65] and antibodies to Epstein-Barr virus (EBV).[59, 60, 64]

Prevalence. It is primarily a disease of adolescents and young adults and rarely occurs in young children or in adults over 40 years of age. In one study of 80 cases it was found that 74 percent of the affected patients were 15 to 25 years of age.[58] In another study, only 3 patients out of 200 were children, 4 were 14 to 16 years old, and only 2 were 29 years of age. The remainder, 191 patients, were 17 to 29 years old.[63]

Etiology. Unknown. However, present evidence implicates the Epstein-Barr virus (EBV) as an etiologic agent.[59, 60, 64] Regardless of the etiology, it has a very low degree of contagion.

Clinical Characteristics. Most of the early symptoms are nonspecific and consist of excessive fatigue, malaise, anorexia, headache and myalgia. Lymphadenopathy is rarely a presenting symptom but develops usually 2 or 3 days after the onset of the first symptoms. By the end of one week palpable lymphadenopathy is present in 70 to 80 percent of all patients; jaundice is present in 8 to 10 percent of patients.

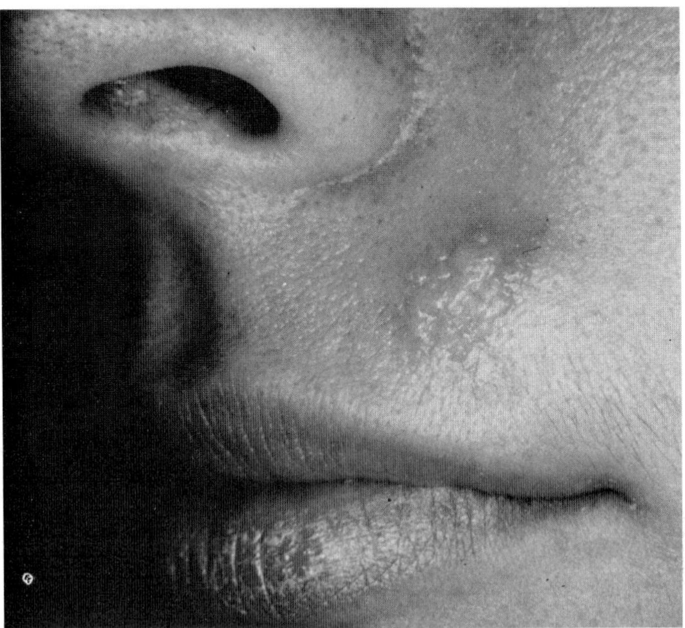

Fig. 3-12. Multiple small vesicles are present on the skin of this patient with acute herpetic gingivostomatitis.

Sore throat is probably the most characteristic symptom and usually develops a few days after the onset of the first symptoms, increasing in severity during the first week and then rapidly subsiding during the next 5 to 7 days.

Palatal petechiae develop in 25 to 35 percent of patients, usually between the fifth and seventeenth day of the illness. The lesions are sharply circumscribed, round petechiae with diameters of from 0.5 to 1.0 mm., and are symmetrically distributed at the junction of the soft and hard palate, or sometimes at the base of the uvula. They tend to turn reddish brown in 24 to 48 hours and may disappear in 3 to 4 days. Recurrent crops of petechiae may develop for the next few days. Such petechiae, however, are not specific for infectious mononucleosis and have been described in rubella and other viral disorders.[56, 57, 62, 66]

Oral lesions in other areas do occur but are not common. These consist of a nonspecific gingivitis or a gingivostomatitis with or without accompanying aphthous ulcerations. It is not clear whether these lesions are actually another symptom of the disease or merely incidental findings: They occur in less than 3 percent of patients.[61]

Treatment. Treatment is symptomatic and supportive. Salicylates may be given for the fever and pharyngitis and sedation for pain when necessary. Secondary infections require appropriate antibiotic therapy.

Prognosis. Generally good. Complete recovery is the rule.

RECURRENT APHTHOUS STOMATITIS

This disease may be defined as recurrent necrotizing ulcerations limited to the oral mucosa.

Etiology. Unknown. The onset of the lesions, however, is frequently associated with trauma or psychic stress[71, 82, 83] and on occasion with the intake of certain foods.[67] Recent investigations suggest that the etiology may involve a delayed type of hypersensitivity to *S. sanguis*[74, 76, 80] or an auto-immune phenomena.[70, 77, 78, 79]

The disease tends to be more common in females,[71, 76] and the highest incidence occurs in the postovulation period prior to

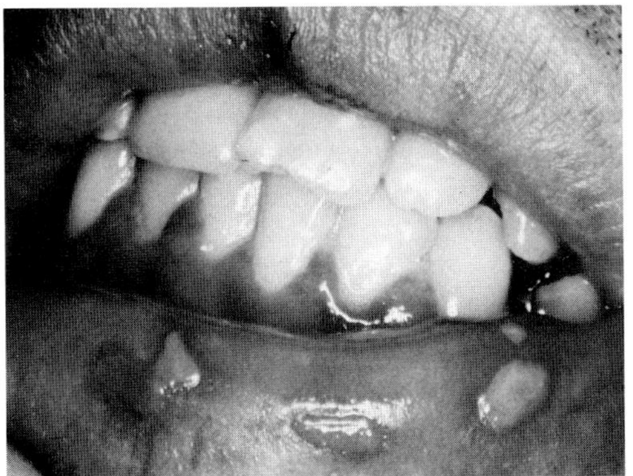

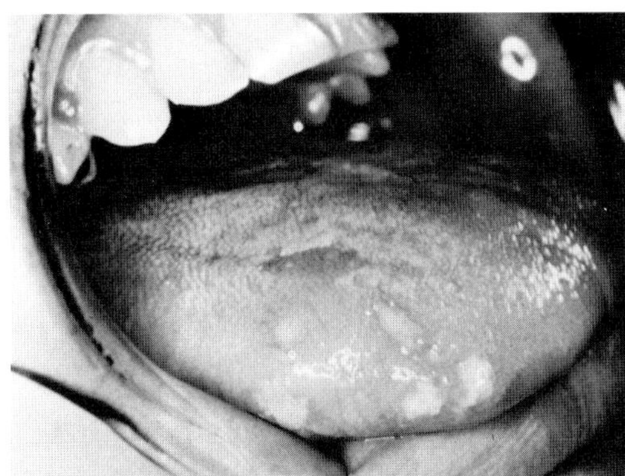

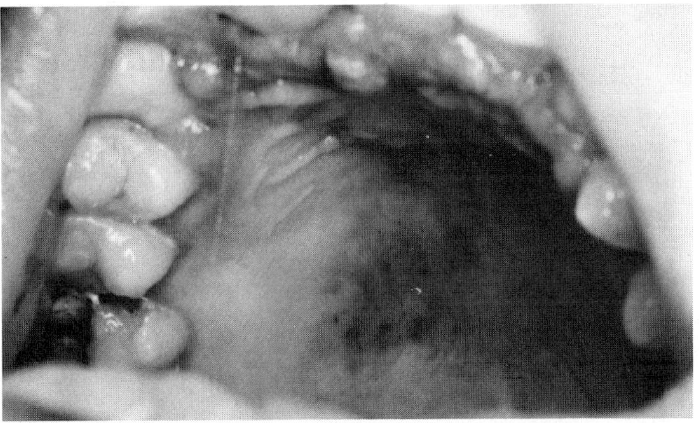

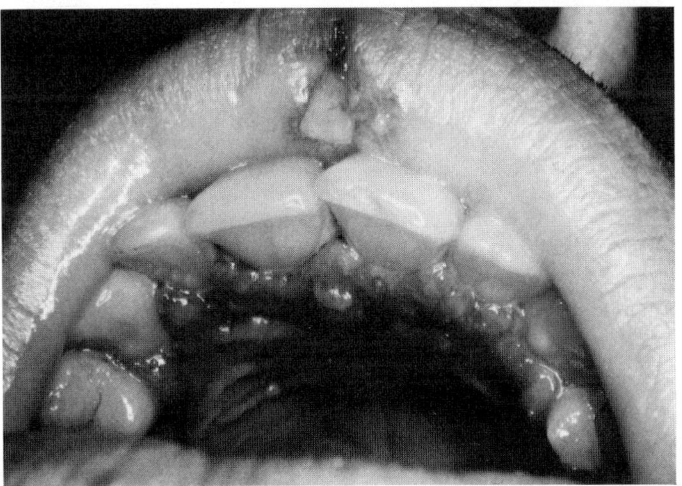

Fig. 3-13. *Top Left.* Shallow painful ulcers are seen on the lip.
Top right. Multiple painful ulcers are present on the tongue.
Center. Small vesicles and ulcers on the hard palate are painful and make swallowing difficult.
Bottom. Ulcerations near the tips of interdental papillae (shown on lingual) resemble those seen in acute necrotizing ulcerative gingivitis. The patient is an adolescent with acute herpetic gingivostomatitis.

menstruation.[68, 69, 73] Numerous studies have demonstrated the familial occurrence of this disease.[72, 75, 81, 83, 84] The aphthous lesions generally have their onset in childhood or adolescence and thereafter tend to recur at frequent intervals throughout life. Complete remissions are uncommon.

Clinical Characteristics. The lesions, which may vary in number from one to several dozen, begin as small localized erosions of the oral epithelium and are not preceded by vesicles. Within a period of 2 to 3 days the ulcerations increase in size and reach a diameter of 1 to 10 mm. The center of these sharply delineated lesions is grayish and the margins may or may not be inflamed. Pain and discomfort are striking clinical features and are the cause for the patient's seeking therapy. Healing occurs in 10 to 14 days without scarring. Prodromal symptoms of burning and tingling may be experienced by the patient 24 to 48 hours preceding clinical ulceration, but there is no systemic involvement (i.e., no fever or regional lymphadenopathy). The lesions are limited to the oral mucous membranes and do not occur cutaneously or at or near the mucocutaneous junction.

Treatment. There is no permanent cure, and in mild cases no treatment is necessary. In patients with severe discomfort, the following regime for symptomatic relief is recommended:[73]

1. Kenalog in Orabase applied topically 4 to 5 times daily.
2. Ascorbic acid, 100 mg. twice daily and ferrous gluconate, 300 mg. every day or twice daily (most useful in females and can be used in conjunction with other forms of therapy).
3. Oral achromycin (Lederle), a 250 mg. suspension used as mouth rinse for 1 minute 4 times a day following meals. Treatment is initiated when lesions first develop and is continued no longer than 5 to 7 days.

HERPANGINA

This is a well-defined clinical entity caused by the Group A Coxsackie[85] virus that occurs in epidemic form in infants and young children during the summer months. Relatively few cases are found in older children and young adults.

Clinical Characteristics. The disease is characterized by the abrupt onset of fever, which peaks in the first 24 to 48 hours and may range as high as 105°F. It is accompanied by anorexia, dysphagia, sore throat, headache, and pain and tenderness in the neck, abdomen and extremities.[85, 86] These symptoms may persist from 3 to 5 days. Objective symptoms are limited to the mouth. Clusters of 2 to 6 grayish white papules or vesicles, ranging in size from 1 to 4 mm., each with a red areola, appear within the first few days on the anterior pillars of the fauces, uvula and soft palate. During the course of 3 to 4 days the surface of the lesions ulcerate, leaving sharply outlined superficial ulcers. The illness is not severe. Healing is rapid, and complete recovery within a week is the rule.

Treatment. None required aside from symptomatic measures. Antibiotics are not indicated, since they have no effect on the etiologic virus and secondary infection is not a problem.

Differential Diagnosis. The infection must be differentiated from herpetic gingivostomatitis. The limitation of the lesions to the posterior pharynx, their small size, the benign course and the seasonal epidemic pattern serve to distinguish this entity from herpetic gingivostomatitis.[85, 86, 87]

In this latter disease the gingiva is hyperemic and ulcerations appear on the gums, lips, tongue and buccal mucosa. In addition, herpetic gingivostomatitis can occur during any time of the year and can be extremely debilitating. These two diseases, in turn, can readily be differentiated from recurrent aphthae, because recurrent aphthae seldom occur in the pharynx and are not accompanied by systemic symptoms.

PERICORONITIS

Pericoronitis refers to an acute inflammatory reaction of the gingiva surrounding a partially or incompletely erupted tooth, most often the mandibular third molar.

Etiology. The cause is generally an accumulation of food debris and bacteria under the gingival operculum of an erupting tooth.

Clinical Characteristics. The gingival operculum—usually overlying a mandibular third molar—becomes red, swollen and painful. With gentle pressure a purulent exudate can generally be discharged. The swollen operculum may interfere with closing of the jaws, and as a result the opposing maxillary tooth may further traumatize the already swollen operculum. The cheek in the area of the angle of the jaw may be swollen and there may be regional lymphadenopathy; in severe cases this may be accompanied by fever and malaise.

Treatment. Gentle debridement under the swollen gingival operculum with a curet to remove debris and permit discharge of the purulent exudate usually relieves some of the acute symptoms. If the swollen operculum is being traumatized by an opposing tooth, the occlusal surface of the offending tooth should be reduced so that it will not cause further injury (Fig. 3-14). The patient should be placed on warm physiologic saline rinses. In addition, if fever and a lymphadenopathy are present, administration of an antibiotic may be necessary.

Once the acute symptoms have subsided one must decide whether to retain or extract the involved tooth. If the third molar is to be retained, it will be necessary not only to surgically remove the operculum but to leave a distal saddle area. If the tooth is so situated in the ramus that it is impossible to obtain a distal saddle area following removal of the operculum, extraction of the tooth is the treatment of choice.

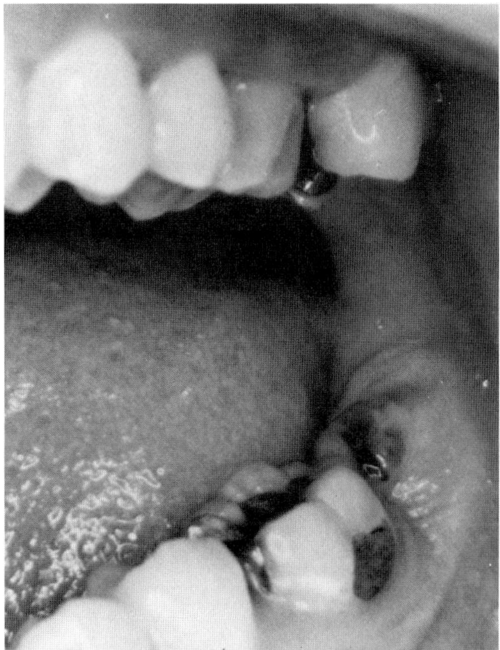

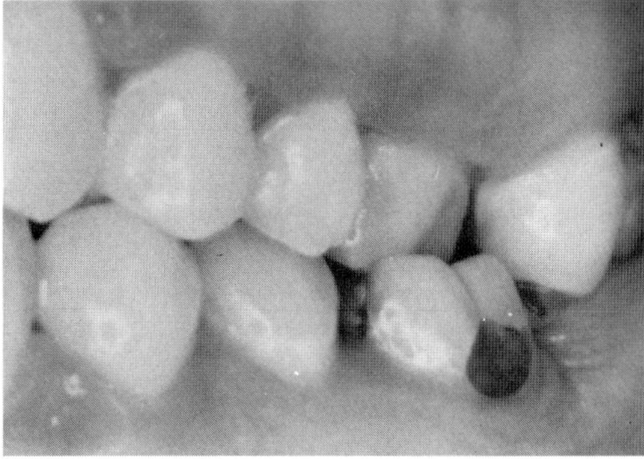

Fig. 3-14. *Top.* Gingiva about the last mandibular molar is swollen and painful. *Bottom.* The opposing maxillary molar tooth is traumatizing the mandibular gingiva. In these instances, part of the treatment consists of reducing the occlusal surface of the offending tooth so that it will not cause further injury to the mandibular gingiva.

ACUTE PERIODONTAL ABSCESS

This is rare in children and adolescents. When a periodontal abscess is present, it most frequently involves a tooth on which an orthodontic band extends below the margin of the gingiva.

Clinical Characteristics. The gingiva in the area of the lesion is swollen, red, smooth, shiny and painful. A purulent exudate can usually be expressed from the margin of the gingiva by the gentle insertion of a curet. The tooth is vital upon pulp testing.

Treatment. Curettage is the treatment of choice in children and adolescents. The response to this method of therapy tends to be very good.

Differential Diagnosis. This lesion should not be confused with the retrocuspid papilla (see chap. 1), a normal structure, nor with a periapical abscess, which is associated with a nonvital tooth.

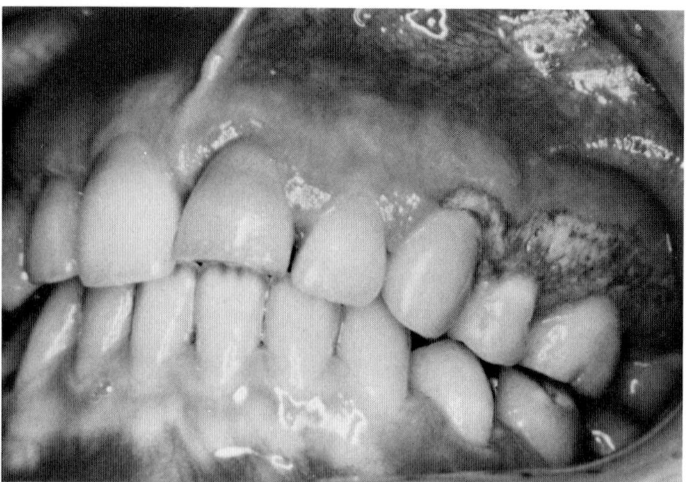

Fig. 3-15. Note the erosion of the buccal attached and free gingiva in the maxillary cuspid-molar region in a 16-year-old female as a result of toothbrush trauma.

MISCELLANEOUS

Acute Gingival Problems. Acute, painful lacerations to the gingiva (Fig. 3-15) can be caused by the improper use of a toothbrush, even in cases where the brush used has soft, polished bristles.

REFERENCES

Eruptive Cyst

1. Clark, C. D.: A survey of eruptive cysts in the newborn. Oral Surg., *15*:917, 1962.

Acute Necrotizing Ulcerative Gingivitis

2. Cahn, L. R.: The penetration of the tissue by Vincent's organism. J. Dent. Res., *9*:695, 1929.
3. Carter, W. G., and Ball, D. M.: Results of a three year study of Vincent's infection at Great Lakes Naval Dental Dept. J. Periodont., *24*:187, 1953.
4. Clark, R. E., and Giddon, D. B.: Body geometry of patients who had recurrent attacks of acute necrotizing ulcerative gingivitis. Arch. Oral Biol., *16*:205, 1971.
5. Courant, P. R., Paunio, I., and Gibbons, R. J.: Infectivity and hyaluronidase activity of debris from healthy and diseased gingiva. Arch. Oral Biol., *10*:119, 1965.
6. Davis, R. K., and Baer, P. N.: Necrotic ulcerative gingivitis in drug addict patients being withdrawn from drugs. Oral Surg., *31*:200, 1971.
7. Emslie, R. D.: Cancrum oris. Dent. Pract. Dent. Rec., *13*:481, 1963.
8. Formicola, A. J., Witte, E. T., and Curran, P. M.: A study of personality traits and acute necrotizing ulcerative gingivitis. J. Periodont., *41*:36, 1970.
9. Gallagher, J. R., Heald, F., and Masland, R. P., Jr.: Recent contributions to adolescent medicine. N. Eng. J. Med., *25*:123, 1958.
10. Giddon, D. B., Clark, R. E., and Varni, J. G.: Apparent digital vasomotor hypotoricity in the remission stage of acute necrotizing ulcerative gingivitis. J. Dent. Res., *48*:431, 1969.
11. Giddon, D. B., Zackin, S. J., and Goldhaber, P.: Acute necrotizing ulcerative gingivitis in college students. J.A.D.A., *68*:381, 1964.
12. Goldberg, H., Ambinder, W. J., Cooper, L., and Abrams, A. L.: Emotional status of patients with acute gingivitis. New York State Dent. J., *22*:308, 1956.
13. Goldhaber, P., and Giddon, D. B.: Present concepts of the etiology and treatment of acute necrotizing ulcerative gingivitis. Inter. Dent. J., *14*:468, 1964.
14. Grupe, I. L., and Wilder, L. S.: Observations of necrotizing gingivitis in 870 military trainees. J. Periont. Dent., *27*:255, 1956.
15. Hampp, E. G., Mergenhagen, S. E., and Omata, R. R.: Experimental infections with oral spirochetes. J. Infect. Dis., *109*:43, 1961.

16. Hampp, E. G., and Mergenhagen, S. E.: Experimental intracutaneous fusobacterial infections. J. Infect. Dis., *112:*84, 1963.
17. Heylings, R. T.: Electron Microscopy of acute ulcerative gingivitis (Vincent's type). Br. Dent. J., *122:*51, 1957.
18. Jiminez, M. L., Ramos, J., Garrington, G., and Baer, P. N.: Familial occurrence of necrotizing ulcerative gingivitis in children in Colombia, South America. J. Periodont., *40:*414, 1969.
19. Lehner, T.: Immunoglobulins in ulcerative gingivitis. Br. Dent. J., *127:*165, 1969.
20. Listgarten, M.: Electron microscopic observations on the bacterial flora of acute necrotizing ulcerative gingivitis. J. Periodont., *36:*328, 1965.
21. MacDonald, J. B., Gibbons, R. J., and Socransky, S. S.: Bacterial Mechanics in Periodontal Disease. Ann. N.Y. Acad. Sci. *85:*467, 1960.
22. MacDonald, J. B., Socransky, S. S., and Gibbons, R. J.: Aspects of the pathogenesis of mixed anaerobic infections of mucous membranes. J. Dent. Res., *42:*529, 1963.
23. MacDonald, J. B., Sutton, P. M., Knoll, M. L., Madlener, E. M., and Grainger, R. M.: Pathogenic components of and experimental fusospirochetal infection. J. Infect. Dis., *98:*15, 1956.
24. Malberger, E.: Acute infectious oral necrosis among young children in the Gambia, West Africa. J. Periodont. Res., *2:*154, 1967.
25. Manson, J. D., and Rand, H.: Recurrent Vincent's survey of 61 cases. Br. Dent. J., *110:*386, 1961.
26. Miller, S. C., and Greene, H. I.: A world wide survey of acute necrotizing ulcerative gingivitis: A preliminary report. J. Dent. Med., *13:*66, 1958.
27. Miller, S. C., and Greenhut, W. N.: Acute necrotic gingivitis (Vincent's infection: seasonal and age relations. J.A.D.A., *31:*910, 1944.
28. Moulton, R., Ewen, S., and Theiman, W.: Emotional factors in periodontal disease. Oral Surg., *5:*833, 1952.
29. Pindborg, J. J.: Tobacco and gingivitis: correlation between consumption of tobacco, ulceromembranous gingivitis and calculus. J. Dent. Res., *28:*460, 1949.
30. Pindborg, J. J.: The epidemiology of ulceromembranous gingivitis showing the influence of service in the armed forces. Parodontologie, *10:*114, 1956.
31. Pindborg, J. J., Bhatt, M., Devanath, K. R., Narayana, H. R., and Ramachandra, S.: Occurrence of acute necrotizing gingivitis in South Indian children. J. Periodont., *37:*14, 1966.
32. Pindborg, J. J., Bhatt, M., and Roed-Petersen, B.: Oral changes in South Indian children with severe protein deficiency. J. Periodont., *38:*218, 1967.
33. Rizzo, A. A., and Mergenhagen, S. E.: Local Schwartzman reaction in rabbit oral mucosa with endotoxin from oral bacteria. Proc. Soc. Exp. Biol. Med., *104:*570, 1960.
34. Schaeffer, E. M.: The effect of drugs in the treatment of necrotizing ulcerative gingivitis. J.A.D.A., *48:*279, 1954.
35. Schaeffer, E. M.: Biopsy studies of necrotizing ulcerative gingivitis. J. Periodont., *24:*22, 1953.
36. Schluger, S.: Necrotizing ulcerative gingivitis in the Army. Incidence, communicability and treatment. J.A.D.A., *38:*174, 1949.
37. Schwartzman, J., and Grossman, L.: Acute gingivostomatitis. Arch. Redist., *58:*515, 1941.
38. Shannon, I. L., Kilgore, W. G., and O'Leary, T. J.: Stress as a predisposing factor in necrotizing ulcerative gingivitis. J. Periodont., *40:*240, 1969.
39. Sheiham, A.: An epidemiological survey of acute ulcerative gingivitis in Nigerians. Arch. Oral Biol., *11:*937, 1966.
40. Sillevius-Smitt, P. A. E.: Some clinical and epidemiological aspects of Vincent's gingivitis. Dent. Pract. Dent. Rec., *15:*281, 1968.
41. Stammers, A. T.: Vincent's infection: observations on the histopathology and their applications to clerical practice. Br. Dent. J., *81:*4, 1946.
42. Tunicliff, R., Fink, E. B., and Hammond, C.: Significance of fusiform, bacilli and sperilli in gingival tissues. J.A.D.A., *23:*1939, 1936.
43. Wilton, J. M. A., Ivanyl, L., and Lehner, T.: Cell-mediated immunity and humoral antibodies in acute ulcerative gingivitis. J. Periodont. Res., *6:*9, 1971.

Acute Herpetic Gingivostomatitis

44. Black, W. C.: Acute infectious gingivostomatitis ("Vincent's stomatitis"). Am. J. Dent. Child., *56:*126, 1938.
45. Black, W. C.: Etiology of acute infectious gingivostomatitis (Vincent's stomatitis). J. Pediatr., *20:*145, 1942.
46. Buddingh, G. J., *et al.*: Studies of the natural history of herpes simplex infections. Pediatrics, *11:*595, 1953.
47. Burnett, G. A., and Scherp, H. W.: Oral Microbiology and Infectious Disease. eds. p. 530. Williams & Wilkins. Baltimore, 1968.
48. Burnett, F. M., and Williams, S. W.: Herpes simplex: new point of view. Med. J. Aust., *1:*637, 1939.
49. Dascomb, H. E., Adair, C. V., and Rogers, N. G.: Serologic investigations of herpes simplex virus infections. J. Lab. Clin. Med., *46:*1, 1955.
50. Dodd, K., Johnston, L. M., and Buddingh, C. J.: Herpetic stomatitis. J. Pediatr., *12:*95, 1938.
51. Haynes, R. E.: Herpesvirus hominis (herpes simplex virus (fatal infections in children). JAMA, *206:*312, 1968.
52. Kelley, V.: Brennemann's Practice of Pediatrics. vol. 3, chap. 2, p. 3. New York, Harper & Row, 1970.
53. Rogers, A. M.: Acute herpetic gingivostomatitis in the adult. N. Eng. J. Med., *241:*330, 1949.
54. Sheridan, P. J., and Herrmann, E. C.: Intraoral lesions of adults associated with herpes simplex virus. Oral Surg., *32:*390, 1971.
55. Ziskin, D. E., and Holden, M.: Acute herpetic gingivostomatitis: report of 15 cases. J.A.D.A., *30:*1697, 1943.

Infectious Mononucleosis

56. Cassingham, J.: Infectious mononucleosis. Oral Surg., *31:*610, 1971.
57. Courant, P., and Sobkov, T.: Oral manifestations of infectious mononucleosis. J. Periodont., *40:*279, 1969.
58. Dunnet, W. N.: Infectious mononucleosis. Br. Med. J., *5339:*1187, 1963.
59. Evans, A. S., Niederman, J. C., and McCollum, R. W.: Seroepidemiologic studies of infectious mononucleosis with EB virus. N. Eng. J. Med., *279:*1121, 1968.
60. Evans, A. S., Niederman, J. C., and McCollum, R. W.: Infectious mononucleosis-role of EBV virus. N. Eng. J. Med., *280:*112, 1969.
61. Finch, S. C.: Clinical symptoms and signs of infectious mononucleosis. *In* Carter, R. L., and Penman, H. G. (eds.): Infectious Mononucleosis. Blackwell Scientific Publication, Oxford and Edinburgh, 1969.
62. Fraser-Moodie, W.: Oral lesions in infectious mononucleosis. Oral Surg., *12:*685, 1959.
63. Hoagland, R. J.: The clinical manifestations of infectious mononucleosis: a report of two hundred cases. Am. J. Med. Sci., *240:*21, 1960.
64. Niederman, J. E., McCollum, R. W., Henle, G., and Henle, W.: Infectious mononucleosis: clinical manifestations in relation to EB virus antibodies. JAMA, *203:*205, 1968.
65. Paul, J. R., and Bunnell, W. W.: The presence of heterophile antibodies in infectious mononucleosis. Am. J. Med. Sci., *183:*90, 1932.
66. Shiver, C. B. Jr., Berg, P., and Frenkel, E. P.: Palatine petechia, an early sign of infectious mononucleosis. JAMA, *161:*592, 1956.

Recurrent Aphthous Stomatitis

67. Alvarez, W. C.: Canker sores. Minn. Med., *20:*602, 1937.
68. Banoczy, J., and Sallay, K.: Comparative cytologic studies in patients with recurrent aphthae and leukoplakia. J. Dent. Res., *48:*271, 1969.
69. Dolby, A. E.: Recurrent Mikulicz's oral aphthae. Br. Dent. J., *124:*359, 1968.
70. Dolby, A. E.: Recurrent aphthous ulcerations: the effect of sera and peripheral blood lymphocytes upon oral epithelial tissue culture cells. Immunology, *17:*709, 1969.
71. Farmer, E. D.: Recurrent aphthous ulcers. Dent. Pract. Dent. Rec., *8:*177, 1958.
72. Forbes, I. J., and Robson, H. N.: Familial Recurrent Orogenital Ulceration. Br. Med. J., *1:*599, 1960.
73. Francis, T. C.: Recurrent aphthous stomatitis and Behcet's disease. Oral Surg., *30:*476, 1970.

74. Francis, T. C., and Oppenheim, J. J.: Impaired lymphocyte stimulation by some streptococcal antigens in patients with recurrent aphthous stomatitis and rheumatic heart disease. Clin. Exp. Immunol., *6:*573, 1970.
75. Getz, I. I., and Bader, H. I.: Recurrent aphthous stomatitis. Oral Surg., *24:*186, 1967.
76. Graykowski, E. A., Barile, M. F., Lee, W. B., and Stanley, H. R.: The clinical, therapeutic and histopathologic aspects of aphthous stomatitis. JAMA, *196:*637, 1966.
77. Lehner, T.: Stimulation of lymphocyte transformation by tissue homogenates in recurrent oral ulceration. Immunology, *13:*159, 1967.
78. Lehner, T.: Autoimmunity and the management of recurrent oral ulceration. Br. Dent. J., *122:*15, 1967.
79. Lehner, T.: Immunoglobulin estimation of blood and saliva in human recurrent oral ulceration. Arch. Oral Biol., *14:*351, 1969.
80. Oppenheim, J. J., and Francis, T. C.: The role of delayed hypersensitivity in immunological processes and its relationship to aphthous stomatitis. J. Periodont., *41:*205, 1970.
81. Pappworth, M. H.: Clinical mucosal ulceration. Br. Med. J., *1:*271, 1941.
82. Ship, I. I., Morris, A. L., Durocher, R. T., and Burket, L. W.: Recurrent aphthous ulcerations and recurrent herpes labialis in a professional school student population. IV. Twelve-month study of natural disease patterns. Oral Surg., *14:*30, 1961.
83. Sircus, W., Church, R., and Kelleher, J.: Recurrent aphthous ulcerations of the mouth. Q. J. Med., *26:*235, 1957.
84. Strandberg, J.: Investigations concerning ulcus neuroticum mucosae oris. Acta. Otolaryngol. (Stockh.), *1:*103, 1918.

Herpangina

85. Parrot, R. H., Ross, S., Burke, F. G., and Rice, E. C.: Herpangina: clincal studies of specific infectious disease. N. Eng. J. Med., *245:*275, 1951.
86. Parrot, R. H., Wolf, S. I., Nudelman, J., Naiden, E., Huebner, R. J., Rice, E. C., and McCullough, N. B.: Clinical and laboratory differentiation between herpangina and infectious (herpetic) gingivostomatitis. Pediatrics, *14:*122, 1954.
87. Wehole, P. F.: The diagnosis and management of oral infections. Pediatr. Clin. North Am. *3*(4):876, 1956.

4

Chronic Lesions Affecting the Gingiva and Oral Mucosa

STURGE-WEBER SYNDROME

Sturge-Weber disease is also known as Sturge-Weber-Dimitri disease, encephalotrigeminal angiomatosis or meningofacial angiomatosis, and is characterized by a venous angioma over the cerebral cortex and an ipsilateral "port-wine" nevus of the face. The facial nevus usually occurs in the area of the skin supplied by the trigeminal nerve (Fig. 4-1). The cerebral angioma frequently causes a contralateral hemiparesis, epilepsy and some degree of mental retardation.[1,4,5,7,9,13] The clinical manifestation, however, can be quite variable. From a dental standpoint these cases are of interest because some of the patients have gingival hemangiomas (Fig. 4-2) occurring generally on the same side as the facial nevus.[2,3,6,8,10,11,12] The clinical picture of the gingival lesion is also variable because most of the patients are on diphenylhydantoin sodium therapy for epilepsy. In some patients the tongue, palatal mucosa and floor of the mouth on the side with the facial nevus have a darker hue than the rest of the oral mucous membranes.[2]

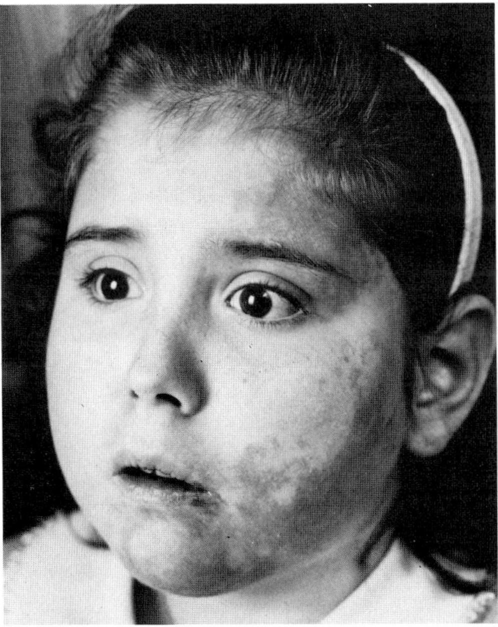

Fig. 4-1. Facial nevus is seen in the area supplied by the trigeminal nerve. (Figs. 4-1 through 4-4 from Baer, P. N., Stanwich, L., Alloy, J., Merritt, A. D., and Lewis, J. R.: Oral Surg., *14:*1383, 1961.)

Etiology. Unknown. There is no evidence of heredity being a factor or of any chromosomal aberrations.

Treatment. Although there is no known treatment for the systemic problem, the gingival hemangioma can readily be removed by electrosurgery. This method is in fact preferable to the use of a scalpel. Hemorrhage has not been a problem. Unfortunately, rapid recurrence of the lesion is common. We have successfully combatted this problem by having the patient wear nightly a "positive pressure appliance"[2] (Figs. 4-3 through 4-7) starting 2 weeks after surgery.

GINGIVAL REPARATIVE GRANULOMAS

These painless, soft, red to purple hyperplastic growths are attached to the gingiva or mucous membrane by a sessile or pedunculated base. They may be smooth or lobulated (Fig. 4-8). Surface ulcerations are common. Histologically the lesions are classified as either pyogenic granulomas or peripheral giant cell reparation granulo-

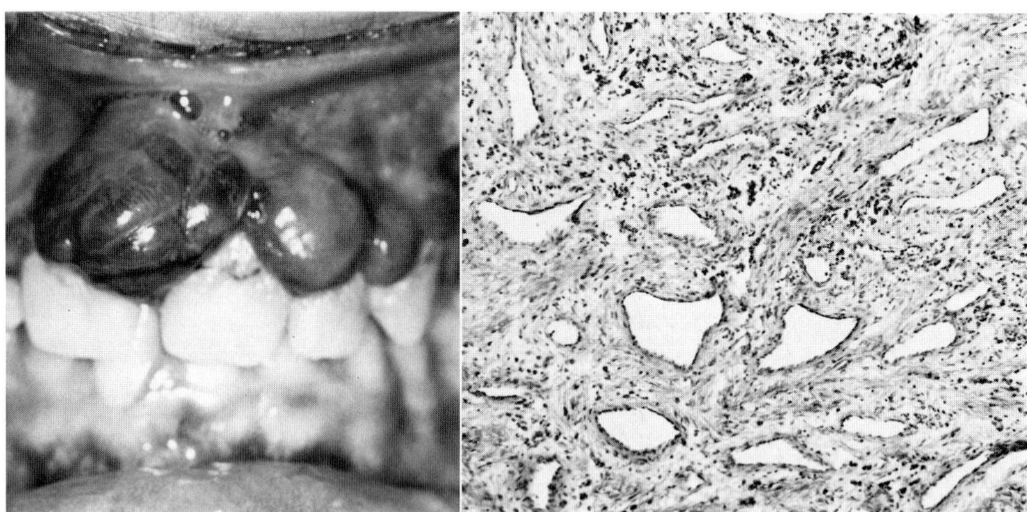

Fig. 4-2. *Left.* A gingival hemangioma appears in the maxillary arch. *Right.* Histologic appearance of hemangioma.

mas,[14,15,16,17,18] although clinically they look alike. There is no sex predilection.

Etiology. Unknown. These lesions, however, are frequently associated with the loss of deciduous teeth, the eruption of permanent teeth or various local irritational factors.

Treatment. Surgical excision of these lesions without accompanying extraction of the associated tooth is the treatment of choice. If there are recurrences a second excision without tooth extraction is indicated because these are innocuous lesions and radical treatment should be avoided.

THE GINGIVOSTOMATITIS SYNDROME

This syndrome consists of a triad of symptoms—an unusual type of gingivitis, an angular cheilitis and a glossitis.[20,21,22] However, all three symptoms need not be present in every case to make the diagnosis; the presence of any two is sufficient. The disease can occur at any age, and has a proclivity for females. The patients complain of burning and sore mouths, a symptom which is exacerbated by the consumption of highly seasoned food. The gingivitis

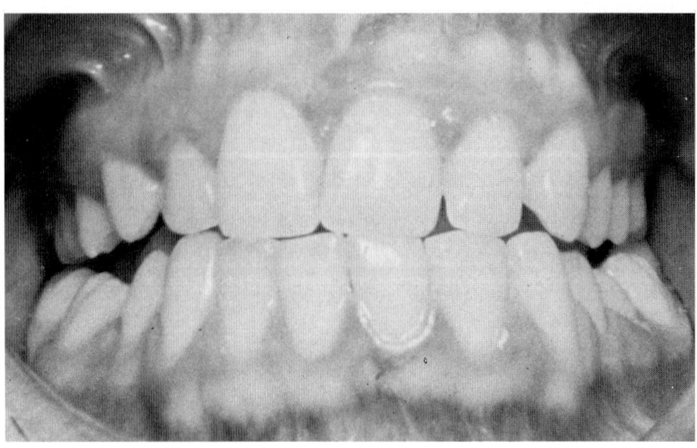

Fig. 4-3. Compare this postoperative appearance with Figure 4-2 *Left.*

is unusual in that it is bright red, edematous and/or hyperplastic, and sharply demarcated (Fig. 4-9). It extends from the margin of the gingiva to the mucogingival junction and is more extensive and severe on the labial and buccal surfaces than on the palatal or lingual aspects, thus giving the gingival lesion the appearance of a highly polished acrylic denture. No evidence of desquamation is present and the Nikolsky sign is negative.

Etiology. Several etiologic factors may precipitate these symptoms, the most common being an allergic reaction to chewing gum, particularly those brands that are mint flavored.[21] Other flavoring agents may produce similar results. Psychiatric factors have also been shown to play a significant role,[20] and there is some evidence of hormonal involvement.[19]

Treatment. Spontaneous remissions of this disease followed by exacerbations are common. Cessation of chewing gum by patients who are chronic chewers can result in immediate and rapid improvement of the lesions and a disappearance of the symptoms (Fig. 4-10). Complete return of the mucous membranes to normal, however, may take several months to more than a year. In patients who deny chewing gum, complete surgical excision of the affected gingival tissues can also result in complete remission.[20,22] In selected cases, successful results have been reported following hormonal therapy.[19]

DESQUAMATIVE GINGIVITIS

There is a great deal of controversy as to whether or not desquamative gingivitis should be considered a clinical entity or whether it represents merely a nonspecific reaction to a number of causes.[27] For instance, desquamation of the gingiva can accompany several dermatologic disorders such as pemphigus, pemphigoid, epidermolysis bullosa or lichen planus. It may also result from a diverse variety of nonspecific causes, such as from the ingestion of extremely hot food or as an allergic response to a mouthwash or toothpaste.

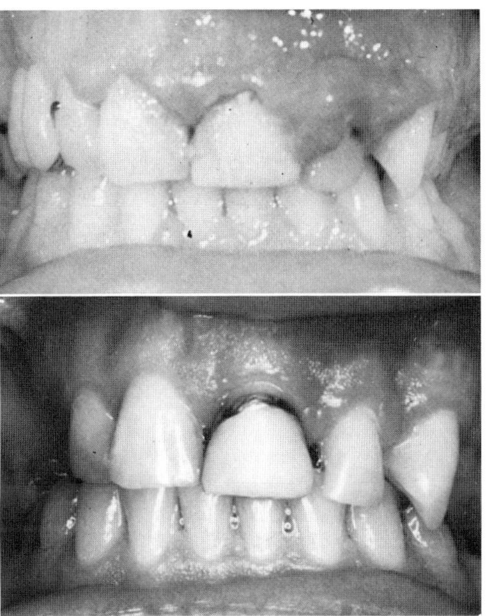

Fig. 4-4. *Top and bottom.* Pre- and postoperative results are shown. Treatment was given with a positive-pressure appliance after surgical removal of hemangioma.

We feel that there *is* a clinical entity known as desquamative gingivitis. It is a disease characterized by being limited entirely to the gingiva. The lesions are bright red and are smooth and glistening. No other mucous membrane or mucosal area is affected. The maxillary anterior labial gingiva is the surface most often affected, but the other labial surfaces may be involved. The attached gingiva on the lingual and palatal surfaces is either not affected or involved to a lesser degree.[24] The pressure caused by rubbing the labial attached gingiva with a finger elicits a positive Nikolsky sign (Fig. 4-11). When the epithelium is sloughed off it leaves a raw, sensitive surface. In some instances the condition is preceded by the formation of small watery blisters.[28] The symptoms that accompany this condition consist of a burning sensation which is aggravated by certain

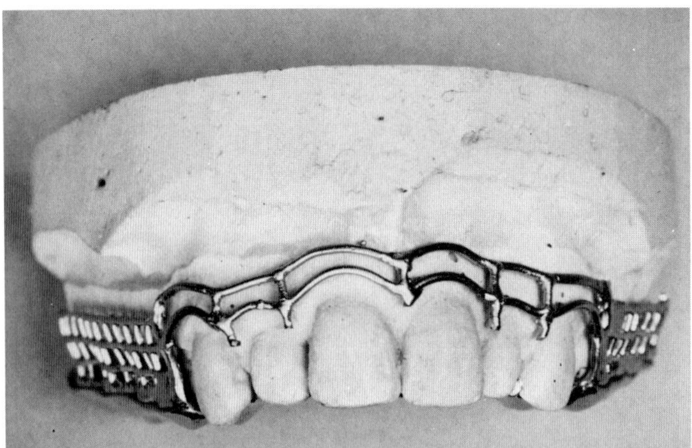

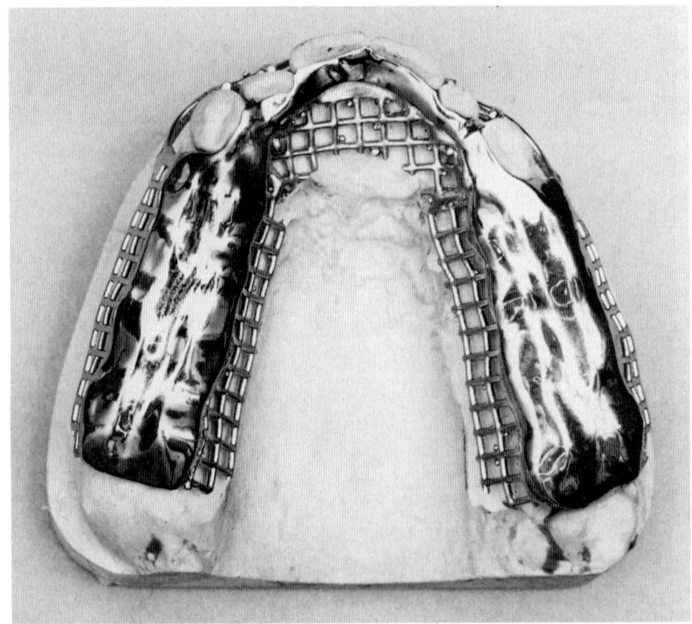

Fig. 4-5. The positive-pressure appliance has a chrome cobalt framework. (Figs. 4-5 through 4-7 from Davis, R. K., Baer, P. N., and Palmer, J. H.: J. Periodont., *34*:17, 1963.)

foods (particularly condiments) and beverages which are acid in nature.

Etiology. Unknown. The disease affects mostly women. Although an estrogen deficiency has been considered as an etiologic factor in postmenopausal women, it does not appear to play a role in the younger age group. This may mean that we are dealing with two very different clinical entities. Histories, physical examinations and laboratory tests indicate that these patients apparently are all healthy. The disease is frequently complicated by the fact that because of the painful gingival condition, these patients have difficulty in maintaining good plaque control, thus further aggravating the already existing gingival problem.

Treatment. Untreated, the disease is apparently of indefinite duration with periods of remission and exacerbation. No spontaneous cures, however, have ever been reported. Some investigators have reported successful results following the application of systemic steroids on an empirical

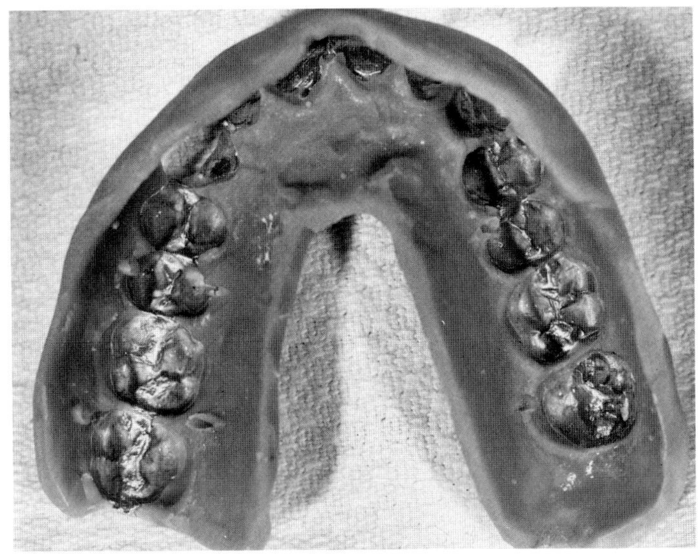

Fig. 4-6. A soft plastic liner is curved over a metal framework.

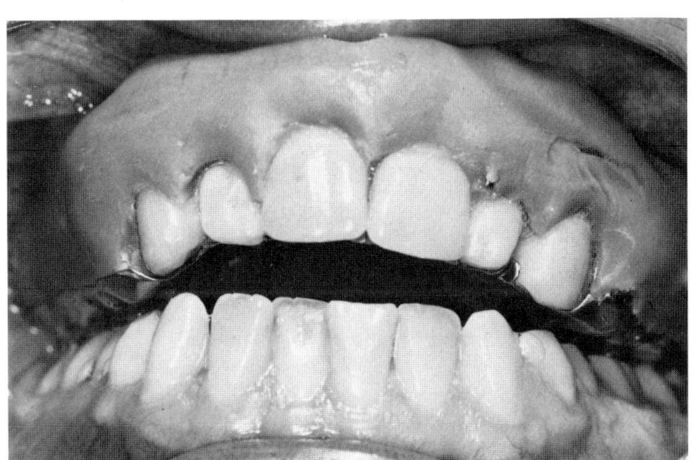

Fig. 4-7. Positive-pressure appliance is seen in position.

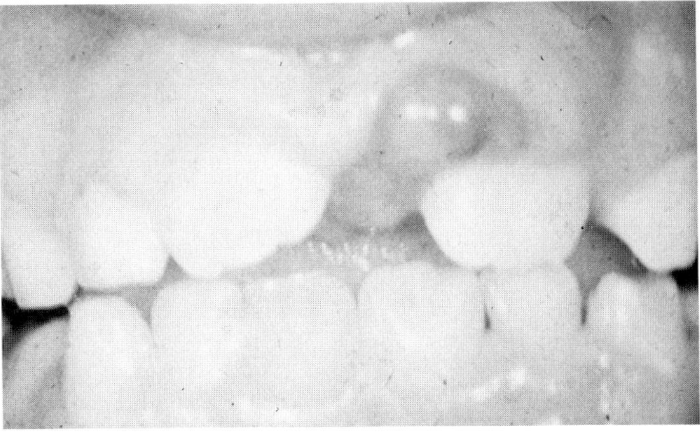

Fig. 4-8. This peripheral giant cell reparative granuloma in a 6-year-old girl was reported to have developed shortly after loss of her primary central incisors. (From Standish, and Shafer.)[18]

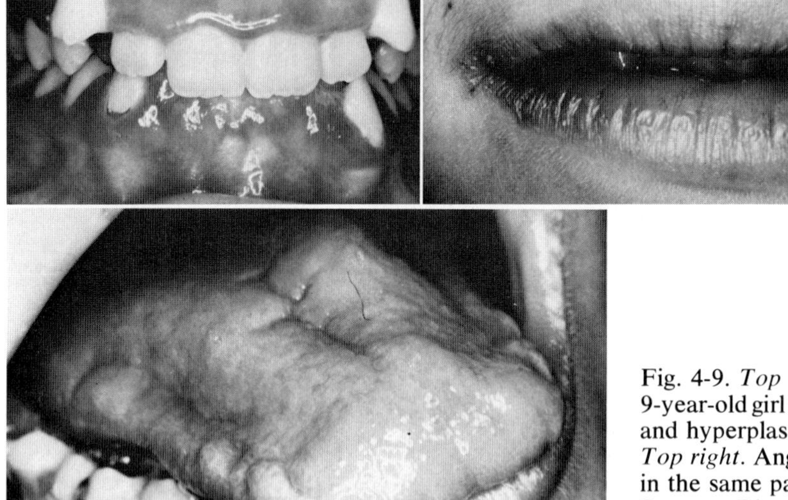

Fig. 4-9. *Top left.* The gingiva in this 9-year-old girl is bright red, edematous and hyperplastic.
Top right. Angular cheilitis is evident in the same patient.
Bottom. Glossitis is seen in the same patient.

basis.[24,25] In many cases, this does afford at least temporary relief of the patient's symptoms and the gingiva may also show clinical improvement. This use of steroids is not recommended for long term therapy, however, and should be avoided, particularly in the younger patients, because of the possibility of adverse side effects. On a short term basis, however, topical steroids appear to reduce the sensitivity of the gingival tissues and permit the establishment of good plaque control. This in turn can sometimes control the disease. When the topical steroids have not been effective, we have achieved success by resecting all the affected gingival tissue. The healing following the gingival resection proceeds at a normal rate and the newly formed tissue tends to be normal in appearance (Fig. 4-12). Resection enables the patient to practice good plaque control and apparently to prevent a recurrence of the disease. If the lesion should recur, however, which may happen on occasion, we have found that patients have fewer symptoms than before the gingival resection.

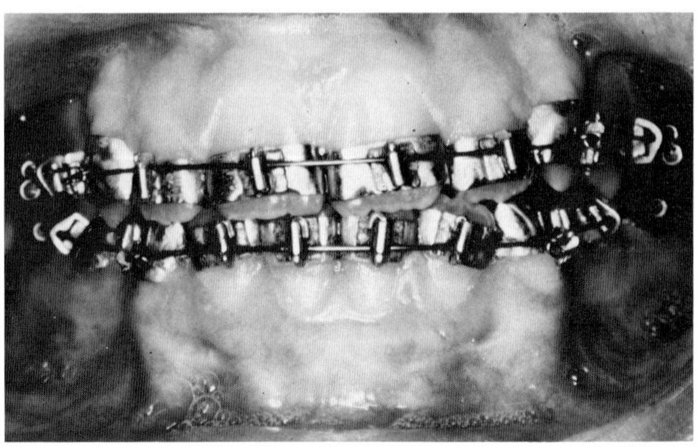

Fig. 4-10. Remission in the patient shown in Figure 4-9 *Top left* followed cessation of chewing a mint-flavored gum. Gum chewing was discontinued because of orthodontic appliances.

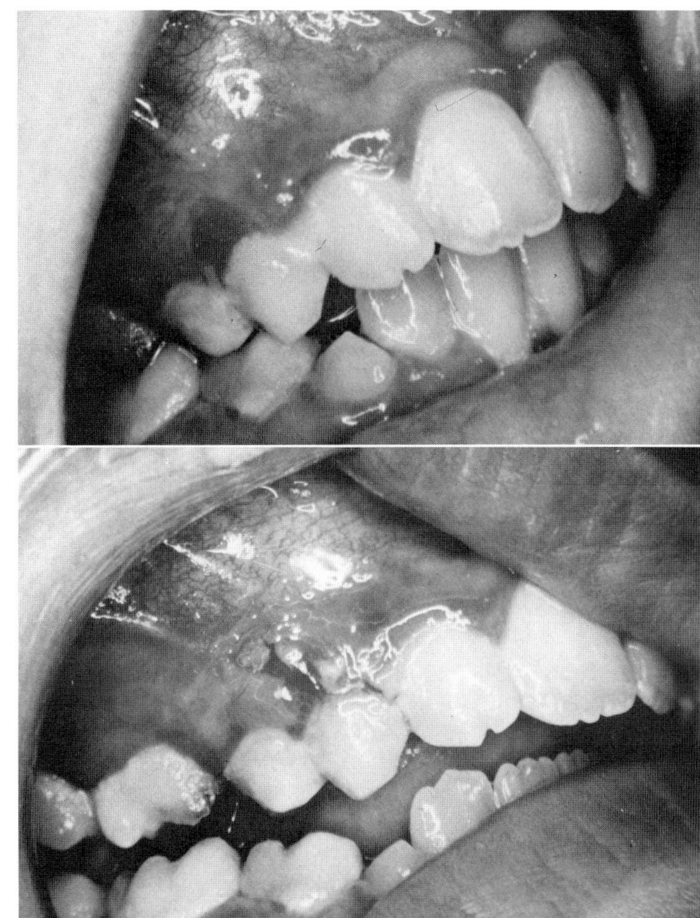

Fig. 4-11. *Top.* Desquamative lesions appeared on the maxillary right cuspid-molar area in a 9-year-old girl. *Bottom.* A positive Nikolsky sign was elicited in the right maxillary cuspid area.

Differential Diagnosis. A biopsy is of little help in diagnosis, since the histologic changes noted are too nonspecific.[24, 25, 27] However, immunofluorescent studies eliminate pemphigus and pemphigoid.[26] If the mucosa of the cheek is involved in addition to the gingival lesion, a form of erosive lichen planus is probably indicated. Thus, by a process of elimination, a diagnosis of desquamative gingivitis can be made.

A newly defined entity in nonmenopausal women has recently been described which appears to be similar to desquamative gingivitis. It is called desquamative inflammatory vaginitis.[23] It has been noted that in this entity the affected areas in the vagina are usually fiery red and have well-delineated margins, although some do have serpiginous configurations. Areas of the epithelium exhibit a grayish pseudomembrane that peels off when the vagina is wiped, exposing an inflamed red surface. Some patients report a mild burning and pruritus. Other striking features of the disease include its persistence if untreated, its poor response to treatment and its tendency to recrudesce. The cause of this vaginitis is unknown.

The treatment tried and the results obtained are also interesting. Estrogen given both orally and intravaginally had little or no effect either clinically or microscopically. This was to be expected, since all the women examined had active ovarian

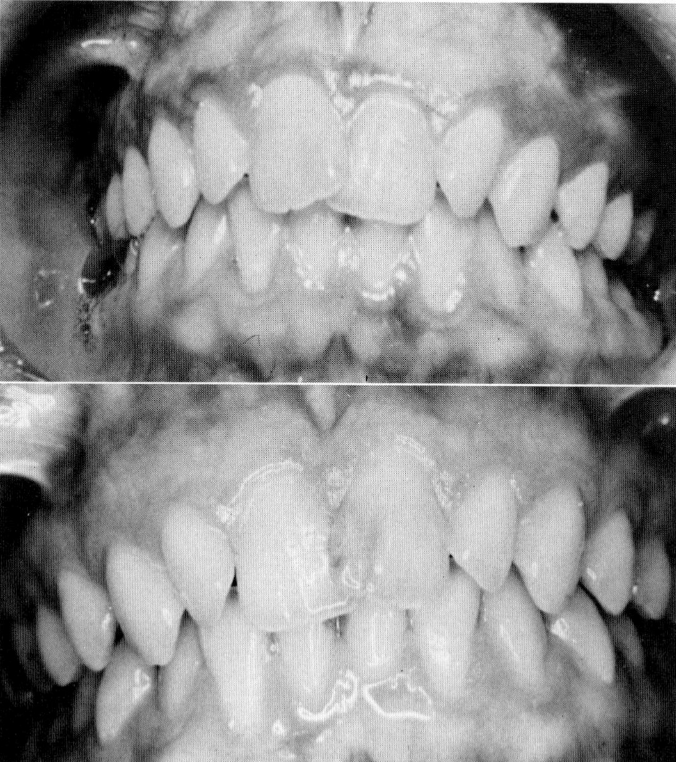

Fig. 4-12. *Top.* Desquamative gingivitis in an 18-year-old female was confined to maxillary labial and buccal gingiva. *Bottom.* Results were obtained following resection of all involved gingival tissue. This case has been in remission for more than five years.

function. The response to antibacterial agents given systemically or locally was also discouraging. However, several patients who were treated by intravaginal applications of corticosteroids alone or combined with antibacterial agents, were benefited. Healing, however, was slow and often incomplete. Finally, "even after improvement or apparent cure, the vaginitis had a tendency to recur."[23]

EPIDERMOLYSIS BULLOSA

This disease of the skin is rare, occurring as either a dominant or recessive mendelian trait, and is characterized by vesicles, bullae and epidermal cysts (milia). It occurs in 4 variants:[29, 31, 35]

1. The simple type—dominantly inherited and usually manifest at birth or shortly thereafter. It is characterized by bullae or vesicles in the skin at the site of trauma. The mucous membranes and nails are usually not involved.[32] The bullae resolve spontaneously, leaving only a temporary residual brown pigmentation. The disease tends to either subside or disappear at puberty.[30] Since there are no oral lesions, this type is of little concern from a dental point of view.

2. The recessive lethal form—associated with skeletal atrophy. This form usually terminates fatally in the first 3 months of life, and is also of no concern from a dental standpoint.

3. The dystrophic type, severe form—recessively inherited and very mutilating. It does have oral manifestations.

4. Dystrophic type—dominantly transmitted has much milder manifestations than the recessively inherited variant. It also has oral manifestations.

Etiology. Unknown. It has been thought that the lesions might be caused by an inherited deficiency in elastic-fibers of the

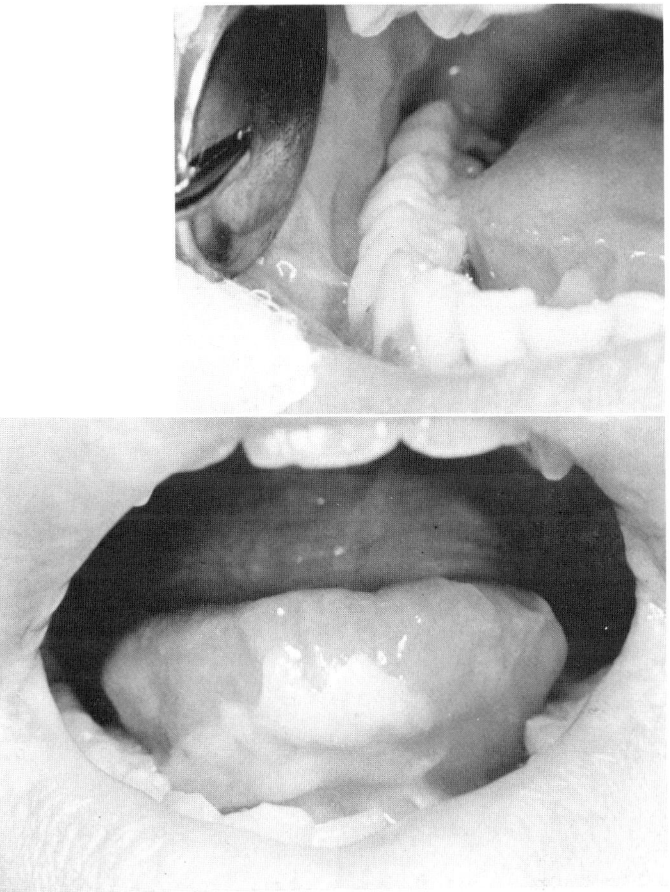

Fig. 4-13. *Top.* Scar formation may fuse the mucosa directly to the marginal area of the gingiva, thereby obliterating the buccal vestibule. *Bottom.* The tongue may be limited in its motion because of scarring.

skin, but the evidence for this is not convincing. Others have explained the lesions as resulting from an inherited defect involving the permeability of the blood vessels or from abnormal vasomotor nerve control.

Clinical Characteristics. Oral lesions occur in approximately 15 percent of the patients with the dystrophic forms.

In the severe dystrophic form the entire oral mucosa may become involved, including the palate, gingiva, cheeks and tongue. Such involvement may lead to the labial and buccal vestibules becoming completely obliterated (Fig. 4-13 *Top*), because scar formation occurs and fuses the mucosa in the vestibular area directly to the marginal area of the gingival tissues.[36] The

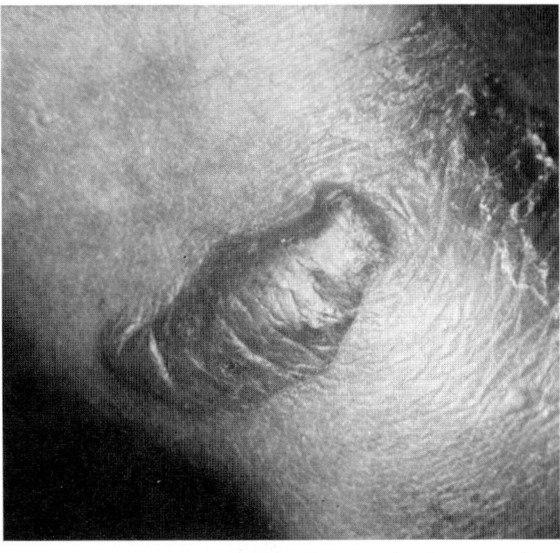

Fig. 4-14. Bullae on the knee of a 9-year-old girl.

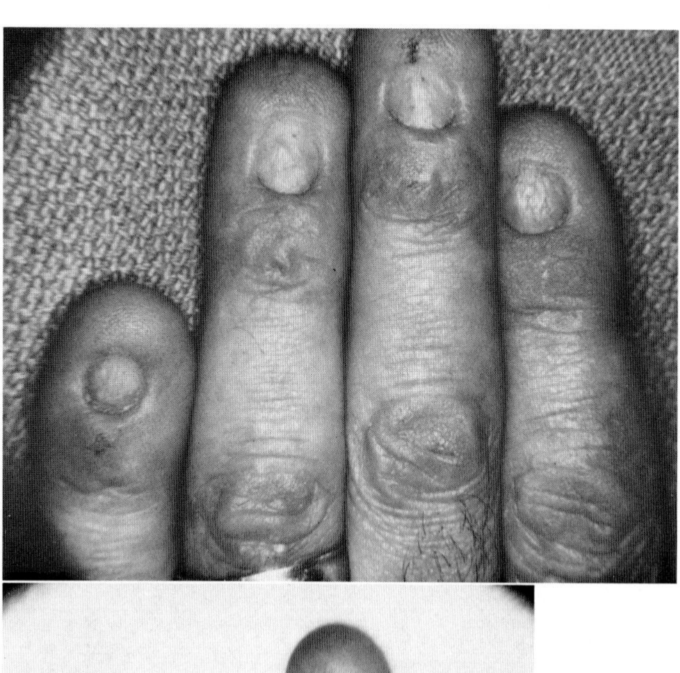

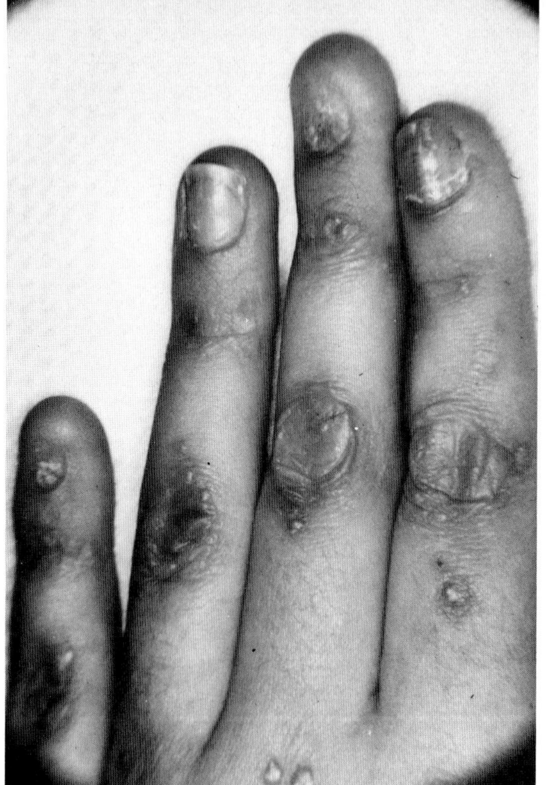

Fig. 4-15. *Top.* Dystrophic fingernails on the father. *Bottom.* Dystrophic fingernails on the daughter as well as milia on her hands.

motion of the tongue may become limited because of scarring (Fig. 4-13 *Bottom*). Opening the mouth may also be difficult because scars form in the cheeks and angles of the mouth. The lesions and resultant scarring can also affect the pharynx, larynx and esophagus and result in stenosis of these structures. On rare occasions, malig-

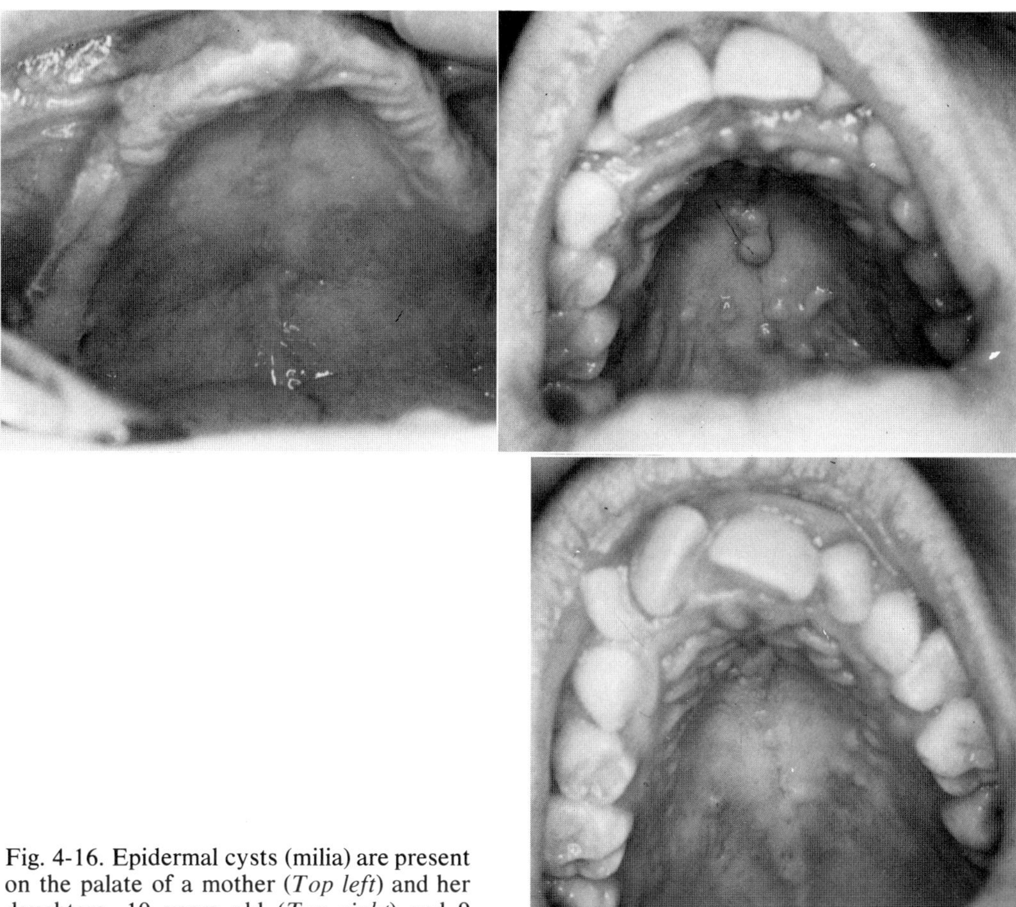

Fig. 4-16. Epidermal cysts (milia) are present on the palate of a mother (*Top left*) and her daughters, 10 years old (*Top right*) and 9 years old (*Bottom*).

nant changes may occur in some of the areas of extensive scarring in the esophagus.[31]

It has been reported that the primary and permanent teeth may erupt in a hypoplastic condition and appear discolored, and be readily prone to erosion and caries.[30, 33, 36]

In addition to bullae and vesicles on the skin, grouped milia are common on the extensors or surfaces of the hands and forearms. The atrophic skin changes on the hands may produce contracture. The loss of fingernails and toenails is frequent. The conjunctiva may also become affected and this may lead to blindness.

In the less severe, dominantly inherited dystrophic form, vesicles and bullae also occur on the areas of the skin which are subjected to trauma (Fig. 4-14). Epidermal cysts or milia are usually present on the dorsal surface of the hands and the exterior aspect of the forearm. The fingernails and toenails (Fig. 4-15) may be dystrophic or missing. The oral lesions that may occur are usually mild and cause no serious permanent scarring. Milia may occur on the palate (Fig. 4-16). The gingival lesions, when present, are red, diffuse and desquamative, clinically eliciting a positive Nikolsky sign and resembling the gingival lesions seen in desquamative gingivitis (Fig. 4-17 *Top*). It should be remembered, however, that even when many members of a family are affected by disease not all will

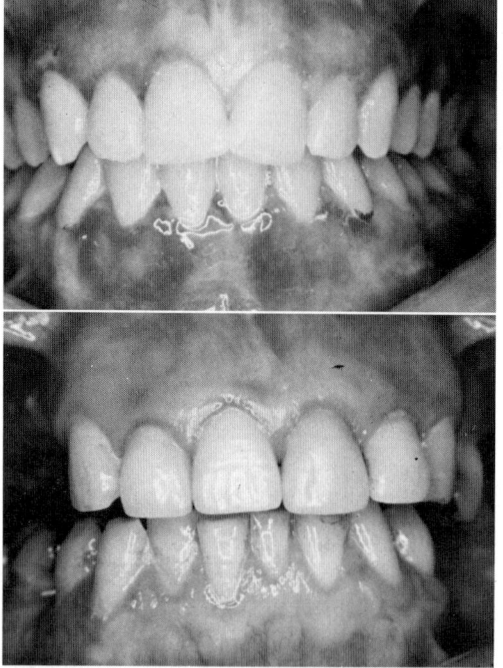

Fig. 4-17. *Top*. These gingival lesions in a 14-year-old female resemble those seen in desquamative gingivitis.
Bottom. The father of the above patient with normal gingiva.

necessarily exhibit oral lesions (Fig. 4-17 *Bottom*).

Treatment. There is no known treatment. Fortunately the simplex type, as mentioned previously, tends to go into spontaneous remission at puberty. The milder dystrophic variety can generally be managed by the patient without too much discomfort. The main problem is usually esthetic, owing to the unsightly lesions on the extremities and the loss or disfigurement of the fingernails. In the more severe forms of the disease, topically applied fluocinolone acetonide 0-2 percent cream affords some relief for the cutaneous lesions.[34]

LICHEN PLANUS

In this disease of the mucocutaneous tissues the cutaneous lesions are polygonal papules which may be discrete or coalesce into larger plaques. The lesions are initially erythematous and covered with glistening, silvery scales. With involution the cutaneous lesions become less red and more violaceous, and then tan and brown. The lesions are associated with considerable pruritus and have a predilection for symmetrical distribution on the flexor surfaces of the wrists, forearms and legs above the ankles. The face, scalp, palms and plantar surfaces are generally spared.

It has been reported that between 30 and 50 percent of patients with dermal lichen planus also have oral lesions.[37,38,43,45,46] However, oral lesions may also appear without cutaneous lesions. In most of these instances, if the patients are followed for a sufficient length of time, it will be found that they will eventually develop both skin and oral mucosal lesions, whether the lesions originated on the skin or on the oral mucosa. There are cases of oral erosive lichen planus, however, in which cutaneous lesions never form.

There is no relationship between the severity of the cutaneous lesions and the severity of incidence of the involvement of the oral mucous membranes.[45,46] Cutaneous lesions are rarely present in patients who consult a dentist.

There is considerable variability in the clinical appearance of the oral lesions. Unlike the cutaneous lesions, the oral lesions are generally grayish white. The most common site for the oral lesion is the buccal mucosa, where 80 percent occur; the lingual involvement accounts for 65 percent and the labial for 20 percent. Lesions of the gingiva, floor of the mouth and palate are rare and occur in less than 10 percent of cases.[45,46]

The lesions have been classed into various morphologic types,[38] the most common being the *reticular lesion* which consists of interlacing white lines forming a latticework, the so-called striae of Wickham. A white elevated dot is characteristically present at the intersections of the striae. When the reticular pattern occurs on the gingiva, it is frequently associated

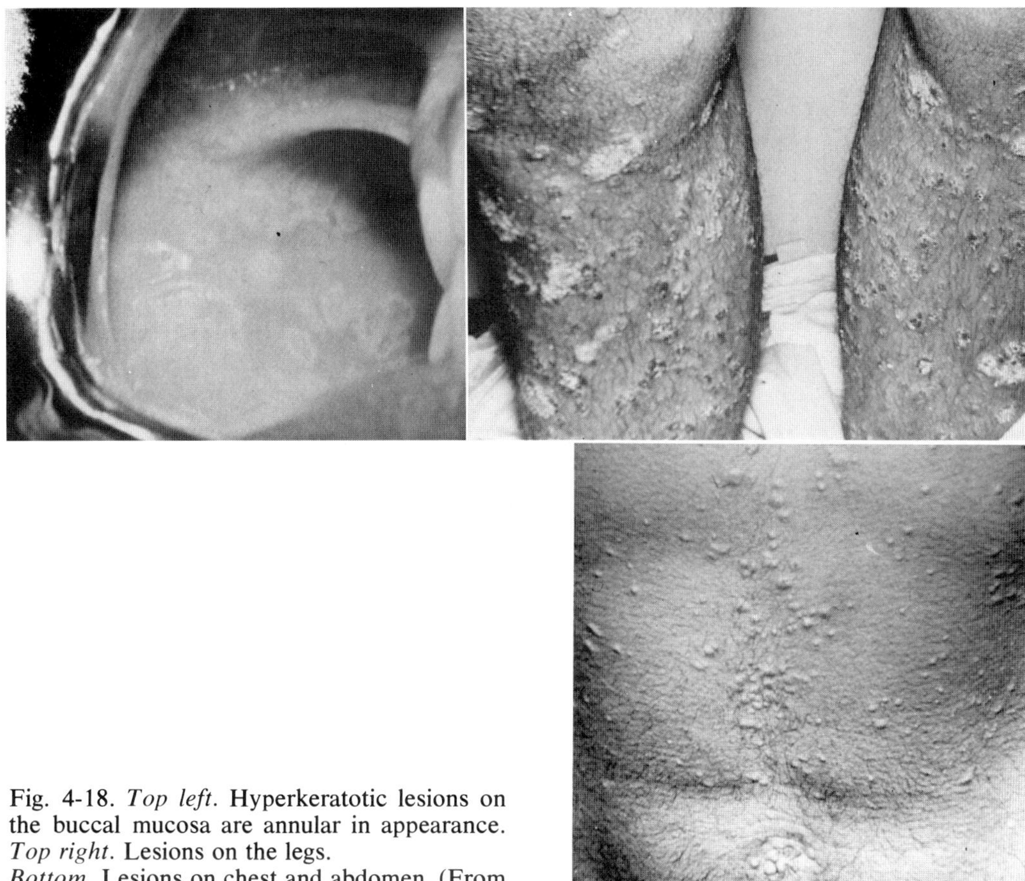

Fig. 4-18. *Top left.* Hyperkeratotic lesions on the buccal mucosa are annular in appearance. *Top right.* Lesions on the legs. *Bottom.* Lesions on chest and abdomen. (From Davis, Baer, Archard, and Palmer.)[58]

with a desquamative gingivitis.[45, 46] An annular arrangement of the white lesion is also quite common.

The other morphologic types found are *papules,* small raised lesions that give the mucosa a grayish white pebbly appearance, and the *plaque form,* consisting of a solid raised white plaque. These latter morphologic types are generally not seen in the adolescent and young adult; neither is the erosive variant, which can count for almost 50 percent of the oral lesions seen in the adult.[46] This absence is probably because the erosive form usually originates in an area of atrophic mucosa.[40] The erosive type begins as such and does not result from a progression of the nonerosive morphologic to an erosive type.

Generally there is no itching or discomfort with most of the nonerosive forms of oral lesions, although they may on occasion elicit a burning sensation or create awareness by their roughness. The erosive or bullous type, on the other hand, is generally accompanied by a considerable degree of pain and discomfort.

Diagnosis. Occasionally when the lesions are confined to the oral cavity some confusion may arise as to whether the lesion is lichen planus or possibly pemphigus or pemphigoid. A biopsy generally settles this question unless secondary infection, which is common in the oral cavity, obscures the histologic features. In these instances the diagnosis can be made by a process of elimination by using immuno-

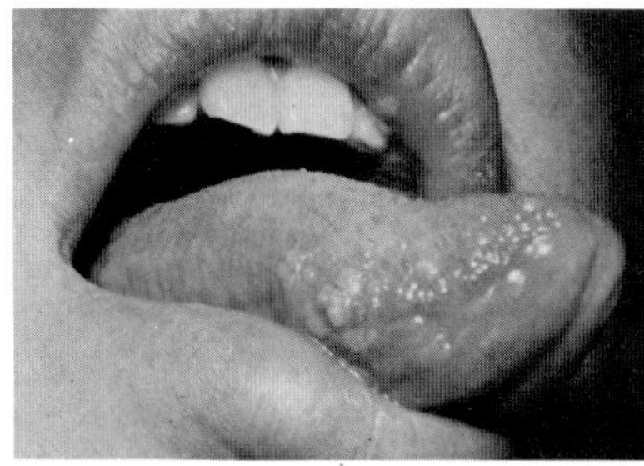
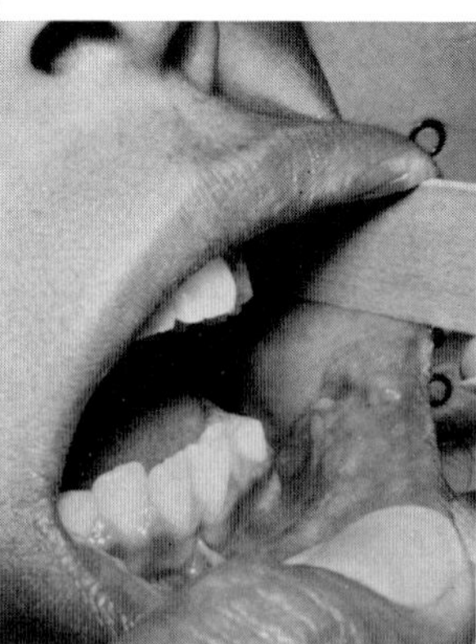
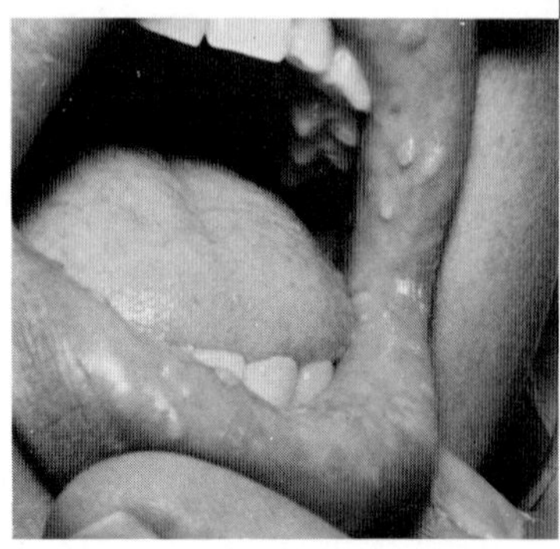

Fig. 4-19. *Top.* Focal epithelial hyperplasia lesions on the tongue. *Center.* Lesion on the buccal mucosa.
Bottom. Lesions on the lips. (Courtesy of Dr. Howell O. Archard.)

fluorescent techniques.[42] Patients with pemphigus demonstrate antibodies to intercellular cementing substance; those with pemphigoid, to basement membrane.[44] If the tests for both of these are negative, then the diagnosis of oral lichen planus can be made with some confidence.

Etiology. Unknown. However, the evidence is very good for attributing this disease, in part at least, to psychosomatic factors. Exacerbations and remissions can generally be correlated with periods of emotional stress and tranquility. There is also a familial aspect to this disease which is not well understood.[39, 41] More women than men tend to be affected.

Treatment. There is no specific treatment. Many patients, however, do have cancerphobia, and reassurance that the lesion is benign and not malignant, or even premalignant, is often helpful.

Remissions may occur spontaneously. In most instances the disease is chronic, with periods of exacerbation and remission following the emotional status of the patient.

CASE HISTORY

A 15-year-old black male was first seen in the dental clinic with several white, annular hyperkeratotic lesions on the buccal mucosa (Fig. 4-18) and soft palate. Dermal lesions were seen

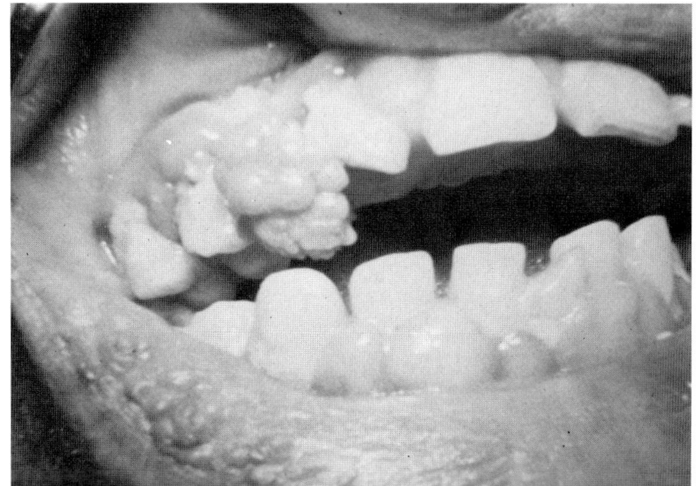

Fig. 4-20. This pedunculated oral lesion extends downward between the upper right cuspid and lateral incisor in patient shown in Figure 4-22. (From Davis, Baer, Archard, and Palmer.)[58]

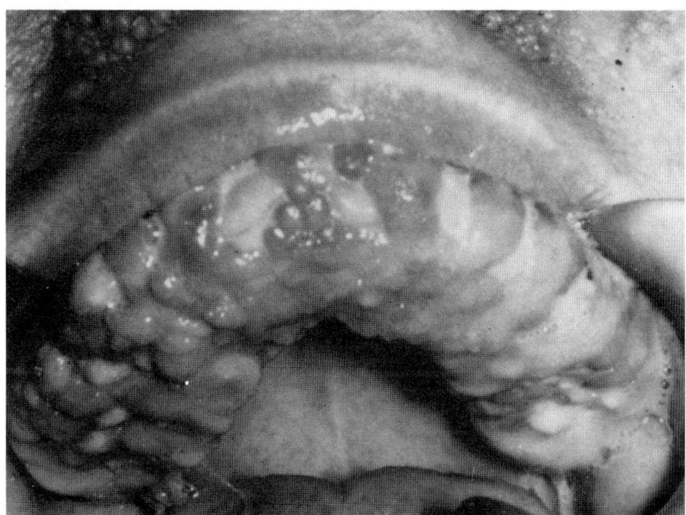

Bottom. Multiple oral fibromatous tumors on the gingiva usually present after puberty. (From Sareen, C. K., Ruvalcaba, R. H. A., Scotvold, M. J., Mahoney, C. P., and Kelley, V. C.: Am. J. Dis. Child., *123*:34, 1972.)

on the extremities, chest, and abdomen and glans penis. A biopsy of the oral lesion was made with a clinical diagnosis of lichen planus.

Medical History. The patient had been delivered normally. One older, mentally retarded male sibling had been a resident of a children's center for several years. Except for a heart murmur the patient had been in good health. He had been institutionalized because of juvenile delinquency. A family history revealed that the patient's father had deserted the family shortly after the birth of his second son and that the mother then began drinking heavily. When the patient reached school age he began to run away from home, often sleeping in hallways or streets. He indicated that he left home because of abuse by his mother's male visitors. He had received very little formal education prior to his admission to the children's center.

Pathologic Report. The rete pegs of a slightly acanthotic epithelium demonstrated both reticulation and the "saw-tooth" characteristic. A dense uniform infiltrate, predominating in lymphocytes, stretched along the lamina propria immediately under the epithelium and filled the papillary projections. This infiltrate began in the section rather abruptly and extended to one end of the specimen. The deeper tissues then revealed only mature collagenous fibers, a minimal vascularity, and skeletal muscle. Despite all the lymphocytes present in the lamina propria, only a few were seen

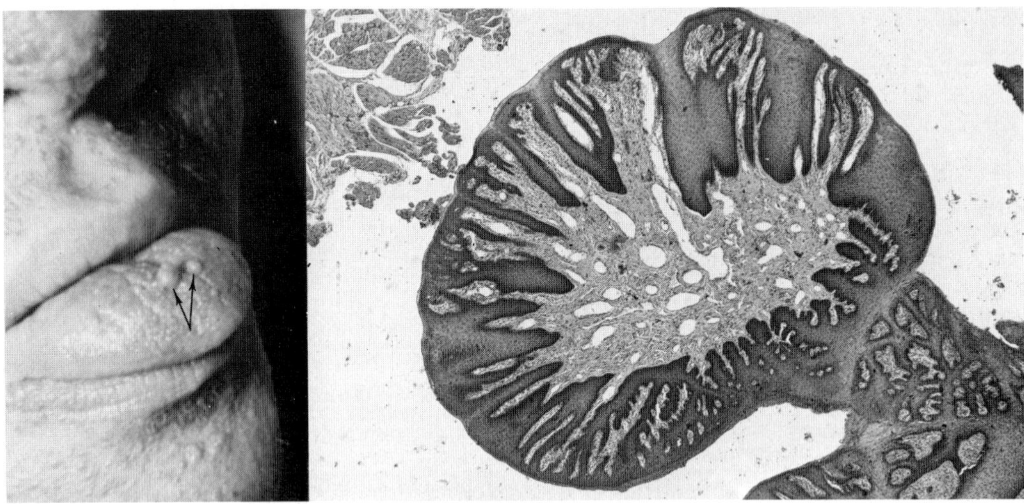

Fig. 4-21. *Left.* Hemangiomas on the tongue. *Right.* A photomicrograph of the hemangioma.

filtering through the epithelium. Liquefaction degeneration of the basal cell layer was evident in a number of areas and on different levels. There was a tendency for it to coalesce with edema of the underlying connective tissue, forming cords in the zone of intense infiltrate.

The epithelium was unremarkable except for the characteristics mentioned above and presented normal maturation with minimal acanthosis and parakeratosis. Atypia was not seen.

Diagnosis. Lichen planus, buccal mucosa.

FOCAL EPITHELIAL HYPERPLASIA

The lesions are asymptomatic and vary in size from 2 to 5 mm. They are multiple, soft, discrete or confluent round to avoid elevations of the same color as the adjacent normal mucosa. The lesions are found in the greatest abundance on the lower lip, but also may involve the tongue, buccal mucosa, upper lip and gingiva (Fig. 4-19). The hard palate and floor of the mouth are rarely, if ever, involved.

Etiology. Unknown. Viral[48] and genetic factors[54] may play a role. Most of the reported cases have occurred in patients who were either Eskimos, and North, Central or South American Indians,[47, 48, 49, 54] although other races on occasion may also be affected.[50, 51, 52] The disease is found almost exclusively in children 6 to 18 years of age.[53]

Treatment. Treatment is unnecessary. The lesions may disappear spontaneously[47] and probably most often do, since they are rarely found in the adult.

TUBEROUS SCLEROSIS
(Epiloia, Bourneville's disease)

This clinical syndrome consists of the triad of epilepsy, mental retardation and adenomas of sebaceous glands, or so-called skin tumors. The cutaneous lesions, rarely evident at birth, develop slowly, usually making their first appearance toward the end of the second or beginning of the third year of life. Epilepsy and mental deficiency usually become evident in infancy or early life. When the disease is fully developed, lesions of an extraordinary diversity may be encountered, with bones, brain, heart, kidneys, lungs and skin being involved in characteristic ways.[61]

Fibrous growths can occur on any surface of the oral mucosa,[60] but are found most frequently on the gingiva and

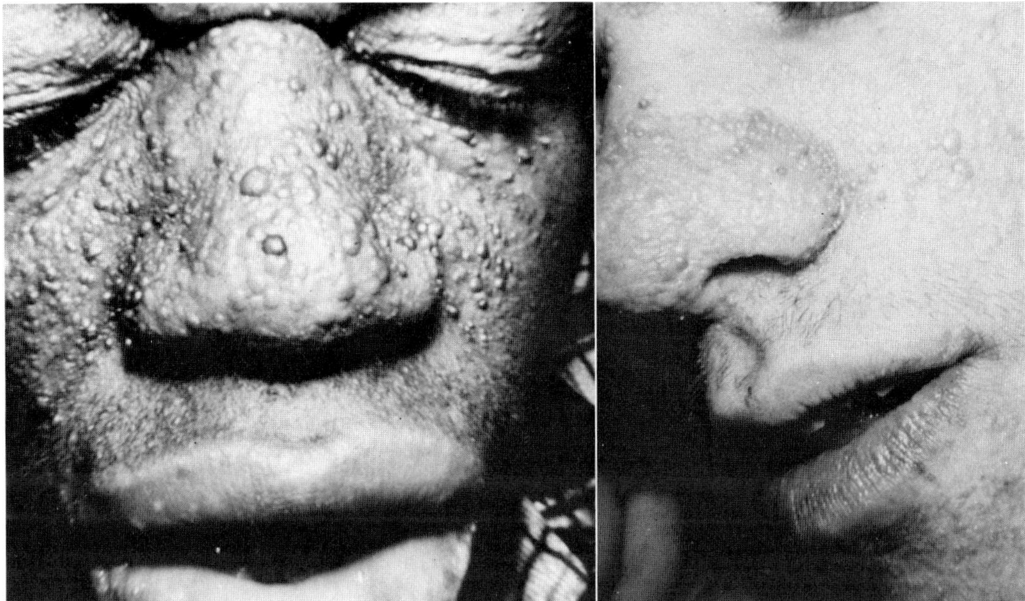

Fig. 4-22. Sebaceous adenomas on the face.

tongue,[57,58] hard palate[57] and upper lip (Figs. 4-20 and 4-21).[59]

Etiology. The disease is inherited as an irregular autosomal dominant trait with a high mutation rate. Both sexes are equally affected.

Clinical Characteristics. The skin lesions are smooth, shiny symmetrically clustered papules or nodules located in the paranasal area and extend over the molar eminences and onto the forehead. The individual adenoma range in size from 0.1 to 1.0 mm. (Fig. 4-22).

The brain lesions consist of areas of malformed cortex with extensive astroglioses and a mixture of glioblasts and abnormal ganglion cells.[56,62] The nodules or tubers may become calcified and roentgenographically observed.

Mental retardation is usually noticed during the early years of life and may vary in degree. Some patients may even have normal IQs. Convulsions are another prominent feature of this disease; however, there may be long periods of remission between seizures. During periods of remission mental deterioration may continue to progress. Focal signs of paresis are common, as are speech defects, spasms and clonus of the muscles of the extremities.[55]

Prognosis. Survival into the third decade is unusual and survival after the age of 40 years is rare.[55] Most die before they are 20 years of age. Death may be due to seizures, associated tumors or intercurrent diseases.

REFERENCES

Sturge-Weber Syndrome

1. Bielawski, J. G., and Tatelman, M.: Intracranial calcification in encephalotrigeminal angiomatosis. Am. J. Roentgenol., *62*:247, 1947.
2. Davis, R. K., Baer, P. N., and Palmer, J. H.: A preliminary report on a new therapy for dilantin gingival hyperplasia. J. Periodont. *34*:17, 1963.
3. DeLapa, R. J., and Blair, A. E.: Juvenile hemangioendothelioma: report of a case. J. Oral Surg., *18*:346, 1960.
4. Green, J. R.: Encephalo-trigeminal angiomatosis. J. Neuropath. & Exp. Neurol., *4*:27, 1945.

5. Greenwald, H. M., and Koota, J.: Associated facial intracranial hemangiomas. Am. J. Dis. Child., *5*:868, 1936.
6. Gyarmati, I.: Oral change in Sturge-Weber's disease. Oral Surg., *13*:795, 1960.
7. Lichtenstein, B. W.: Sturge-Weber-Dimitri syndrome; cephalic form in neurocutaneous hemangiomatosis. A.M.A.Arch. Neurol. Psychiat., *71*:291, 1954.
8. Malkin, M., and Bethoney, T.: Sturge-Weber disease: report of a case. J.A.D.A., *69*:443, 1964.
9. Peterman, A. F., Hayles, A. B., Docketry, M. B., and Love, J. G.: Encephalotrigeminal angiomatosis (Sturge-Weber disease). JAMA, *167*:2169, 1958.
10. Protzel, M. A.: Sturge-Weber disease. Oral Surg., *10*:388, 1957.
11. Spruyt, J. L. L.: Encephalotrigeminal angiomatosis. Dent. Pract., *15*:140, 1964.
12. Thoma, K. H.: Sturge-Kalischer-Weber syndrome with pregnancy tumors. Oral Surg., *5*:1124, 1952.
13. Wohlwill, F. J., and Yakovlev, P. I.: Histopathology of meningofacial angiomatosis (Sturge-Weber's disease). J. Neuropath. Exp. Neurol., *16*:341, 1957.

Gingival Reparative Granulomas

14. Bhaskar, S. N., and Jacoway, J. R.: Pyogenic granuloma-clinical features, incidence, histology, and result of treatment, report of 242 cases. J. Oral Surg., *24*:391, 1966.
15. Giansanti, J. S., and Waldron, C. A.: Peripheral giant cell granuloma: review of 720 cases. J. Oral Surg., *27*:787, 1969.
16. Kerr, D. A.: Granuloma pyogenicum. Oral Surg., *4*:158, 1951.
17. Lee, K. W.: The fibrous epulis and related lesions. Periodontics, *6*:277, 1968.
18. Standish, S. M., and Shafer, W. G.: Gingival reparative granulomas in children. J. Oral Surg., *19*:367, 1961.

The Gingivostomatitis Syndrome

19. Allen, E. P., Varon, H. H., and Kingsley, W. B.: Effect of ovarian therapy on degenerative gingival disease. Oral Surg., (in press).
20. Epstein, R. S., Archard, H. O., Griffin, J. W., and Baer, P. N.: Psychiatric and histologic findings in an unusual type of chronic gingivitis. J. Periodont. *43*:110, 1972.
21. Kerr, D. A., McClatchey, K. D., and Regezi, J. A.: Idiopathic gingivostomatitis. Oral Surg., *32*:402, 1971.
22. Owings, J. R.: An atypical gingivostomatitis: A report of four cases. J. Periodont. *40*:538, 1969.

Desquamative Gingivitis

23. Gardner, H. L.: Desquamative inflammatory vaginitis: a newly defined entity. Am. J. Obstet. Gynec., *102*:1102, 1968.
24. Glickman, I., and Smulow, J. B.: Chronic desquamative gingivitis—its nature and treatment. J. Periodont., *35*:397, 1964.
25. Goldman, H. M., and Ruben, M. P.: Desquamative gingivitis and its response to topical triamcinolone therapy. Oral Surg., *21*:579, 1966.
26. Jordan, R. E., Triftshauser, C. T., and Schroeter, A. L.: Direct immunofluorescent studies of pemphigus and bullous pemphigoid. Arch. Derm., *103*:486, 1971.
27. McCarthy, F. P., McCarthy, P. L., and Shklar, G.: Chronic desquamative gingivitis: a reconsideration. Surgery, *13*:1300, 1960.
28. Merritt, A. H.: Chronic desquamative gingivitis. J. Periodont., *4*:30, 1933.

Epidermolysis Bullosa

29. Allen, A. C.: The Skin, ed. 2, pp. 303-305. New York, Grune & Stratton, 1967.
30. Boyer, H. E., and Owens, R. H.: Epidermolysis bullosa. A rare disease of dental interest. Oral Surg., *14*:1170, 1961.
31. Gorlin, R. J., and Goldman, H. M.: Thoma's Oral Pathology. ed. 6, pp. 679-680. St. Louis. C. V. Mosby, 1970.
32. Gorlin, R. J.: Epidermolysis bullosa. Oral Surg., *32*:760, 1971.
33. Kaslick, R. S., and Brustein, H. C.: Epidermolysis bullosa. Oral Surg., *14*:1315, 1961.
34. Severin, G. L., and Farber, M.: The management of epidermolysis bullosa in children. Arch. Derm., *95*:302, 1967.
35. Shafer, G. W., Hine, M. K., and Levy, B. M.: Oral Pathology. ed. 2, p. 703. Philadelphia, W. B. Saunders, 1963.

36. Winstock, D.: Oral aspects of epidermolysis bullosa. Br. J. Dermatol., *74*:431, 1962.

Lichen Planus

37. Altman, J., and Perry, H. C.: The variation and course of lichen planus. Arch. Derm., *84*:179, 1961.
38. Andreasen, J. O.: Oral lichen planus. Oral Surg., *25*:31, 1968.
39. Bloom, D.: Lichen planus of the mucous membrane in two sisters. Arch. Derm. Syph., *45*:328, 1942.
40. Cooke, B. E. D.: The oral manifestations of lichen planus: 50 cases. Brit. Dent. J., *96*:1, 1954.
41. Epstein, S.: Lichen planus confined to the oral cavity in twins. Arch. Derm. Syph., *45*:382, 1942.
42. Jones, R. E., Triftshauser, C. T., and Schroeter, A. L.: Direct immunofluorescent studies in pemphigus and bullous pemphigoid. Arch. Derm., *103*:486, 1971.
43. Kutscher, A. H., and Zegarelli, E. U.: Oral and dermal lichen planus. New York State Dent. J., *23*:128, 1957.
44. Peck, S. M., Osserman, K. E., Weiner, L. B., Lefkovits, A., and Osserman, R. S.: Studies in bullous diseases. N. Eng. J. Med. *279*:951, 1968.
45. Shklar, G., and McCarthy, P. L.: The oral lesions of lichen planus. Oral Surg., *14*:164, 1961.
46. Shklar, G.: Erosive and bullous oral lesions of lichen planus. Arch. Derm., *97*:411, 1968.

Focal Epithelial Hyperplasia

47. Archard, H. O., Heck, J. A., and Stanley, H. R.: Focal epithelial hyperplasia: an unusual oral mucosal lesion found in Indian children. Oral Surg., *20*:201, 1965.
48. Clausen, F. P.: Histopathology of focal epithelial hyperplasia. Tandlaegebladet, *73*:1013, 1969.
49. Decker, W. G., and DeGuzman, M. N.: Focal epithelial hyperplasia. Oral Surg., *27*:15, 1969.
50. Hettwer, K. J., and Rodgers, M. S.: Focal epithelial hyperplasia (Heck's disease) in a Polynesian. Oral Surg., *22*:466, 1966.
51. Phillips, H., and Williams, A.: Focal epithelial hyperplasia. Oral Surg., *26*:619, 1968.
52. Severin, I.: Focal epithelial hyperplasia. Tandlaegebladet, *72*:610, 1968.
53. Tan, K. H., Medak, H., and Cohen, L.: Focal epithelial hyperplasia in a Mexican Indian. Arch. Derm., *100*:474, 1969.
54. Witkop, C. J., Jr., and Nisworder, J. D.: Focal epithelial hyperplasia in Central and South American Indians and Ladinos. Oral Surg., *20*:213, 1965.

Tuberous Sclerosis

55. Allen, A. C.: The skin. ed. 2 New York, Grune & Stratton, 1967.
56. Beeson, P. B., and McDermott: Cecil-Loeb Textbook of Medicine ed. 13. pp. 310-311. Philadelphia, W. B. Saunders, 1971.
57. Butterworth, F., and Wilson, M. C.: Dermatologic aspects of tuberous sclerosis. Arch. Derm. Syph., *43*:1, 1941.
58. Davis, R. K., Baer, P. N., Archard, H. O., and Palmer, J. H.: Tuberous sclerosis with oral manifestations. Oral Surg., *17*:395, 1964.
59. Good, C. K., and Garb, J.: Symmetric nevi of face, tuberous sclerosis, epilepsy and fibromatosis growth on scalp with abnormal encephalograms of members of the family. Arch. Derm. Syph., *47*:197, 1943.
60. Gorlin, R. J. Chaundry, A. P., and Kelln, E. E.: Oral manifestations of the Fitzgerald-Gardner, Pringle-Bourneville, Robin, adrenogenital, and Hunter-Pfaundler syndromes. Oral Surg., *13*:1236, 1963.
61. Pillsbury, D. M., Shelley, W. B., and Klingman, A. M.: A Manual of Cutaneous Medicine. Philadelphia, W. B. Saunders Co., 1961.
62. Wintrobe, M. M.: Harrison's Principles of Internal Medicine. ed. 6 pp. 1840-1841. McGraw-Hill, New York, 1970.

5

Fibrous Hyperplasia of the Gingiva

DILANTIN GINGIVAL HYPERPLASIA

Diphenylhydantoin sodium is widely used in the control of epilepsy. Unfortunately, one of the side effects of this drug is a tendency to produce extreme gingival hyperplasia.[15]

Prevalence. The frequency of hyperplasia that occurs following the initiation of diphenylhydantoin sodium therapy varies considerably. Reports range from a low of 3 to 6 percent of cases studied[3,15] to a high of 62 percent. Most investigators place the frequency at about 50 percent of all patients treated, with about 30 percent of patients having a severe enough gingival hyperplasia to warrant surgical correction.[1] No race or sex[6,17] differences have been reported.

Onset. In individuals prone to develop these gingival changes, the onset can occur anywhere from 2 weeks to 3 months or more.[6,14,22] The age of the patient at the time that the diphenylhydantoin sodium therapy is initiated is significant. In general, children and adolescents experience more hyperplasia than adults.[1,7] However, duration of therapy and size of dose appear to be of doubtful significance.[7,10,17]

Pathogenesis. The exact mechanism of action of the drug has not been established. Several theories of action have been proposed such as the creation of a vitamin C deficiency,[8] but this has not been verified.[16] Other speculations concerning the mode of action are based on the alteration and ability of the salivary flow,[2] but that seems unlikely, since the most pronounced effect of the drug appears on the facial surfaces.

An allergic mechanism has been suggested as a cause of the hyperplasia[9] predicted upon the success of antihistamine therapy, but this has not been confirmed.[4,12,13]

Possibly the most logical explanation is that of an exaggerated connective tissue response owing to an alteration of the adrenocortical function, as proposed by Staple.[21] This would be in keeping with the findings of some others that a greater degree of hyperplasia is produced in those areas in which local irritating factors are greatest.[17,22,23,24] Other investigators have been equivocal about the role of plaque in the production of the hyperplasia, suggesting that the lack of oral hygiene might be a secondary factor to the altered contour of the tissues.[7,10,12] However, in keeping with the finding of greater hyperplasia in areas in which local factors exist, it seems reasonable to conclude that poor oral hygiene plays a role.

The direct influence of dilantin on fibroblastic activity and collagen synthesis has been shown in tissue culture studies,[18] in the more rapid healing of wounds in normal patients receiving dilantin,[20] and in an increased tensile strength in healing wounds in rats.[19] It has also been suggested that the wounding acts as a local irritating factor and thus duplicates the exaggerated response of an already metabolically primed tissue. Biochemical studies, however, indicate no increased collagen synthesis. Histologically most specimens show some signs of gingival inflammation.[1,11]

The characteristic histologic features of this disease, namely the subepithelial fibrosis and elongated rete pegs, are even

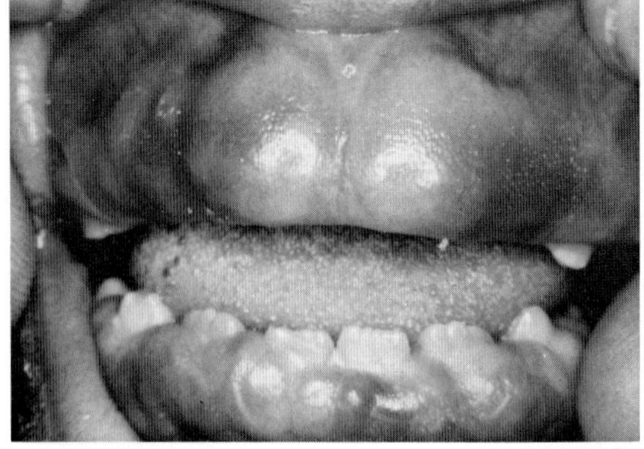

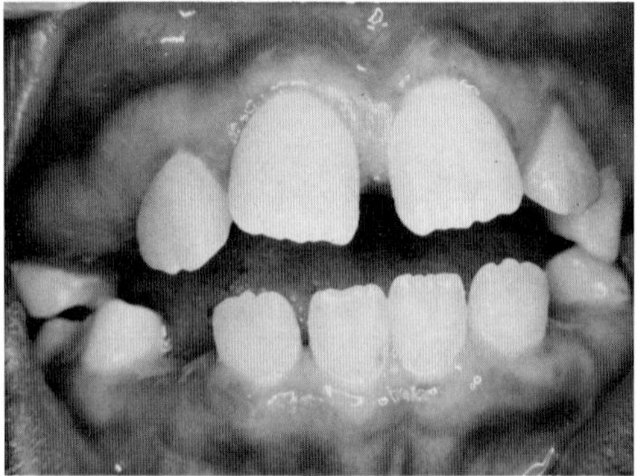

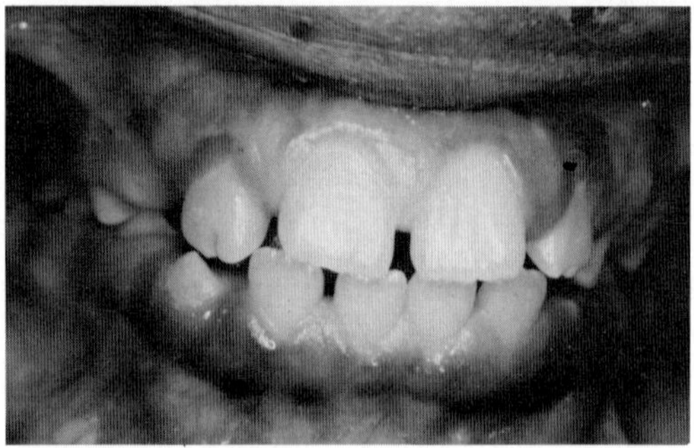

Fig. 5-1. *Top.* Dilantin therapy was started in this 8-year-old before eruption of the permanent incisors, resulting in a delayed passive eruption.
Center. An open bite occurred following surgical removal of fibrous gingival tissue.
Bottom. Spontaneous closure of the open bite occurred in the same patient two years later.

present in those patients whose gingiva appears to be clinically normal.[5A]

Clinical Characteristics. The gingiva in dilantin sodium hyperplasia is extremely fibrous and its clinical appearance varies,

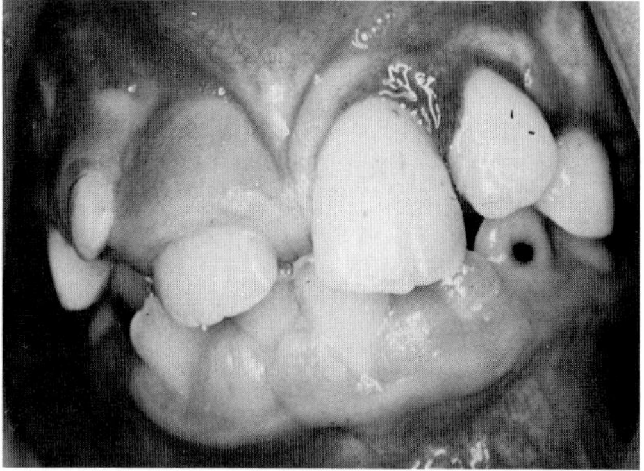

Fig. 5-2. Passive eruption was delayed as a result of dilantin sodium therapy. The gingiva about the maxillary right central and lateral incisors has been surgically excised.

depending upon the age at which the dilantin therapy is initiated. Treatment which is started in children before eruption of their permanent teeth may cause a delay of eruption of the permanent dentition and an open bite owing to the bulk and fibrocity of the gingival tissue (Fig. 5-1). In other instances the teeth may erupt normally from the alveolus, but the fibrous nature of the tissue may result in a delayed passive eruption of the gingiva. As a consequence, there is only partial exposure of the anatomical crowns of one or more teeth, and they look "small" (Figs. 5-2 and 5-3). When the dilantin therapy is started in

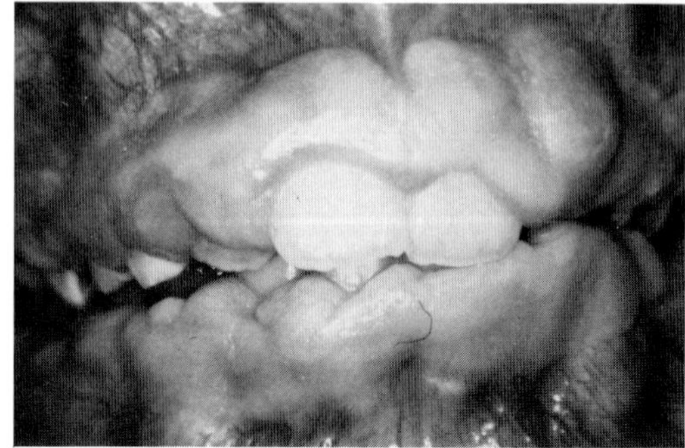

Fig. 5-3. Dilantin sodium therapy started in childhood may delay eruption of some of the permanent teeth or result in a delayed passive eruption.

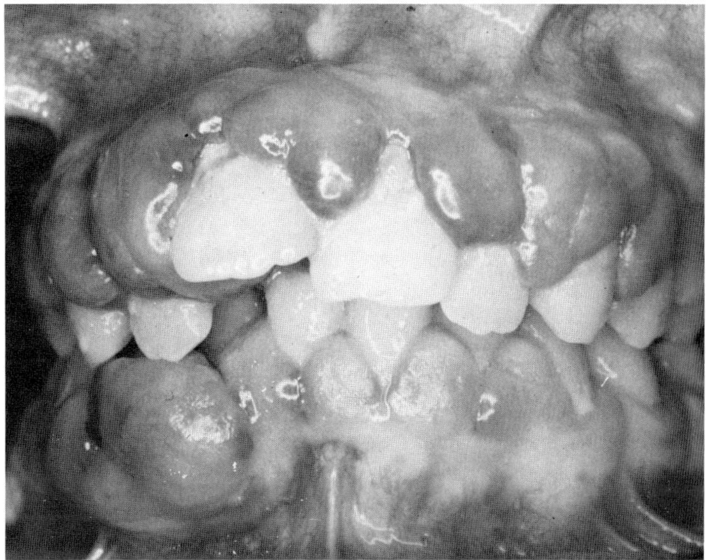

Fig. 5-4. Gingival enlargement is present in an adolescent on dilantin sodium therapy. Compare the gingival contour with that seen in young children (Figs. 5-1 and 5-2).

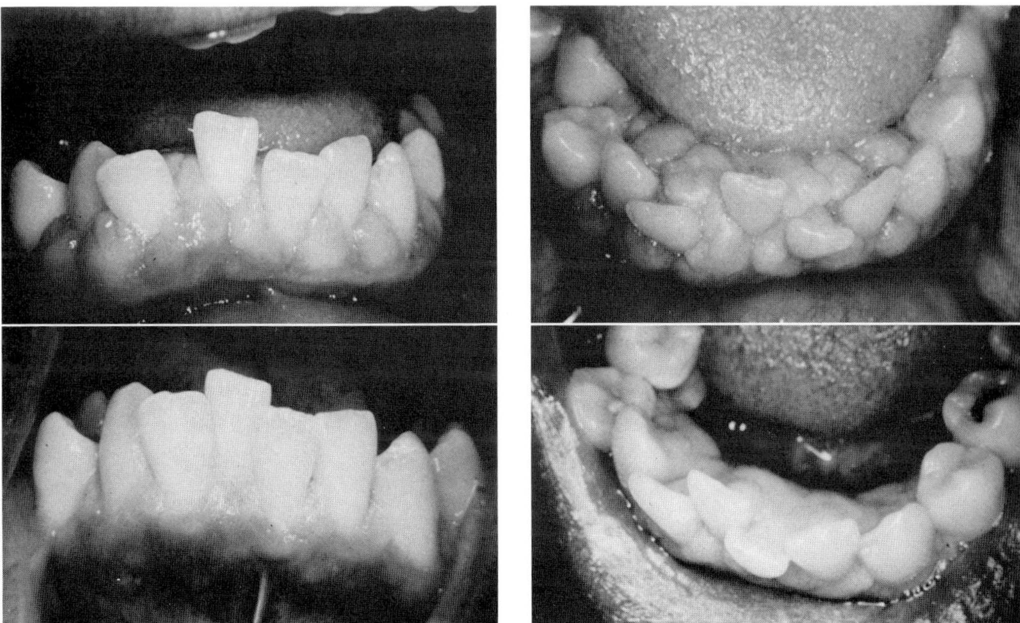

Fig. 5-5. *Top left* and *right*. The gingival tissue may become so bulky and fibrous that it may act as an orthodontic appliance and move and rotate teeth out of alignment.
Bottom left and *right*. The same case shows spontaneous realignment of the teeth following surgical resection of the enlarged fibrous gingival tissue.

adolescence, the lesions assume a completely different form. At this age the lesions usually arise at the interdental papillae and the free gingival margin, and tend to be granular and lobulated in appearance (Fig. 5-4). In some adolescents the interdental papillae become so enlarged that they meet at the facial surfaces of the teeth, creating

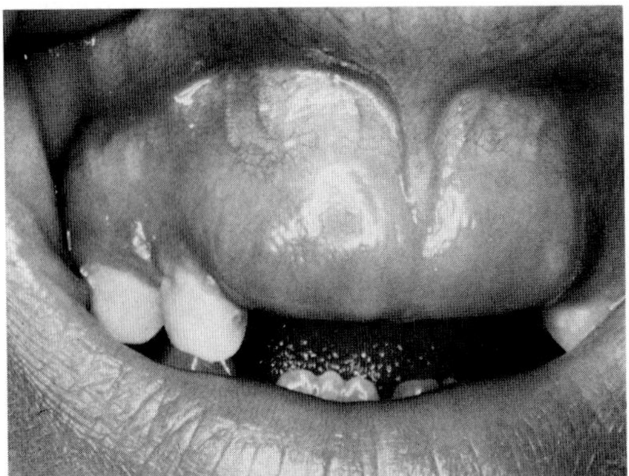

Fig. 5-6. Idiopathic gingival fibromatosis limited to the maxillary central incisor region has retarded eruption of these teeth and is unsightly to the patient.

the appearance of a pseudocleft. In others the gingiva may become so enlarged that it virtually obscures the teeth and, because of its bulk and fibrous nature, may act as an orthodontic appliance and move and rotate the teeth out of their proper alignment (Fig. 5-5). When plaque control is poor, secondary inflammatory changes occur and the granular and stippled appearance of the gingiva may be lost.

The areas in the mouth most frequently affected, in order of severity of involvement, are the maxillary anterior facial surfaces, the mandibular anterior facial surfaces, the maxillary posterior facial surfaces and the mandibular posterior facial surfaces.[17]

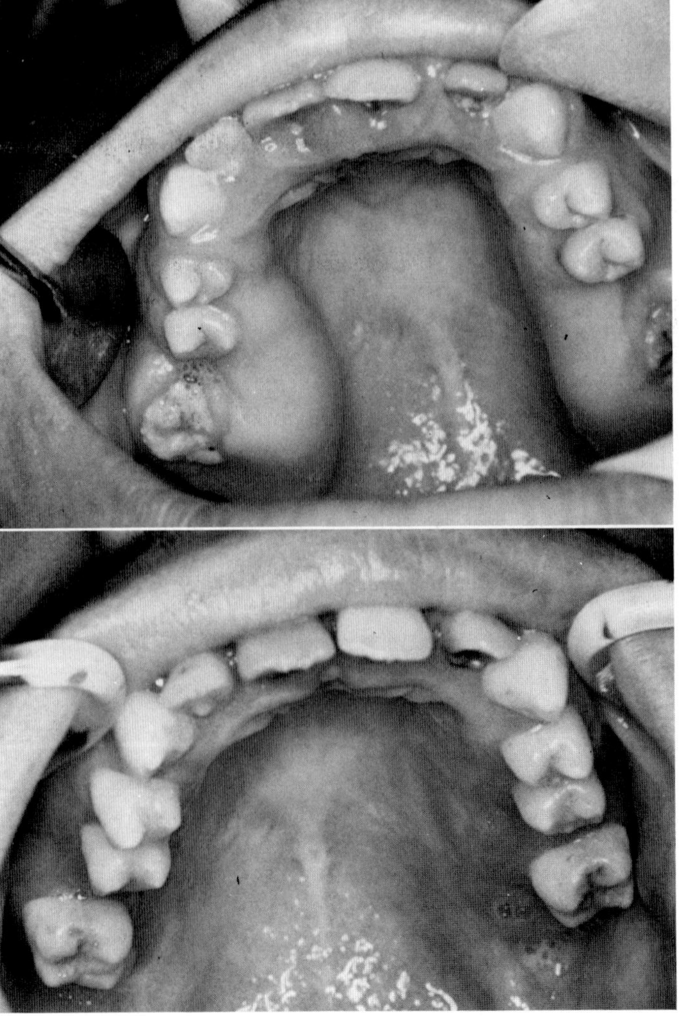

Fig. 5-7. *Top.* A localized form of gingival fibromatosis. *Bottom.* The postoperative result following surgical excision of the fibrous gingival tissue.

Treatment. Treatment depends on the degree of severity of the hyperplasia. Plaque control and elimination of local irritating factors is essential in preventing or retarding regrowth of tissue.

Surgical intervention is necessary when either eruption of the dentition is impaired or severe cosmetic deformities result. Often, especially in the nonretarded patients, one finds an emotional difficulty owing to the appearance of the gingival tissues, and even though recurrence is highly probable, the cosmetic improvement on a short term basis warrants surgical intervention in retarding the rate of regrowth of the gingiva. In such patients a positive pressure appliance (see Chap. 4) has been found to be quite a successful aid in retarding regrowth of the hyperplastic gingival tissue.[5]

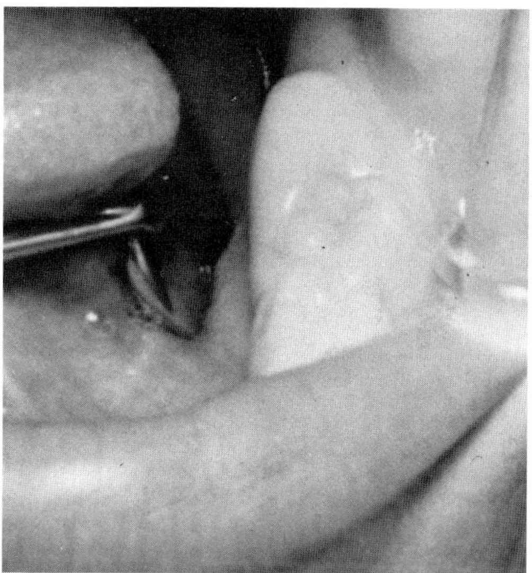

Fig. 5-8. Localized fibrous enlargements in the mandibular molar region tend to extend further lingually than buccally.

GINGIVAL FIBROMATOSIS

Idiopathic or hereditary gingival fibromatosis is a rare condition of the gingival tissues, characterized by enlargement of the free and attached gingiva. In some cases the gingiva can become so firm and dense as to feel on palpation like bone. The enlargement is painless and may extend up to the mucogingival junction but does not affect the alveolar mucosa. The color of the gingiva is normal or slightly paler than normal. The only complaint of the patient is the deformity it causes (see Fig. 5-6).

The fibrous enlargement is usually symmetrical but may be unilateral, and may be generalized or localized. The localized form usually affects the maxillary molar and tuberosity area, particularly on the palatal surface (Fig. 5-7). When the fibrous enlargements affect the mandibular molar region they are usually smaller than in the maxillary arch and extend farther lingually than buccally (Fig. 5-8).

Prevalence. In a survey of 100,000 cases seen in over a 20-year-period at Columbia University Medical Center in New York, Zegarelli and Kutscher reported finding only 20 well-documented cases of fibromatosis.[39]

There is no sex predilection for the occurrence of this disease.

Onset. In some individuals the fibrous gingival enlargement is initiated by the eruption of the first primary teeth, in others by the anterior permanent teeth and in still others by the posterior permanent teeth. This could explain why in some persons the fibrous hyperplasia is generalized, whereas in some others it is localized to the molar and tuberosity areas. The fibrous enlargement may become so firm and resilient as to actually retard the eruption of the teeth into the oral cavity, although there is normal eruption of the teeth from the alveolus. Roentgenographs show a normal relationship between the tooth and the alveolar bone even though the tooth is still completely covered with the fibrous gingival tissue. Factors preventing the tooth's breaking through the soft tissue into the mouth are unknown. It is also unknown how the soft tissue covering the crowns of the teeth is able to withstand the force of mastication without apparent ulceration or pain. In time

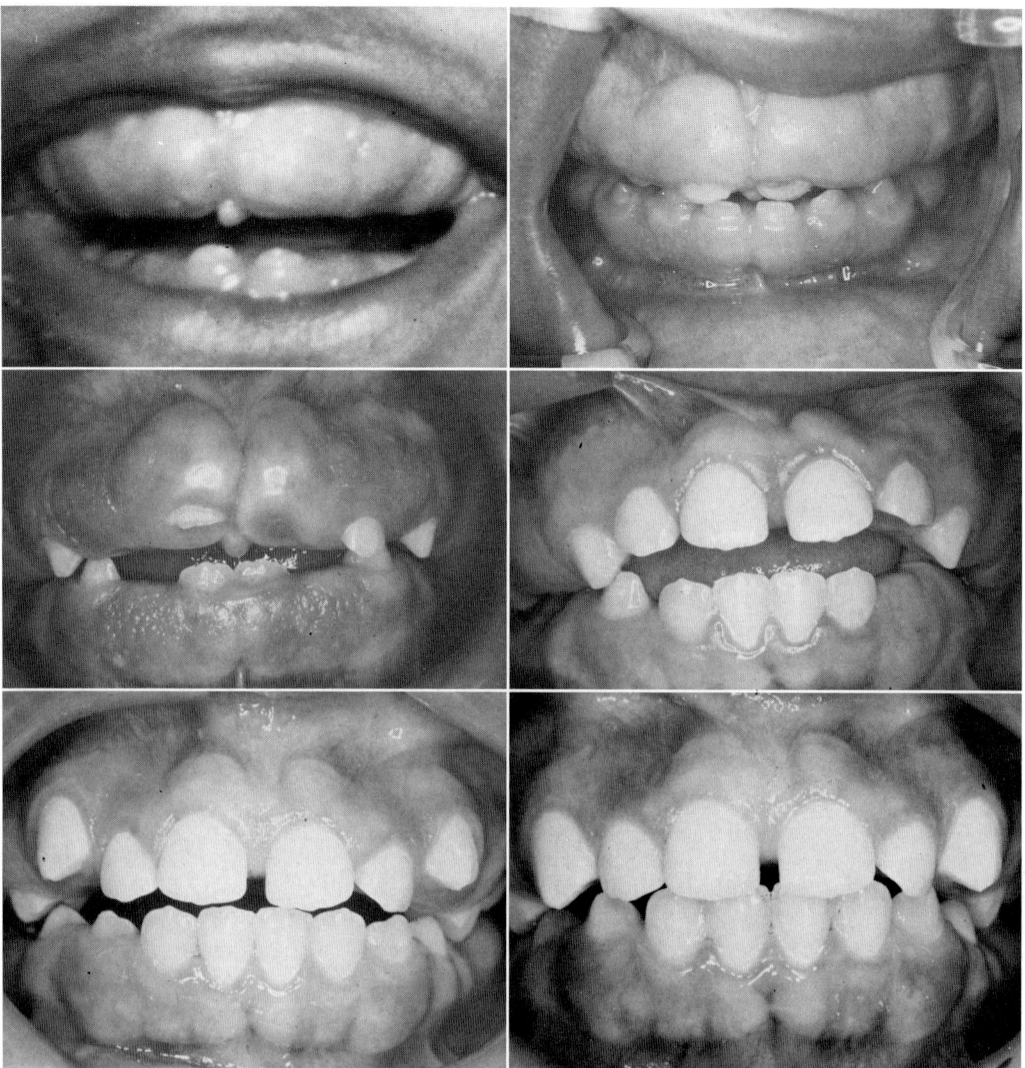

Fig. 5-9. *Top left.* Gingival fibromatosis in a 14-month-old female.
Top right. Appearance of patient at 3 years of age.
Center left. Appearance of patient at 7 years of age just prior to surgical removal of the maxillary and mandibular fibrous gingival tissue.
Center right. The two-month postoperative result. Note the anterior open bite.
Bottom left. The patient at 9 years of age. Note the spontaneous closure of the anterior open bite.
Bottom right. At 11 years of age further closure of the bite occurred.

the occlusal surfaces of the posterior teeth invariably become exposed as a result of mastication, although the buccal, lingual and interproximal tissues extend up to the occlusal surface.

The enlargement of the fibrous gingival tissue tends to be restricted to the growth period of the individual. Nevertheless, there are a few persons who continue to experience slow enlargement into adult life.

Etiology. The inherited form of the disease is transmitted by an autosomal dominant gene with variable expression and possible incomplete penetrance.[29,30,31,36] Envi-

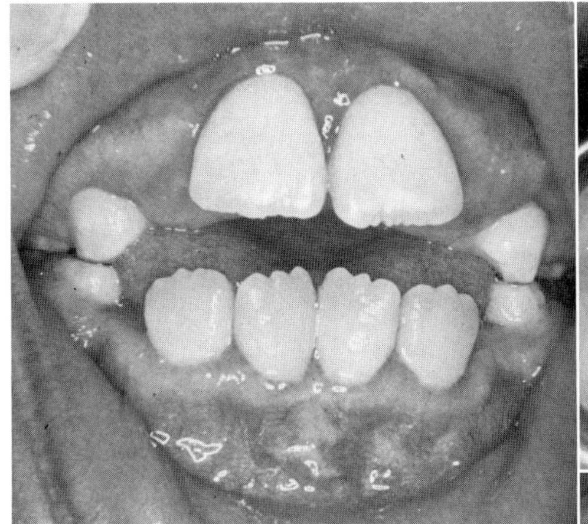

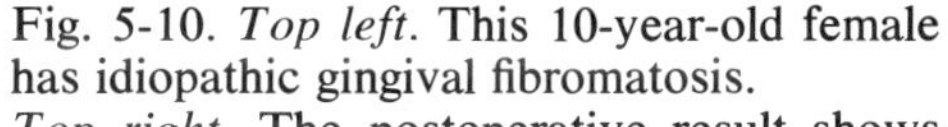

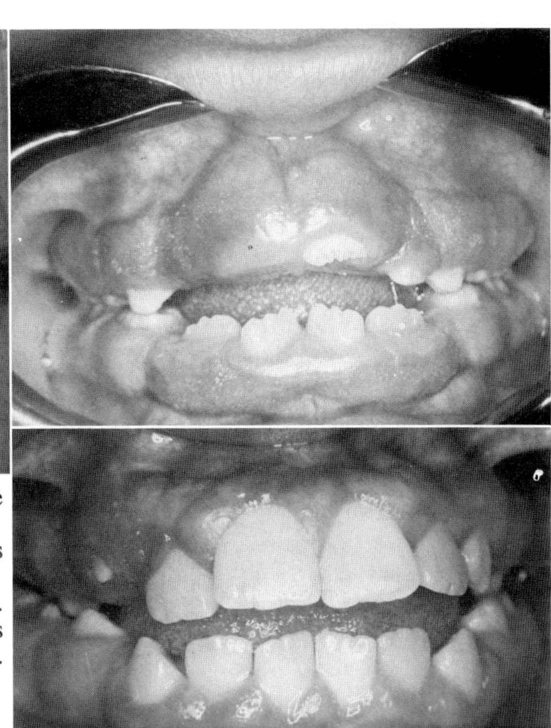

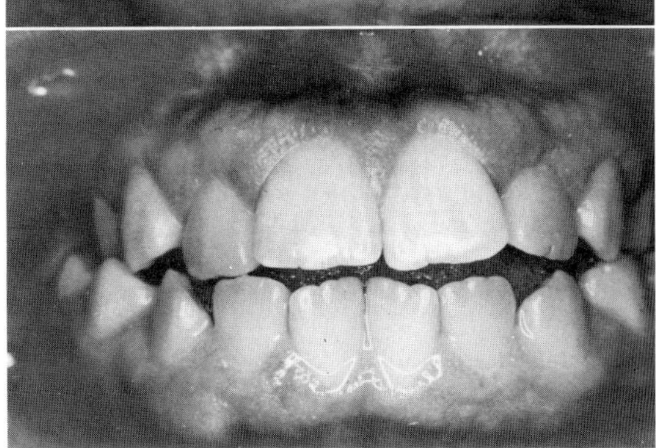

Fig. 5-10. *Top left.* This 10-year-old female has idiopathic gingival fibromatosis.
Top right. The postoperative result shows an anterior open bite.
Center. The same patient at 15 years of age.
Bottom. The patient at 18 years of age shows spontaneous closure of the anterior open bite.

ronmental influences are probably responsible for the variable expressions.[30] Several investigators have traced the disease through succeeding generations.[25,37,38] When one is unable to trace either a familial or hereditary pattern, however, the disease is termed idiopathic gingival fibromatosis.

Local factors, while present, appear to be secondary rather than primary etiologic agents.

Treatment. In the severe generalized cases, in which the teeth are retarded in their active eruption through the thickened fibrous gingival tissue into the oral cavity, a decision must be reached as to the proper time to operate. If the surgery is postponed too long, a permanent anterior open bite may result. On the other hand, it can be argued that since the most growth of fibrous gingival tissue occurs in areas in which teeth are actively erupting, the later the operation is done, the more unlikely recurrences will be. To help resolve this dilemma the following guidelines may be used:

1. Wait until 1 to 2 years after the teeth concerned would normally have been ex-

pected to penetrate the gingiva before operating.[36]

2. Take a roentgenograph of the involved area. If this shows that the teeth have completely erupted through the alveolar bone and are covered only by soft tissue, the overlying fibrous tissue should be excised immediately.[32]

We have found the following procedure to be successful. Operate on the incisor teeth when a roentgenograph demonstrates that the crowns are only covered by soft tissue—generally when the patient is about 7 to 8 years of age. In this manner an acceptable esthetic result can be obtained at an early age and the anterior open bite, which frequently is present immediately following surgery, will tend to correct itself spontaneously (Figs. 5-9 and 5-10). Then wait until the second molars are in the correct line of occlusion, which is reached when the patient is approximately 14 years of age, before operating on the posterior segments. With this technique we have had minimal problems with rapid and excessive regrowth of tissue.

In patients in whom the fibrous overgrowth of gingival tissue is limited largely to the palatal and tuberosity region of the maxillary arch, there may also be concomitant overgrowth of alveolar bone. In these instances, either osseous surgery is required to obtain proper physiologic gingival contour, or gingival form is compromised.

Prognosis. Long-term follow-up studies indicate that whether the case is generalized or localized in nature, some individuals over the years experience a slow regrowth of fibrous gingiva in the treated areas.

Contrary to some reports in the literature, we have found that this regrowth can occur even in cases in which all the teeth have been extracted and the patient is wearing full dentures. The tendency for regrowth is probably genetically predetermined and is different for different persons. In any event, considering the innocuous nature of the regrowth, there seems little justification for such radical methods of treatment as tooth extraction, excision of the alveolus or removal of all deciduous buds.[34]

Associated Anomalies. Many abnormalities have been associated with hereditary generalized gingival fibromatosis,[28,33,35,36] although hypertrichosis is the most common.[27,36] Not every patient, however, has an abnormality, and some patients are free of abnormalities at birth and during childhood, developing a deformity 10 or more years after the gingival fibrosis is first noticed.[26]

REFERENCES

Dilantin Gingival Hyperplasia

1. Aas, E.: Hyperplasia gingiva diphenylhydantoinea. Acta. Odontol. Scand. (Suppl.), *34:*1963.
2. Babcock, J. R.: Incidence of gingival hyperplasia with Dilantin therapy in a hospital population. J.A.D.A., *78:*1447, 1965.
3. Blair, D., Bailey, K. C., and McGregor, J. S.: Treatment of epilepsy with Epanutin. Lancet, *2:*363, 1939.
4. Breg, W. R., and Falcetti, J. P.: Ineffectiveness of antihistamine therapy for gingival hyperplasia due to diphenylhydantoin sodium. N. Eng., J. Med., *257:*1128, 1957.
5. Davis, R. K., Baer, P. N., and Palmer, J. H.: A preliminary report on a new therapy for Dilantin gingival hyperplasia. J. Periodont., *34:*17, 1963.

5A. Donnenfeld, O. W., and Stanley, H. R.: Effect of plaque in patients following gingivectomy for dilantin hyperplasia. J. Dent. Res., *52:*97, 1973.

6. Dummett, C. O.: Oral tissue reactions from Dilantin medication in the control of epileptic seizures. J. Periodont., *25:*112, 1954.
7. Esterberg, H. L., and White, P. H.: Sodium Dilantin gingival hyperplasia, J.A.D.A., *32:*16, 1945.
8. Frankel, S. I.: Dilantin sodium in the treatment of epilepsy. J.A.M.A., *114:*1320, 1940.
9. Gailard, R. A.: Antihistaminic therapy for gingival hyperplasia acetate as an adjunct in its treatment. J. Oral Surg., *13:*280, 1955.
10. Glickman, I., and Lewitus, M.: Hyperplasia of the gingivae associated with Dilantin (sodium diphenylhydantoinate) therapy. J.A.D.A., *28:*199, 1941.

11. Han, S. S., Hwang, P. J., and Lee, O. H.: A study of the histopathology of gingival hyperplasia in mental patients receiving sodium diphenylhydantoin. Oral Surg., *23:*774, 1967.
12. Ingle, J. I., Howard, W. L., and Zwick, H. H.: Effects of antihistaminic therapy on diphenylhydantoin sodium (Dilantin) gingival hyperplasia. J.A.D.A. *58:*65, 1959.
13. Holowach, I., Thurston, D. L., and Gilster, J. E.: Antihistamine therapy for gingival hyperplasia due to diphenylhydantoin. N. Eng. J. Med., *259:*180, 1958.
14. Kimball, O. P.: The treatment of epilepsy with sodium diphenylhydantoinate. JAMA, *112:*1244, 1939.
15. Merritt, H. H., and Putnam, T. J.: Sodium diphenylhydantoinate in treatment of convulsive disorders. JAMA, *111:*1068, 1938.
16. Milhon, J. A., and Osterberg, A. E.: Relationship between gingival hyperplasia and ascorbic acid in the blood and urine of epileptic patients undergoing treatment with sodium diphenylhydantoinate. J.A.D.A. *29:*207, 1942.
17. Panuski, H. J., Gorlin, R. J., Bearman, J. E., and Mitchell, D. F.: The effect of anticonvulsant drugs upon the gingiva-A series of analysis of 1048 patients. I. J. Periodont. *31:*336, 1960; II. J. Periodont., *32:*15, 1961.
18. Shafer, W. G.: Effect of Dilantin sodium and on growth of human fibroblast like cell cultures. Proc. Soc. Exp. Biol. Med., *104:*198, 1960.
19. Shafer, W. G., Beatty, R. E., and Davis, W. B.: Effect of Dilantin sodium on tensile strength of healing wounds. Proc. Soc. Exp. Biol. Med., *98:*348, 1958.
20. Shapiro, M.: Acceleration of gingival wound healing in non-epileptic patients receiving diphenylhydantoin sodium (Dilantin, Epanutin). Exp. Med. Surg., *16:*41, 1958.
21. Staple, P. H.: The adrenal glands and gingival hyperplasia due to phenytoin sodium. Lancet, *2:*600, 1953.
22. Staple, P. H.: Some tissue reactions associated with 5:5-diphenylhydantoin (Dilantin) sodium therapy. Br. Dent. J., *95:*289, 1953.
23. Stern, L., Eisenbud, L., and Klatell, J.: Analysis of oral reactions to Dilantin sodium. J. Dent. Res., *22:*157, 1943.
24. Ziskin, D. E., Stowe, R., and Zegarelli, E. V.: Dilantin hyperplastic gingivitis. 1. Its cause and treatment. 2. Differential appraisal. Am. J. Orthodont. *27:*350, 1941.

Gingival Fibromatosis

25. Becker, W., Collings, C. K., Zimmerman, E. R., De La Rosa, M., and Singdahlsen, D.: Hereditary gingival fibromatosis. Oral Surg., *24:*313, 1967.
26. Byars, L. T., and Jurkiewicz, M.: Congenital macrogingivae and hypertrichosis with subsequent giant fibroadenomas of the breasts. Plast. Reconstr. Surg., *27:*608, 1961.
27. Byars, L. T., and Sarnat, B. G.: Congenital macrogingivae (fibromatous gingivae) and hypertrichosis. Am. J. Orthodont. Oral Surg. *31:*48, 1945.
28. Chaikin, B. E.: Report of a case of fibromatosis of the gingiva associated with a hypothyroidism. Periodontics, *3:*306, 1965.
29. Emerson, T. G.: Hereditary gingival hyperplasia. Oral Surg., *19:*1, 1965.
30. Fletcher, J. P.: Gingival abnormalities of genetic origin: a preliminary communication with special reference to hereditary generalized gingival fibromatosis. J. Dent. Res. (Suppl. 3), *45:*597, 1966.
31. Gorlin, R. J., and Pindborg, J. J.: Syndromes of the head and neck. pp. 312-316. New York, McGraw-Hill, 1965.
32. Henefer, E. P., Kay L. A.: Congenital idiopathic gingival fibromatosis in the deciduous dentition. Oral Surg., *24:*65, 1967.
33. Hine, M. K.: Fibrous hyperplasia of gingiva. J.A.D.A. *44:*681, 1952.
34. McIndoe A., and Smith, B. O.: Congenital familial fibromatosis of the gums with teeth as a probable aetiological factor. Br. J. Plast. Surg., *11:*63, 1958.
35. Laband, P. F., Habib, G., and Humphreys, G. S.: Hereditary gingival fibromatosis. Oral Surg., *17:*339, 1964.
36. Rushton, M. A.: Hereditary or idiopathic hyperplasia of the gums. Dent. Pract., Dent. Rec., *7:*136, 1957.
37. Savara, B. S., Suher, T., Everett, F. G., and Burns, A. G.: Hereditary gingival fibrosis: study of a family. J. Periodont., *25:*12, 1954.
38. Weski, H.: Elephantiasis gingivae hereditaria. Dtsch. Monatschr. Zahn., *38:*557, 1920.
39. Zegarelli, E. V., Kutscher, A. H., Hyman, G. A.: Diagnosis of the Diseases of the Mouth and Jaws. pp. 196-7. Philadelphia Lea & Febiger, 1969.

6

The Frenums

MAXILLARY LABIAL FRENUM

The importance of the maxillary labial frenum as a cause of a midline diastema has been overestimated largely because of uncertainty as to what constitutes a true abnormal frenum as opposed to a harmless enlarged variation of a normal frenum. That there is a similarity between the two cannot be denied; however, experience has shown that surgical correction based on an incorrect diagnosis leads to failure. The elimination of an enlarged labial frenum does not automatically result in the closure of a midline diastema.

DEVELOPMENT

Fetal Development. The frenum originates in a fold of tissue known as the tectolabial frenum, which develops in approximately the third month of fetal life. During early embryonic life it connects the palatine papilla with a prominence in the center of the maxillary lip, the tuberculum. Thus, the tectolabial frenum of the fetus simulates the abnormal frenum of postnatal life, in that it extends as a continuous band of tissue from the inner aspect of the upper lip over and across the alveolar ridge and is inserted in the palatine papillae (Fig. 6-1).[19,21,22]

Postnatal Development. In later stages, as a result of the increase in size of the alveolar process, the tectolabial frenum becomes separated from the palatine papilla and persists as the upper labial frenum. The frenum also becomes reduced in size and, although it is separated from the papilla, it gives the illusion of being continuous with it. The labial frenum usually retains this position until the teeth erupt. Upon the eruption of the primary teeth, the vertical height of the alveolar bone is increased. At the same time the frenum attachment usually moves more apically and tends to atrophy. This creates a further division between the frenum and the incisal papilla. There are certain circumstances, however, in which a very large maxillary labial frenum will persist and remain in a more coronal position. The tendency to remain in this position may be enhanced by the appearance of the developmental space in the primary maxillary anterior teeth.

Permanent Teeth. With the eruption of the permanent central incisors, further vertical growth occurs in the maxillary arch. If there has been no interruption in the recessive tendencies of the frenum up to this point, this structure usually assumes a normal position well apical to the interdental gingival tissue. It does not *always* assume this more normal position however.

The permanent maxillary central incisors erupt at approximately 7 years of age in crypts separated by a well-defined bony suture (Fig. 6-2). Inevitably, they erupt with a space between them (Fig. 6-3) which in turn favors the continued existence of the frenum. Therefore, when an enlarged lower attached variation of a normal maxillary labial frenum exists after the eruption of the permanent central incisors it would tend to remain until after the eruption of the lateral incisors. If the pressure of the erupting lateral incisors fails to close the space (Fig. 6-4), the cuspids ordinarily can be depended upon to do so when they erupt.

Therefore, the presence of any midline diastema may be considered a normal condition from infancy to the age of 12 years, or until the time that a full complement of maxillary teeth have erupted and are in

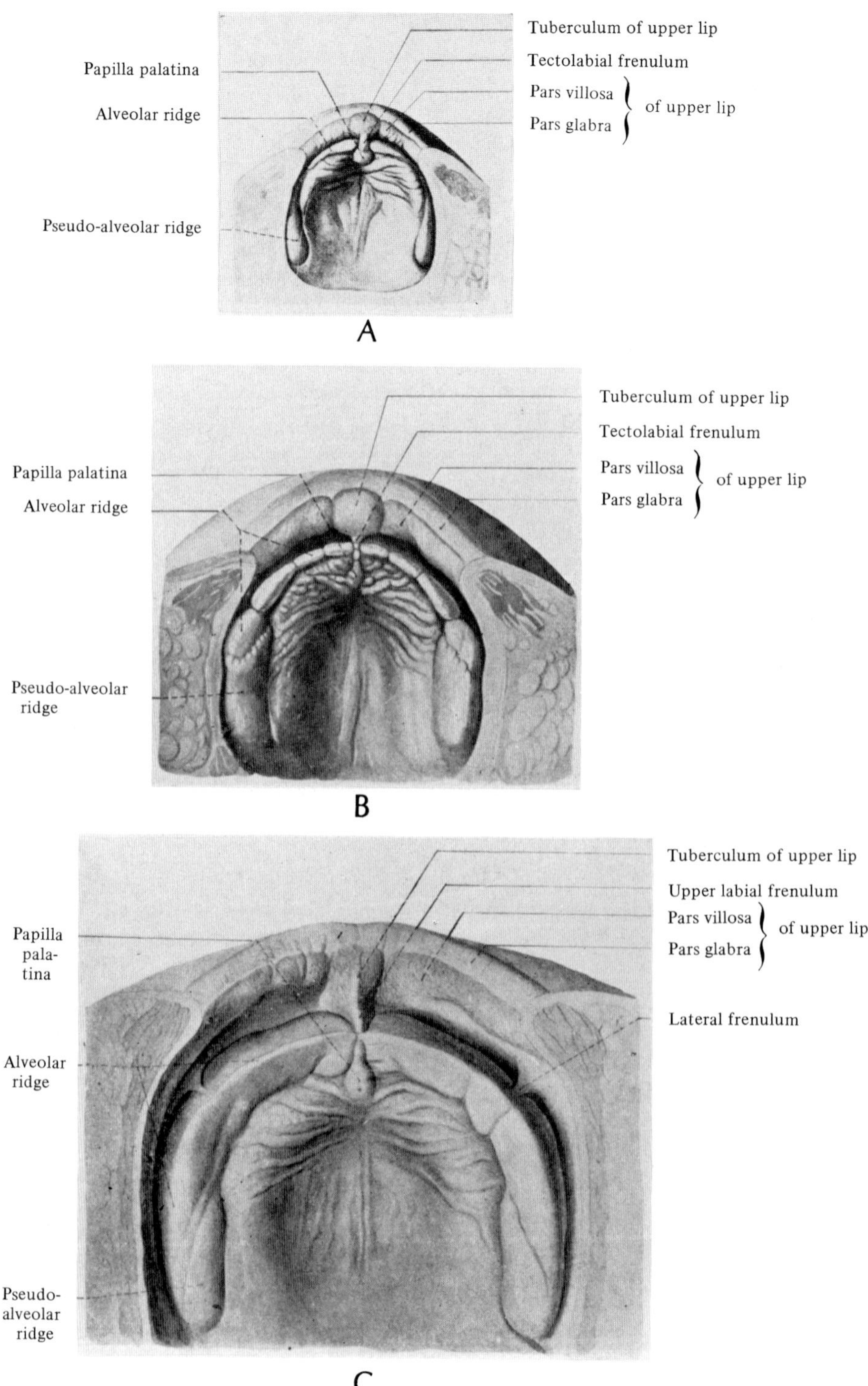

Fig. 6-1. *A*. The tectolabial frenulum of the human fetus at 3 months. *B*. The frenum of the fetus at 4 months. *C*. The frenum of the newborn infant. (From Sicher and Tardler.)[22]

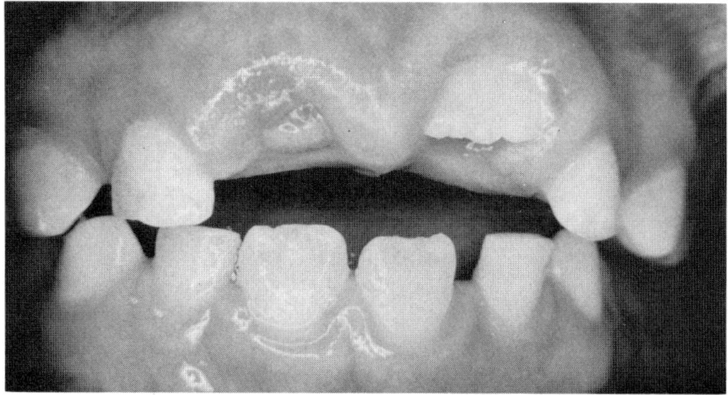

Fig. 6-2. The maxillary incisor erupting at approximately 7 years of age.

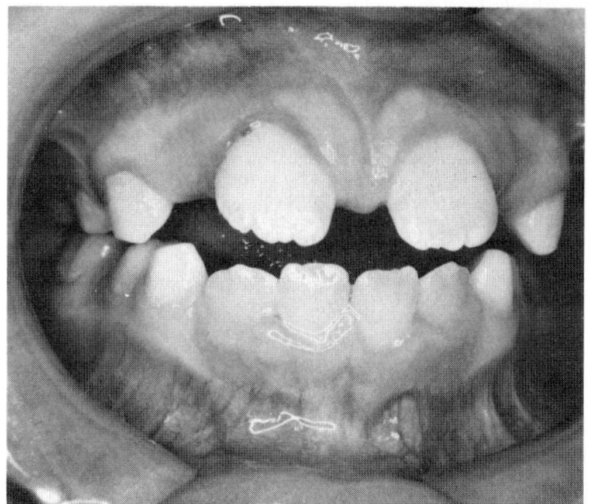

Fig. 6-3. Note the large diastema in the same patient one year later.

good proximal contact with one another. It should also be remembered that a large frenum may be associated with, but not the cause of, a midline diastema. Actually there is a tremendous variation in the size, shape and position of the normal maxillary labial frenum. In general the frenum tends to be much larger in children, and therefore

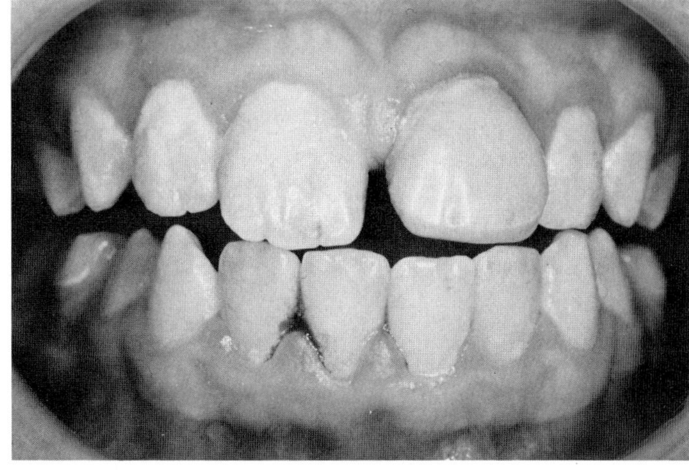

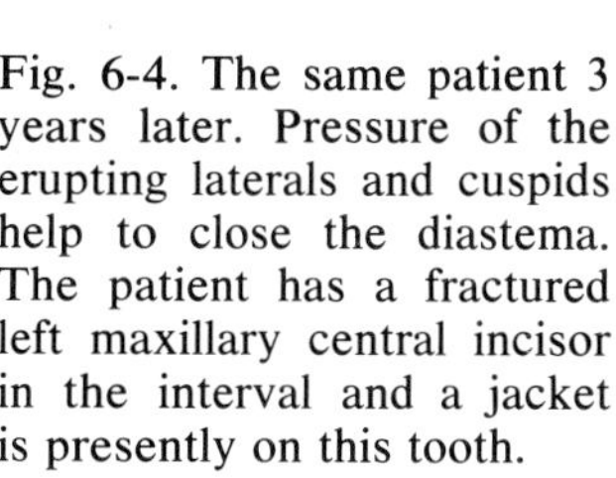

Fig. 6-4. The same patient 3 years later. Pressure of the erupting laterals and cuspids help to close the diastema. The patient has a fractured left maxillary central incisor in the interval and a jacket is presently on this tooth.

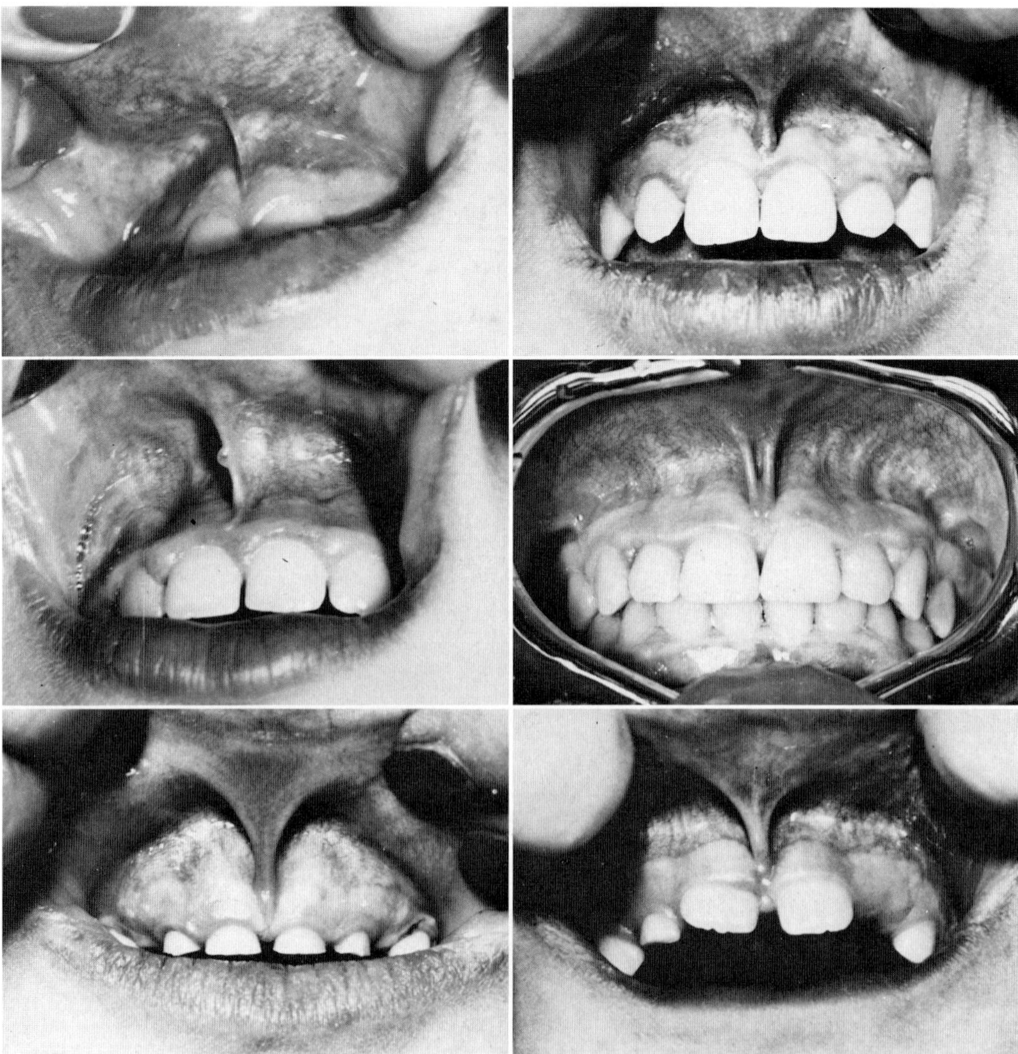

Fig. 6-5. Variations of the normal frenum. The range is from a thin, almost nonexistent slip of tissue to a broad, sturdy structure. Small harmless nodules, as frequently seen along the crest of the frenum, and bifurcated frenums are not uncommon. In children, the frenum normally is wider and longer than in adults. Occasionally, the frenum may appear to be depressed in a shallow groove between the roots of a currently erupting central incisor. Further alveolar development can be anticipated labially as well as vertically. (Courtesy of Dr. B. F. Dewell.)[14]

is frequently diagnosed as abnormal when it is not (Figs. 6-5 and 6-6). A maxillary frenum that requires surgical correction is actually quite rare. Most often a large frenum associated with a diastema exists because there was insufficient pressure stimulation from the central incisors to cause it to atrophy. Thus, most enlarged maxillary frenums are the result, not the cause, of a midline diastema between the maxillary central incisors.[1,5,12,13,14,15]

Etiology of Midline Diastema. In a study involving 1000 patients Clark[9] noted that one or both of the parents of 60 percent of the patients had labial diastema, and that in 5 percent the diastema was associated with

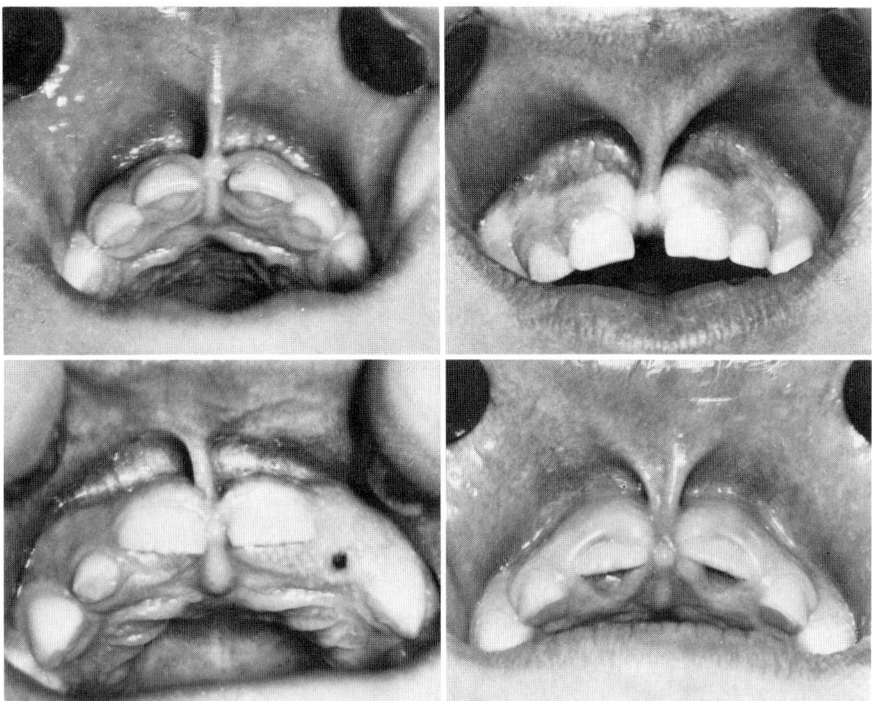

Fig. 6-6. These four questionable frenums in deciduous and early mixed dentition require frequent observations. Note in particular the palatine papillae which can be as effective as the frenum in perpetuating a midline diastema. Future development will determine whether the frenum resection is indicated or whether they will respond more favorably to active orthodontic treatment. (Courtesy of Dr. B. F. Dewell.)[14]

supernumerary teeth in the midline. Other causes were congenitally missing lateral incisors, tongue (Fig. 6-7) or other habits, and a cleft of the interseptal alveolar bone (Fig. 6-8). This latter condition enables an abnormal frenum to persist, since it prevents the transseptal fibers of the periodontal ligament from running from the cementum of one central incisor to the other. A histologic investigation of the interdental tissues at the maxillary midline region[3] has shown that the tissues in this area are different from those found in other interdental regions. A group of connective tissue fibers were found in the area (designated the supracrestal sutural fiber groups), which originate on the cementum of the central incisors and pass over the crest of the alveolar bone to insert into the tissues of the intermaxillary suture (Fig. 6-9). This results in a reduction in the quantity of the transseptal fibers between the central incisors, and probably causes a decrease in the strength of the tissue bond between these teeth.

Destructive periodontal disease, which causes so-called tooth migration, is another cause of diastema formation in the maxillary anterior region, and is dealt with separately in Chapter 10.

Relationship of the Midline Diastema and the Maxillary Labial Frenum. There is usually no relationship between the size of a diastema and the size of the frenum. In other words, enlarged frenums may be found when the central incisors are contacting or when they are separated, though in the latter case the frenums atrophy and become normal in size following eruption of the lateral incisors.[8] The independent char-

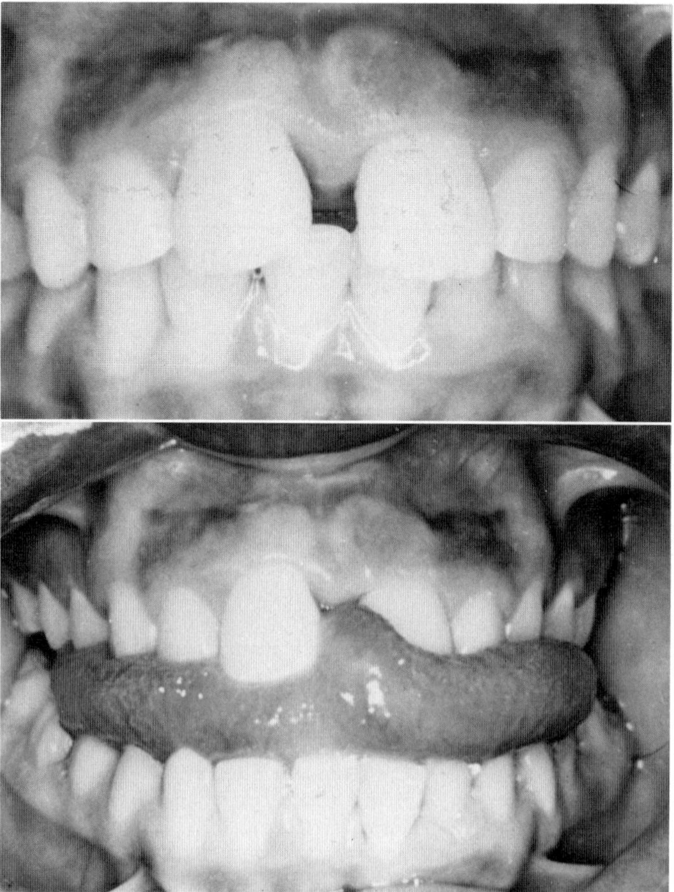

Fig. 6-7. *Top.* A diastema due to a tongue habit.
Bottom. The tongue inserted between the maxillary central incisor.

acter of the frenum and a midline diastema, and their lack of correlation, are shown in Table 6-1.

Similarly, there is no correlation between the shape of the alveolar septum between the maxillary central incisors, the approximation or lack of approximation of the premaxillary bone at the intermaxillary suture, and the midline diastema.[3]

Treatment. It is almost universally held that surgical removal of the maxillary labial frenum is rarely indicated.[8, 12, 13, 14, 15] In any event surgical correction should not be instituted until the maxillary permanent cuspids have fully erupted. Actually, it probably would be better to wait until the upper permanent second molars have fully erupted in order to more fully take advantage of the effect of growth and development upon closure of the midline space. If the midline diastema is still present at that age, the first attempt should be to close the space orthodontically. If tissue hyperplasia instead of pressure atrophy of the frenum results from the orthodontic procedure, or if the diastema returns, it is convincing evidence that surgical correction is needed. At that time, with the orthodontic appliance in place, surgical resection should be accomplished.[9] This inevitably results in rapid and permanent closure of a midline diastema.

ANTERIOR MANDIBULAR FRENUMS

Frenum attachments that insert into the margin of the free gingiva and that cause

TABLE 6-1. LACK OF CORRELATION BETWEEN FRENUM AND MIDLINE DIASTEMA

	No Diastema			Diastema Present			
	Attach. Ht., mm.	Frenum Width, mm.	Age Yr.	Attach. Ht., mm.	Frenum Width, mm.	Diastema Width, mm.	Age Yr.
	4.5	2.0	9	6.5	1.5	1.5	9
	6.5	1.5	12	5.5	2.0	1.5	9
	5.0	1.5	10	8.0	1.0	1.0	17
	4.0	2.0	12	6.5	2.0	1.5	16
	6.5	2.0	14	8.0	2.0	3.0	9
	7.0	1.5	14	5.0	2.0	1.0	14
	5.0	1.5	13	3.0	1.5	1.5	7
	8.5	2.0	13	6.0	1.5	1.0	13
	6.0	1.5	11	5.0	2.5	1.5	19
	7.0	1.0	13	5.5	1.5	1.5	10
	6.0	1.5	15	4.0	2.0	2.5	15
	7.0	1.0	12	4.5	1.0	2.5	8
	5.0	1.5	15	4.5	1.5	1.0	11
	7.0	1.5	12	3.0	1.0	1.0	9
	9.0	2.0	12	5.0	2.0	2.5	9
	9.5	2.0	6	5.0	1.5	1.5	10
	3.5	1.5	10	4.0	1.5	2.0	9
Aver.	6.3	1.6		5.2	1.7	1.7	
Range	3.5–9.5	1.0–2.0		3.0–8.0	1.0–2.5	1.0–3.0	

* (After Ceremello)[8]

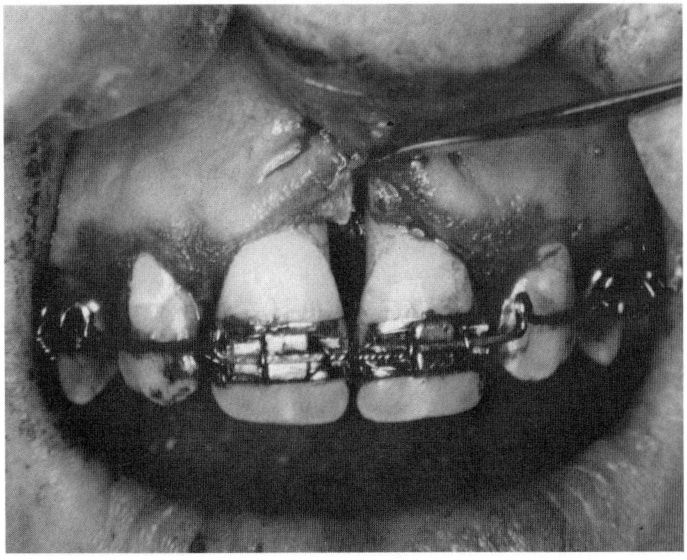

Fig. 6-8. A cleft in the interseptal alveolar bone.

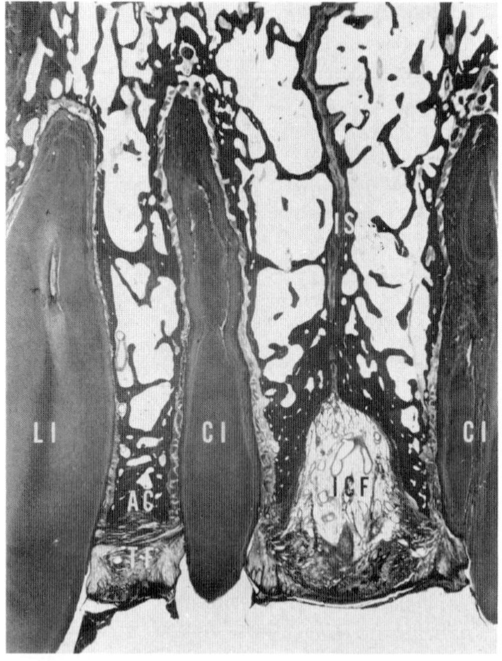

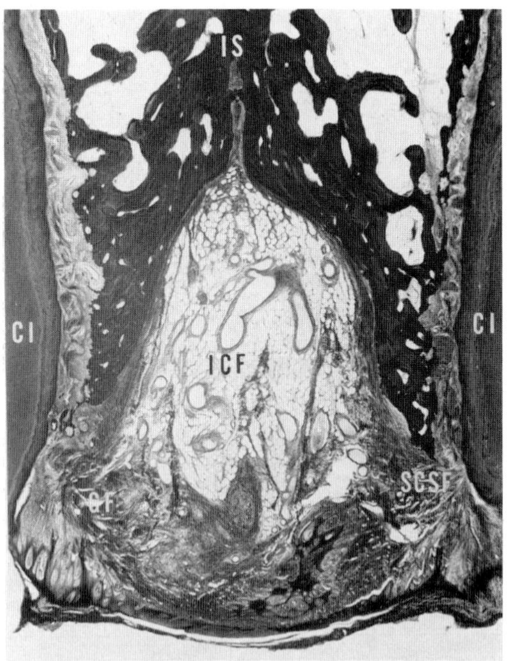

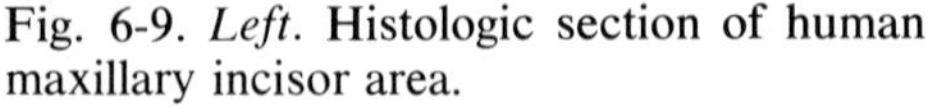

Fig. 6-9. *Left.* Histologic section of human maxillary incisor area.
ICF is the incisor canal and foramen,
CI is the central incisor tooth,
LI is the lateral incisor.
Right. Higher magnification of the above figure.
CI is the central incisor,
ICF is the incisive canal and foramen,
SCSF is the supracrestal-sutural fiber bundles.
(Courtesy of Dr. R. B. Allman, Jr.)

movement of the free gingiva during movements of the lips or cheeks also cause of gingival recession (see Chap. 7). A diagnosis of this condition can be made by applying tension to the lip (Fig. 6-10), causing the margin of the gingiva to retract from the tooth. In advanced lesions, gingival recession may be associated with a frenum and complicated by the presence of a

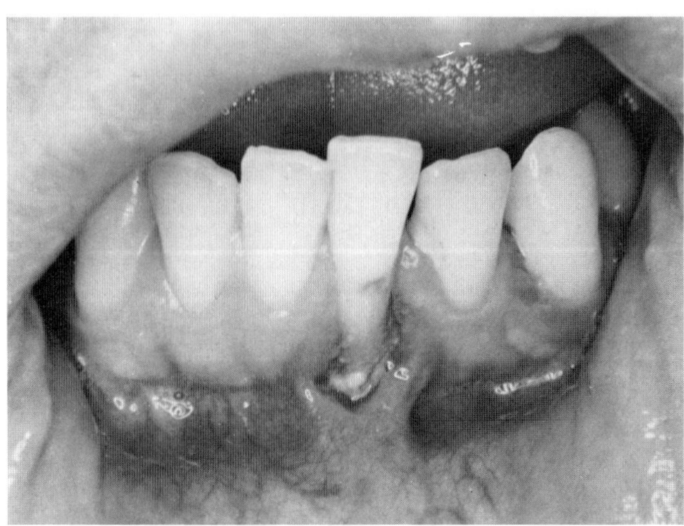

Fig. 6-10. Retraction of gingival margin due to frenum pull.

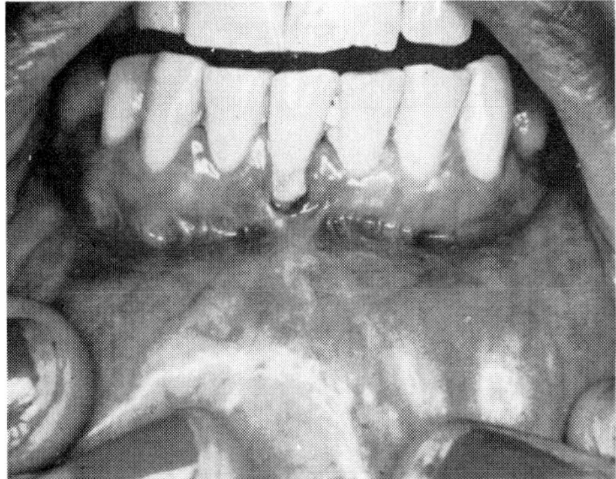
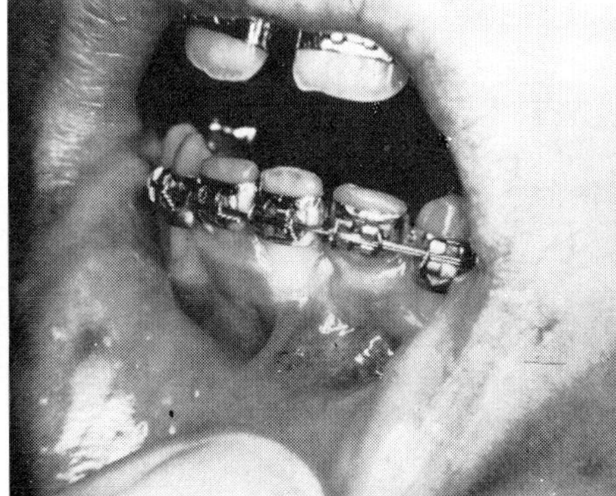

Fig. 6-11. Note the similar frenum insertions in mother (*left*) and teenage daughter (*right*).

shallow vestibule. The end result of such a situation may be the total lack of attached gingiva over the labial surface of the root. Similarly, frenums that insert near the margin of the gingiva but not at it, and that are associated with true periodontal pockets, may result in gingival recession. The reason for this is that tensional movements associated with movements of the mouth generally cause distension of the coronal portion of the pocket, with resulting inflammatory changes and deepening of the pocket. There are times when it is difficult to decide whether mucogingival surgery is or is not indicated. In such situations it is helpful to examine the patient's parents to determine whether the position of the anterior mandibular frenum follows a familial tendency (Fig. 6-11).

Treatment. Mucogingival surgery is indicated in such situations as those mentioned above. Excellent results can usually be obtained by a variety of surgical techniques (Fig. 6-12).[4, 10, 11, 17, 18] In cases in which root coverage is desired and a frenum problem exists, it is suggested that the frenum problem be resolved first. The plastic surgical procedure for root coverage can be done at a later date as a secondary surgical procedure if it is needed.

A high anterior labial frenum attachment and a small amount of attached gingiva is a common and normal finding in children. The presence of a high labial frenum attachment and a narrow band of attached gingiva per se is not an indication for surgical intervention. The mean width of the attached gingiva increases from the primary to the adult dentition.[2, 7] Therefore, it is generally more desirable to postpone surgery until the late teens or early twenties. In other words, full advantage should be taken of all growth and development in the area of the chin as well as the completion of all possible passive eruption and normal apical movement of the frenum. Even then, surgery should only be done when it has been proven beyond a reasonable doubt that the patient, despite all instruction, cannot maintain proper oral hygiene because of the anatomical configuration of the area. Many patients are capable of maintaining good oral hygiene even with a relatively high frenum attachment, shallow vestibule and minimum amounts of attached gingiva.

THE LINGUAL FRENUM

In newborns the lingual frenum extends all or most of the way to the tip of the tongue. Only as a result of postnatal apical growth of the tongue does the frenum recede, so that in the normal child by 2 to 5 years of age the tongue tip extends well beyond the frenum.[6] In circumstances of

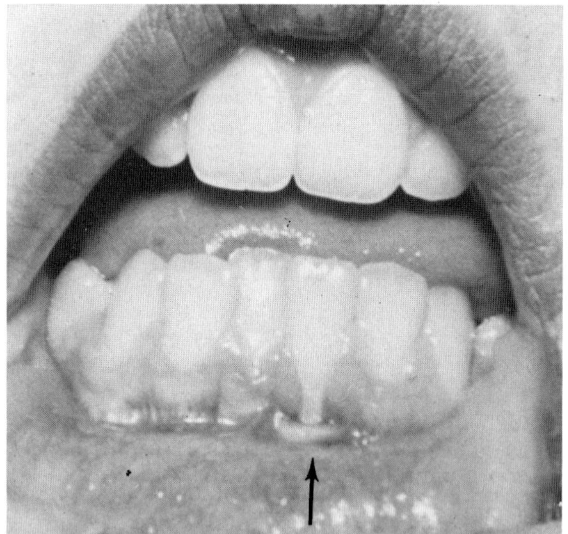

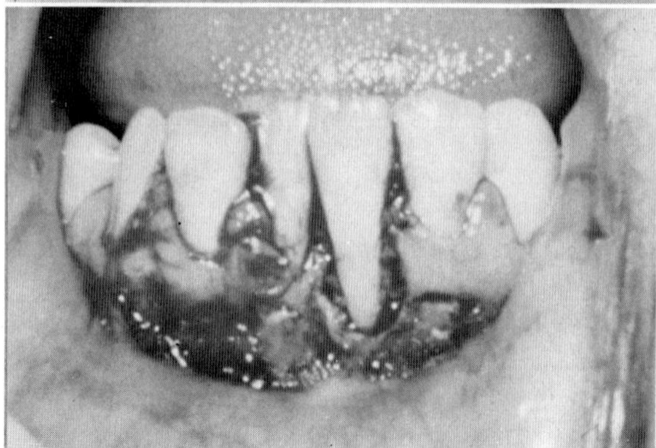

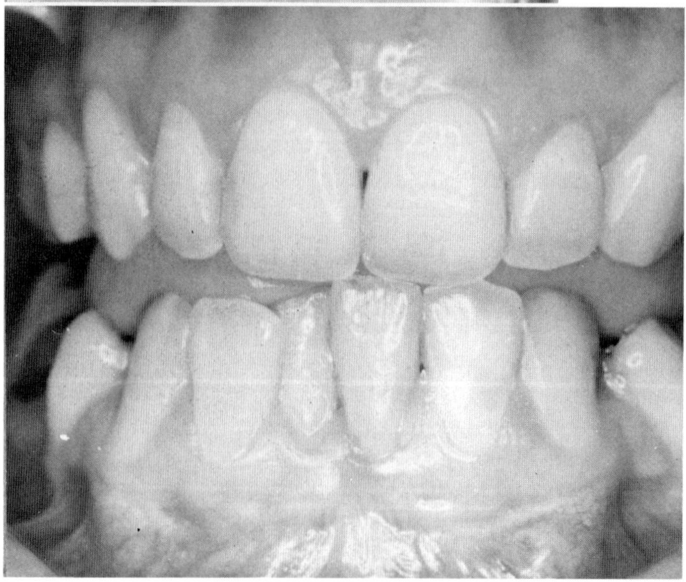

Fig. 6-12. *Top*. Frenum insertion and a shallow vestibule in a 16-year-old female. *Center*. Note the amount of alveolar destruction.
Bottom. The postoperative result 7 years later.

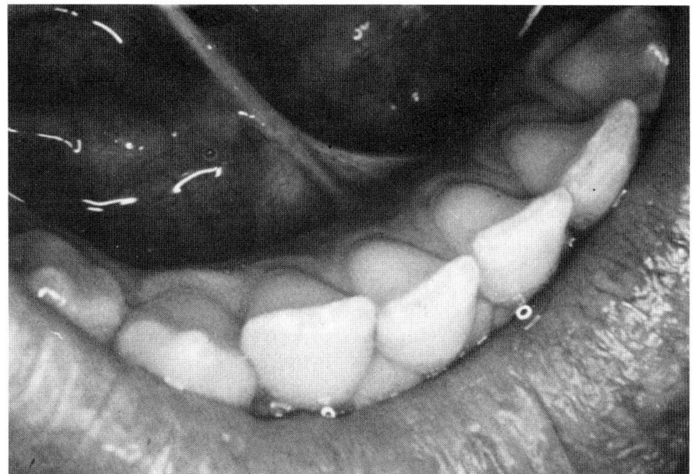

Fig. 6-13. Lingual frenum.

impaired development of the tongue, a short frenum (tonguetie) may occur.

In the infant, the normally mobile tongue is unconfined by teeth and extends outward between the maxillary and mandibular arches. When swallowing, the infant keeps his jaws parted and his tongue placed between the occlusal gum pads to produce a vacuum for sucking. With the eruption of teeth, the tongue is confined within the oral cavity. At approximately 2½ years of age, when all primary teeth have erupted and are in occlusion, the "infantile swallow" is replaced by the "adult swallow." In the adult swallow, the lips are closed, the teeth held in occlusion, and the tip of the tongue raised and pressed against the anterior portion of the palate, sealing the anterior portion of the mouth. At the same

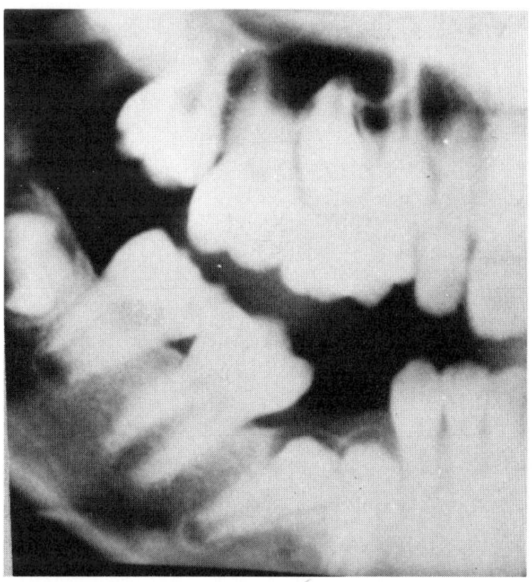

Fig. 6-14. A roentgenograph demonstrating impaction of the mandibular right bicuspids.

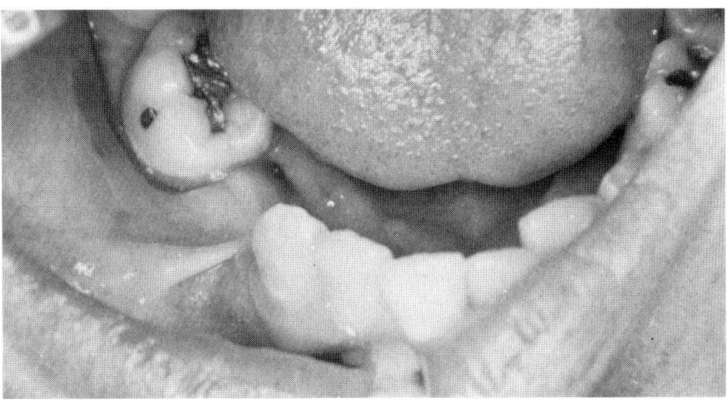

Fig. 6-15. A frenum in this patient inserting into the alveolar crest.

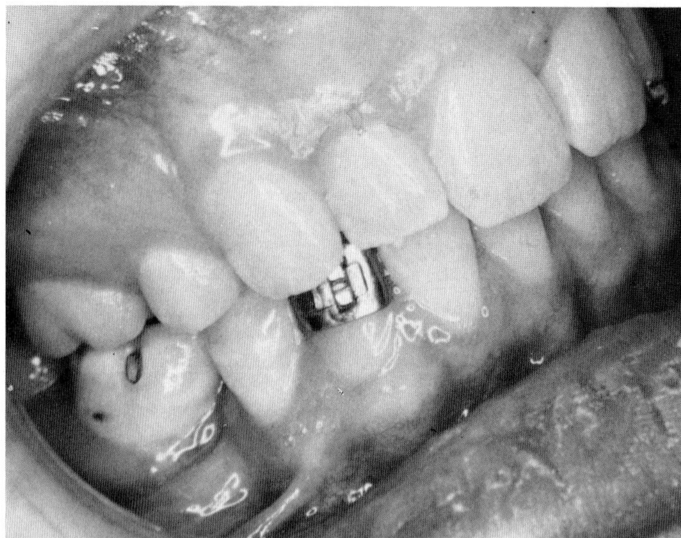

Fig. 6-16. The postoperative results following orthodontic treatment. (Compare with Fig. 6-15.)

time, the hyoid bone and larynx are elevated, while the nasal cavity and respiratory openings are sealed.[16]

There is little evidence, however, to substantiate a common belief that lisping or other speech defects result from tonguetie.[16] Clipping the lingual frenum at birth, a common practice in former years, is no longer favored, and in fact is definitely contraindicated, because it establishes a pathway for possible bacterial infection of the submaxillary glands.[20]

The lingual frenum may on occasion insert onto the attached gingiva of the lingual surface (Fig. 6-13), but it has almost never been reported to insert into the margin of the free gingiva. Therefore, it rarely is a problem in periodontics.

THE FRENUM IN OTHER LOCATIONS

On occasion, owing to noneruption of certain teeth, such as the mandibular bicuspids (Fig. 6-14), there is a lack of vertical growth of the mandible in that region. As a result, the frenum in such an area may insert directly onto the ridge of the edentulous area (Fig. 6-15). Following surgical exposure and orthodontic treatment to encourage eruption of these teeth, they may be brought into the proper plane of occlusion. Vertical growth of the alveolar process accompanies the eruption of these teeth and results in the more apical position of the frenum (Fig. 6-16).

REFERENCES

1. Adams, C. P.: The relation of spacing of the upper central incisor to abnormal frenum labia and other features of the dentofacial complex. Dent. Rec., *74*:72, 1954.
2. Ainamo, J., and Loe, H.: Anatomical characteristics of gingiva. A clinical and microscopic study of the free and attached gingiva. J. Periodont., *37*:5, 1966.
3. Allman, R. B., Jr.: A histologic investigation of the interincisal tissues at the maxillary midline. Thesis. University of Southern California, School of Dentistry. Los Angeles, June, 1966.
4. Ariaudo, A.: Problems in treating a denuded labial root surface of a lower incisor. J. Periodont., *37*:274, 1966.
5. Bedell, W. R.: Non-surgical reduction of the labial frenum with and without orthodontic treatment. J.A.D.A., *42*:510, 1951.
6. Bosma, J. F.: Personal communication.
7. Bowers, G. M.: A study of the width of attached gingiva. J. Periodont., *34*:201, 1963.

8. Ceremello, P. J.: The superior labial frenum and its orthodontic considerations. Am. J. Orthodont., *39:*120, 1953.

9. Clark, D.: Immediate closure of labial diastema by frenectomy and maxillary ostectomy. J. Oral Surg., *23:*273, 1968.

10. Cohen, D. W., and Ross, S. E.: The double papillae repositioned flap in periodontal therapy. J. Periodont., *39:*65, 1968.

11. Corn, H.: Technique for repositioning the frenum in periodontal problems. Dent. Clin. North Am., p. 79, 1964.

12. Curran, M.: Superior labial frenectomy. J.A.D.A., *41:*419, 1950.

13. Dewel, B.F.: The labial frenum, midline diastema, and palatine papilla: a clinical analysis. Dent. Clin. North Am., p. 175, 1966.

14. Dewel, B. F.: The normal and the abnormal labial frenum: clinical differentiation. J.A.D.A., *33:*318:1946.

15. Gibbs, S. L.: The superior labial frenum and its orthodontic considerations. N.Y. State Dent. J., *34:*550, 1968.

16. Horton, C. E., Crawford, H. H., Adamson, J. E., and Ashbell, T. S.: Tongue-tie. Cleft Palate J., *6:*8, 1969.

17. Nabers, J.: Extension of the vestibular fornix utilizing a gingival graft. Periodontics, *4:*77, 1966.

18. Nabers, J.: Free gingival grafts. Periodontics, *4:*243, 1966.

19. Noyes, H. J.: The anatomy of the frenum labii in new born infants. Angle Orthodont., *5:*3, 1935.

20. Parmelee, A. H., Sr.: The mouth of the newborn. Pediat. Clin. North Am., *3:*849, 1956.

21. Sicher, H.: Orban's Oral Histology and Embryology. ed. 6, p. 11. St. Louis, C. V. Mosby, 1966.

22. Sicher, H., and Tandler, J.: Anatomie fur Zahnarzte. Berlin, Julius Springer, 1928.

7
Gingival Atrophy

Gingival recessions may be caused by a number of factors, such as inflammatory periodontal disease, tooth position, a high frenum attachment, trauma from a habit, improper brushing, or factitial disease. In some instances, however, the cause of gingival recession or atrophy remains an enigma, particularly in those cases in which the crevicular depth is shallower and the plaque control better in the area of gingival recession than in other areas. That gingival recession is a common phenomenon, regardless of the cause, has been proved by many epidemiologic studies.

A high frenum attachment may also be responsible for gingival atrophy. Problems of this nature are discussed in more detail under problems associated with mandibular frenums (Chap. 6).

Epidemiological Studies

Ervin and Bucher studies. In a study of 1,252 patients, Ervin and Bucher[2] found that 80 percent had root exposure of 1 mm. or more. The incidence varied with age from 60 percent in the 20- to 29-year-olds to 95 percent for those over 50 years of age. The average number of teeth exposed per person increased from 4.8 percent in the 20- to 29-year age group to 10.2 percent in those over 50 years old. Trott and Love,[14] in a study limited to the labial surfaces of the mandibular incisor teeth, reported an incidence of 13.1 percent in a group of young people 14 to 19 years of age.

Malposed teeth. They also noted that recession was frequently associated with malposed teeth. However, it was difficult to ascertain from their report whether they had observed true recession, since they did not record the distance from the cemento-enamel junction to the margin of the gingiva. Instead they recorded any abnormal apical exposure of the buccal aspect of a mandibular incisor tooth which differed from the average height of the adjoining marginal gingiva. In other words, it is possible that in some instances they were not reporting true gingival recession. (This problem will be discussed in more detail under tooth position.)

Gorman study. Gorman,[5] in a study at the Ohio State University dental school clinics, reported on 4,453 teeth which he examined in 164 patients aged 16 to 86. Of these, he found that 22 percent, or 979 teeth, exhibited root exposure, while of the total number of people examined, 129 or 78 percent, showed tooth root exposure of 0.5 mm. or more. The gingival recessions varied from 54 percent in the 16- to 25-year age group to 100 percent in the 48- to 86-year age group. He also noted that pocket depths were shallower in patients with good plaque control than in those with fair or poor plaque control. His final conclusion was that, in general, as the periodontal pocket or crevicular depth decreased, the amount of gingival recession increased and that the decrease was greater in older persons.

O'Leary study. O'Leary *et al.,*[10] in a study on gingival recession in 529 males, ages 18 to 22 years, found that 27.7 percent had recession, occurring more frequently in the maxillary posterior segments than in

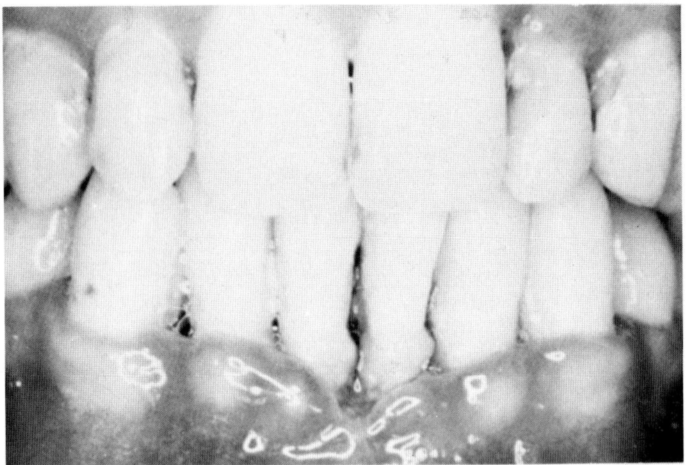

Fig. 7-1. Gingival recession about mandibular incisors as a result of repeated attacks of necrotizing ulcerative gingivitis.

the mandibular posterior segments. This was attributed to the fact that the buccal alveolar plate in the maxillary molar region is considerably thinner than in the corresponding mandibular segments. While the authors could neither prove nor disprove the hypothesis that gingival recession was the result of incorrect or too vigorous brushing, the result of their investigation did reveal that the individual with recession did have significantly lower mean gingival and mean plaque segment scores. This suggests that individuals with recession brush more thoroughly than individuals without recession. Unfortunately, it was not the purpose of their study to investigate or to try to correlate the type of brush used, the method of brushing, and/or the frequency of brushing with the presence or absence of gingival recession.

Increased time. In a further study[11] it was found that the incidence of recession increased with time. The existence of a relationship between the occurrence of recession coupled with a healthier gingival state and lower plaque scores, which was

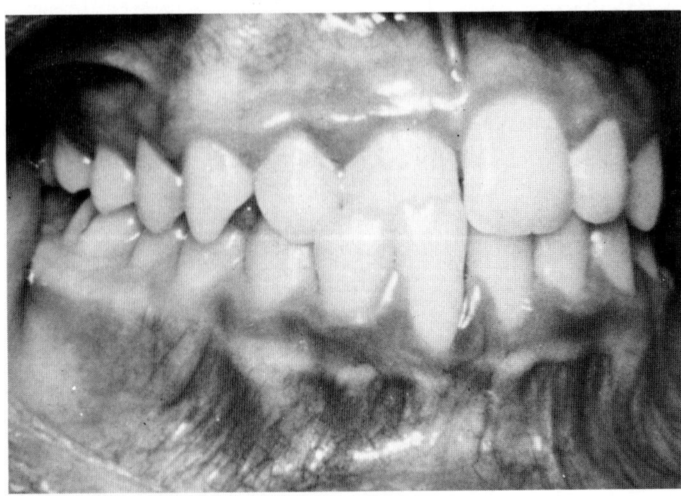

Fig. 7-2. Gingival recession on a labially placed tooth in mandibular arch. The maxillary central incisor in the lingual version has gingival margin high on its anatomical crown, resulting in a small clinical crown.

found in their earlier studies, was corroborated. Although there were no real or statistical differences between groups, it appeared that the percentage of men affected by recession, and the mean amount of recession per man and per tooth, increased with added care. The increase in recession was confined primarily to the facial surfaces of the maxillary posterior teeth. In particular, the maxillary first molars were the teeth most frequently affected. Considering the age of this group, the rate of increase in incidence was rather striking. In a 32-month period the incidence of recession increased from 29.4 percent (138 men) at the first examination to 41.3 percent (194 men) at the end of the 32 months. The maxillary molars continued to show the largest increase in recession. The data also confirmed earlier findings—that the mean gingival plaque scores for subjects with recession, in any area of the mouth, were significantly lower than the scores for subjects with no recession.

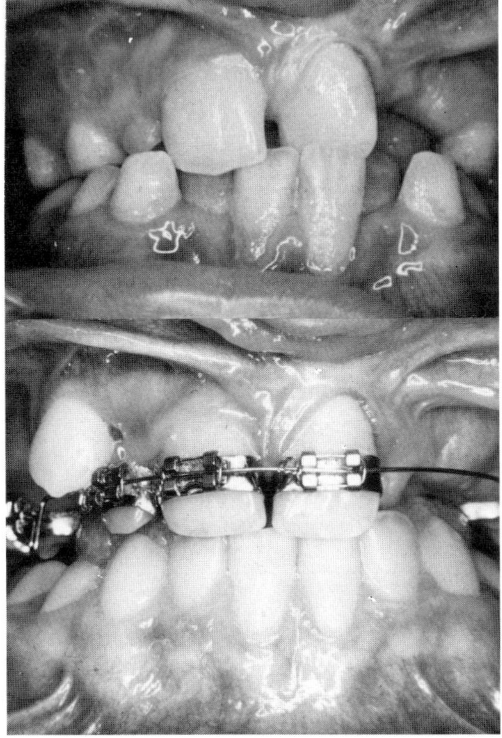

Fig. 7-3. *Top*. Note the labial version of the left mandibular central incisor and the position of the marginal gingiva. (Courtesy Dr. Peter J. Coccaro.)
Bottom. Gingival margins are now at the correct level following malalignment which was corrected orthodontically.

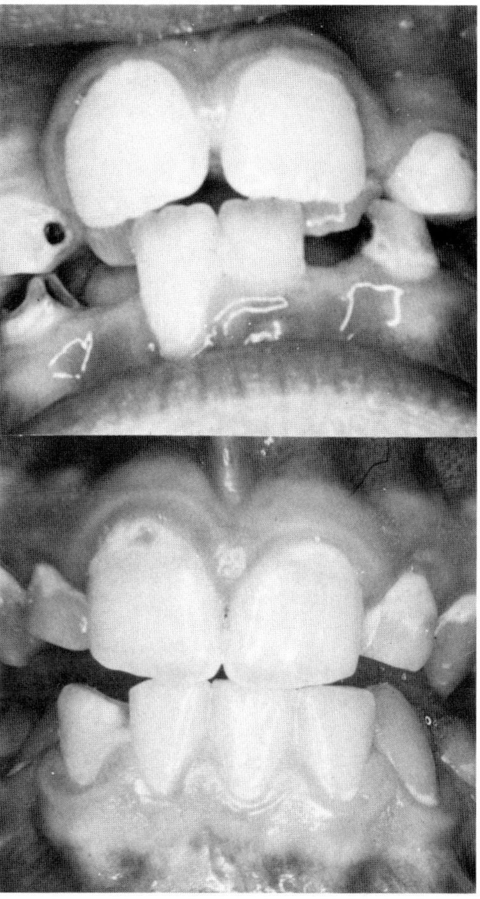

Fig. 7-4. *Top* Note the uneven gingival margin about mandibular incisors. (Courtesy Dr. Peter J. Coccaro.)
Bottom. The realignment of the mandibular incisor coupled with the completion of normal passive eruption has resulted in good physiologic gingival form.

INFLAMMATORY PERIODONTAL DISEASE

Inflammatory hyperplastic gingivitis with the formation of gingival or pseudopockets is the usual type of gingival reaction to local irritants during the adolescent period and is dealt with separately in Chapter 2. Gingival recessions are not the usual sequelae from such a process in this age group, with two exceptions. Repeated attacks of an acute necrotizing ulcerative gingivitis over a period of several years, which may result in considerable root exposure (Fig. 7-1) and an unusual form of periodontosis in which, in addition to a rapid generalized loss of alveolar bone, there occurs a concomitant rapid, generalized, circumferential gingival recession with extensive exposure of the roots of the teeth.

ROLE OF TOOTH POSITION

Gingival recession is frequently associated with labially placed teeth[6,9] for a number of reasons. A labially placed tooth is more susceptible to trauma from food and brushing and is more likely to have a very thin labial cortical plate, a fenestration and/or a dehiscence. Teeth in lingual version, on the other hand, tend to have thickened buccal cortical plates. As a result the gingival margin in the labial surface of such a tooth is placed high on its anatomic crown, resulting in a small clinical crown (Fig. 7-2).

There are other situations when, because of the position of the tooth in the arch, the level of the adjacent gingival margin varies in its height on adjacent teeth and creates the illusion that gingival recession has occurred. In such cases the cause is usually a reduction in arch length which causes a crowding of the mandibular incisors. The treatment of choice in these patients is serial extraction at the proper time and in the proper sequence, followed by orthodontic treatment to realign the incisor teeth.[1] The following case reports will illustrate this point.

CASE HISTORY 1

The mandibular left central incisor in this 10-year-old boy was in labial version (Fig. 7-3). The margin of the gingiva about this tooth was slightly above the cemento-enamel junction. However, because of the presence of both mandibular primary cuspids, the lingual position of the right mandibular lateral incisor and the position of the gingiva about the right central incisor, an illusion was created that gingival recession was present on the labial surface of the mandibular left central incisor. The tooth malalignment was corrected orthodontically. Figure 7-3 shows the patient 3 years later. A combination of tooth realignment, eruption of the permanent cuspids and continued growth and development in the area of the chin has resulted in a good physiologic contour to the marginal gingiva and increased vestibular depth and increased width of the gingiva. No surgery was required.

CASE HISTORY 2

This patient was approximately 11 years of age when first seen. Because of a delay in passive eruption, the position of the margin of the gingiva about the mandibular left central incisor (Fig. 7-4), gave the illusion that there was gingival recession about the labial surface of the mandibular right central incisor. In reality, a careful clinical examination revealed that the margin of the gingiva about this tooth was at its correct physiologic level. Orthodontic treatment was instituted. Figure 7-4 was taken 6 years later. Realignment of the mandibular incisor teeth, coupled with the completion of normal passive eruption, resulted in the establishment of good physiologic form to the gingival tissues. No periodontal surgery was required.

CASE HISTORY 3

This boy was first seen at 9 years of age. The mandibular right central incisor was in labial version (Fig. 7-5). Passive eruption had not yet been completed, and the primary cuspids were also still in position. Figure 7-5 was taken when the patient was 15 years of age. A combination of factors, such as orthodontic treatment, completion of passive eruption and the eruption of the permanent cuspids, lead to the establishment of good physiologic gingival form without surgery.

ROLE OF TOOTH ERUPTION

In some cases of tooth eruption the margin of the gingiva in one tooth may be near or at the cemento-enamel junction while the gingival margin on the adjacent tooth is still high up on the anatomical crown (Fig. 7-6). This situation may create the illusion that there is an existing gingival recession about the tooth where the gingival margin is at the lower level, when in reality the gingival margin may be at its correct physiologic level. With increase in the patient's age, further normal passive eruption of the gingiva occurs and the condition in such cases generally shows marked spontaneous improvement.

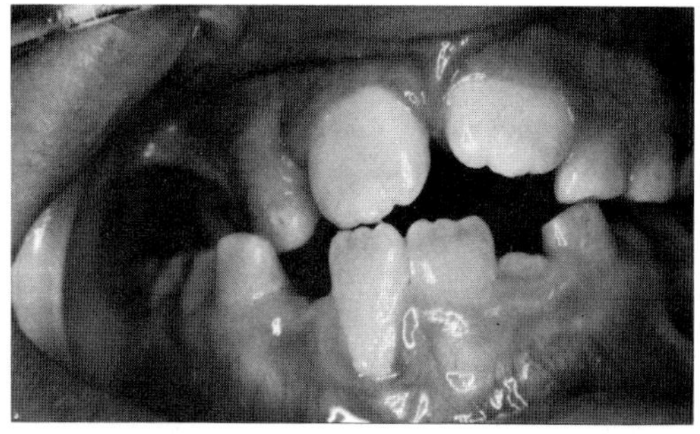

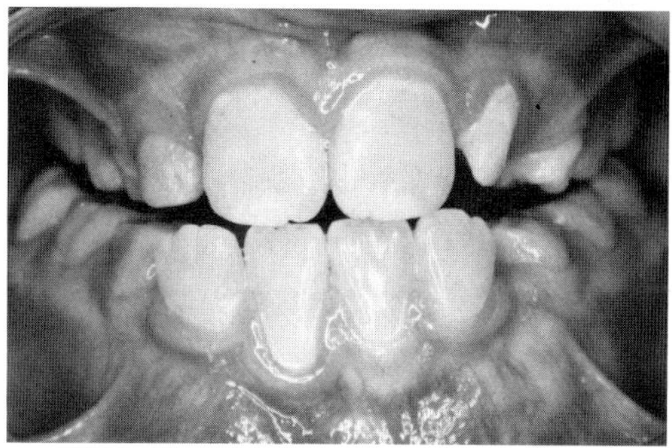

Fig. 7-6. *Top.* This illusion of gingival recession about the mandibular right central incisor is due to the high position of the gingival margin in the adjacent tooth.
Bottom. The gingival margin two years later.

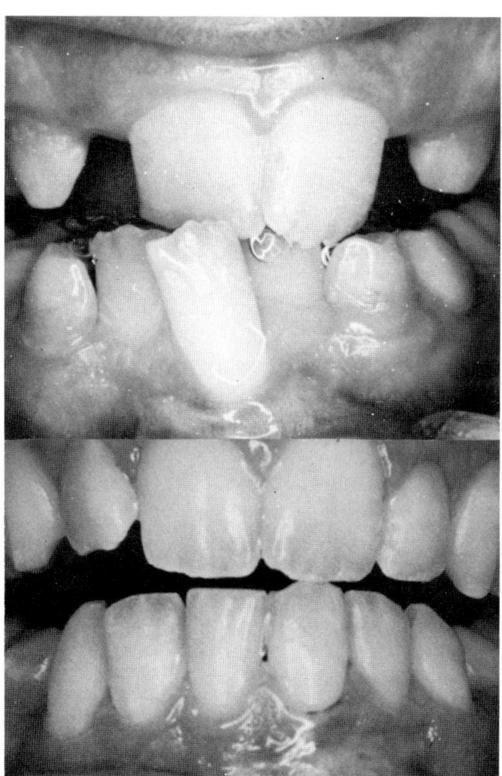

Fig. 7-5. *Top.* Note the gingival margin before orthodontic therapy.
Bottom. Establishment of good physiologic gingival form after completion of orthodontic therapy. (Courtesy Dr. Peter J. Coccaro.)

Factitial (Self-Induced) Gingival Disease

Bizarre-appearing gingival recessions which do not correspond to any known gingival disease, or oral manifestation of any known systemic disease are an entirely different problem (Fig. 7-7). These are usually self-induced lesions, or so-called factitial disease. Psychological factors play an important role in their etiology.[7] While it has long been known that patients with psychological problems may attempt to mutilate themselves, a description of gingival mutilation by children is not too well known. With one exception[7] most case reports have devoted no attention specifically to psychological factors, although a few reports do contain some hints that difficulties in family psychodynamics might underlie the problem.[3,4,8,12,13,15] The following report of a case illustrates this point.

CASE HISTORY

When Judy was referred for evaluation, she had been living with adoptive parents, Mr. and Mrs. C, for 6 months. Mr. and Mrs. B, her natural parents, were married when they were 22. Mr. B drank heavily before he was married, and this pattern had continued. Mrs. B, frequently overwhelmed and depressed by her unhappy life, felt that she had to mother her spendthrift, alcoholic husband. There were 5 children ranging in age from 3 years to 16 years of age.

Mrs. B was described as a very passive, ineffectual woman. She did not seek psychiatric treatment but leaned heavily on her family. Her marriage was stormy and chaotic for all of its 17 years.

One of the sources of the strife in the family was the continual financial difficulty that resulted from Mr. B's drinking. Mrs. B felt that her one anchor of security was their house, which was heavily mortgaged. In August, 1965, Mr. B decided that he must sell the house in order to make ends meet. His wife objected vigorously and a long fight ensued. Informants reported that she seemed quite depressed after she finally succumbed to his wishes. A few weeks later, Mrs. B hanged herself in the basement of their home. She was discovered by her children. It is unknown whether Judy, age 3 at the time, was present, but it is extremely likely.

Immediately following the suicide, Mr. B took two of his children to Florida. He left Judy and two other children with a friend, and then later sent for them. In Florida they were all living in one motel room. They lived a marginal existence. The children were malnourished and poorly cared for. Judy went to school, but only because a neighbor at the motel took some interest in her. Shortly after they arrived in Florida, Mr. B was admitted to a hospital because of a long-standing circulatory problem complicated by his alcoholism. He underwent a series of amputations and died a few months later without ever leaving the hospital. The children were literally abandoned in Florida. Mrs. C, Judy's paternal aunt, and other aunts and uncles as well, decided that steps had to be taken to rescue the children. The C's flew to Florida and managed to secure rapid court action so that they could assume legal responsibility for the children. They took Judy, and the other aunts and uncles each took custody of one of the other children.

When Judy came to live with Mr. and Mrs. C, she showed signs of malnutrition, had impetigo, and had a severe case of what was probably herpetic-gingivo-stomatitis. It was at this time that the family noted that Judy was excoriating her gums. She also showed other signs of being under tension. She was enuretic, had many nightmares, and was fearful of being left alone; she would not allow the family out of her sight and continually asked for reassurance that they would not abandon her. Her gingival problem was acute, and although she was treated adequately with antibiotics, the lesions did not abate. She was finally referred to us for diagnosis and treatment.

The C family was referred for psychiatric consultation. Mr. and Mrs. C showed considerable concern about Judy's gingival problems, and realized that she had been mutilating her gums by constantly "picking at them with her fingernail." When her gums finally started to heal, the C's felt much relieved. Mr. and Mrs. C appeared to be sensitive people, empathetic to Judy's problem and needs. They stated that they genuinely wanted her to live with them and that they took great pride in the strides she had made toward regaining her physical and psychological stability.

The C's had three children of their own, one of whom was married. They had been somewhat apprehensive when they first took Judy into their home but soon were pleased by the ease with which Judy became incorporated into their family. They legally adopted her and are called "Mommy" and "Daddy."

When Judy was brought into the consultation, she appeared lively and somewhat coquettish; she was friendly but appropriately apprehensive. Of note was her feigning helplessness in order to elicit a reaction from Mr. C. He appeared to perceive the gambit and responded appropriately. Following this, she dropped this form of interaction.

When Mrs. C was seen 6 months later in follow-up, she stated that Judy was continuing to do well. She reported that Judy had had a recent gum flareup after a fever and that she had picked her gums for a short time, but that she had recognized the fact that she was doing this and with encouragement from Mr. and Mrs. C had stopped.

Mr. and Mrs. C seemed to be able to set limits. They commented that they now found that spanking Judy was helpful, whereas at first they had been somewhat hesitant about spanking her because of their fear that she might perceive it as rejection. They felt that Judy was well on her way to making a successful recovery from her extreme traumatic deprivation. Mrs. C volunteered that she felt the mutilation had stopped because "Judy now feels she belongs somewhere."

The psychiatrist predicted that Judy would make a good adjustment. The patient was followed for 6 years and Judy has become a well-adjusted girl. The gingival mutilation has stopped and the gingiva is presently within normal limits (Fig. 7-8; compare with Fig. 7-7, top.)

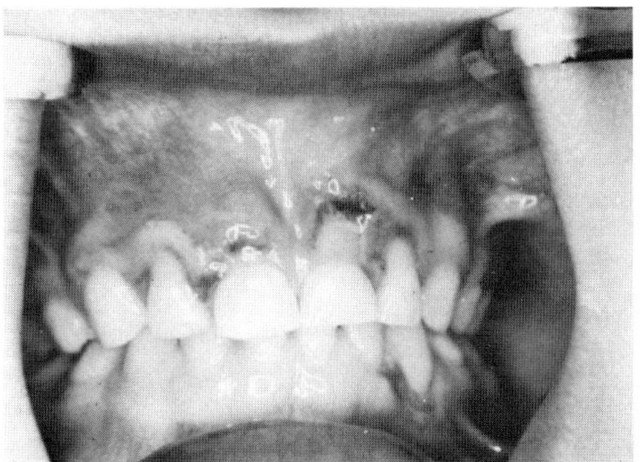

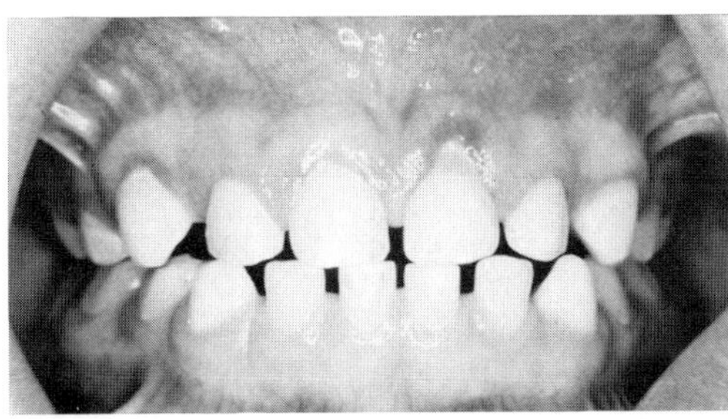

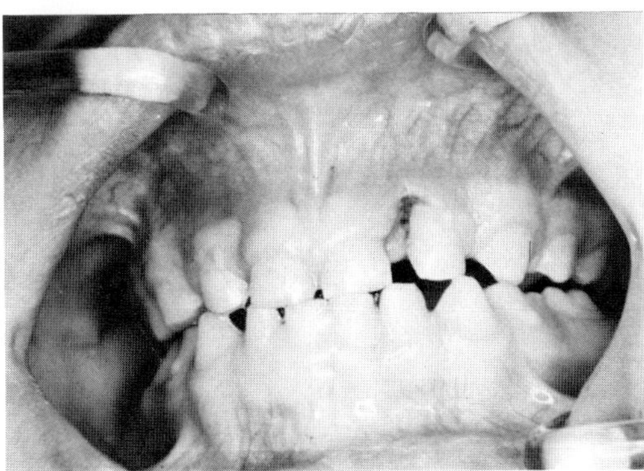

Fig. 7-7. These bizarre appearing gingival recessions were caused by self-induced gingival mutilation. These children were all approximately 3 years of age.

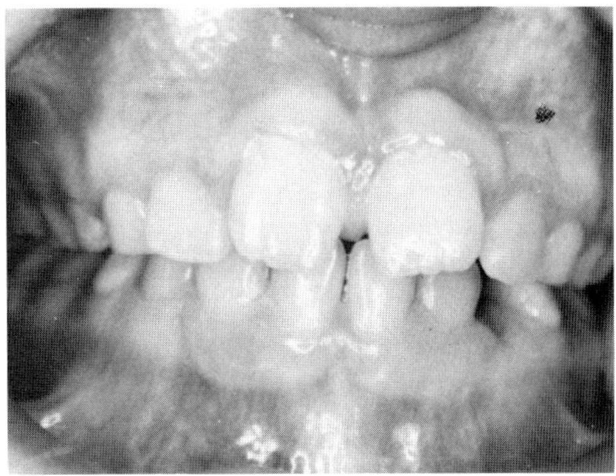

Fig. 7-8. The child shown in Figure 7-7 *Top* at 9 years of age (i.e., 6 years later).

COMMENT

In reviewing this and several other cases of gingival mutilations, several factors stand out as being consistently present: (1) Prior to the onset of the oral problem, the affected child was experiencing a sense of deprivation. (2) In all instances a documented organic lesion had occurred during the time the child was experiencing stress associated with the frustration of his dependency needs. (3) A marked shift in the family dynamics occurred as a result of the oral pathology. Much anxiety was generated and the affected child became the center of his environment. It seems reasonable to hypothesize from this that at a time of extreme stress, if a child has an organic oral pathologic condition which significantly alters his environment, this may meet his dependency needs albeit in a regressive way. Reacting to the new behavior constellation, the child may continue to aggravate his oral lesions by excoriating and denuding his gingiva. In this manner, the gingival mutilation becomes a way of handling the anxiety generated by experiencing unmet dependency needs.

REFERENCES

1. Dewel, B.F.: Serial extraction in orthodontics: indications, objectives, and treatment procedures. Amer. J. Orthodont., *40*: 906, 1954.
2. Ervin, J. C., and Bucher, E. M.: Prevalence of tooth-root exposure and abrasion among dental patients. Dental Items of Interest, *66*:760, 1944.
3. Golden, S., and Chosock, A.: Oral manifestations of a psychological problem. J. Periodont., *35*:349, 1964.
4. Goldstein, I. C., and Dragan, A. I.: Self-inflicted oral mutilation in a psychotic adolescent. Report of a case. J.A.D.A., *74*:750, 1967.
5. Gorman, W. J.: Prevalence and etiology of gingival recession. J. Periodont., *38*: 316, 1967.
6. Hirschfeld, I.: A study of skulls in the American Museum of Natural History in relation to periodontal disease. J. Dent. Res., *5*:241, 1923.
7. Hoffman, H. A., and Baer, P. N.: Gingival mutilation in children. Psychiatry, *31*: 380, 1968.
8. Lewis, T. M.: Gingival traumatization—a habit. J. Periodont., *33*:353, 1962.
9. Morris, M. L.: Position of the margin of the gingiva. Oral Surg., *11*:969, 1958.
10. O'Leary, T. J., Drake, R. B., Jividen, G. J., and Allen, M. F.: The incidence of recession in young males: relationship of gingival and plaque scores. Periodontics, *6*:109, 1968.
11. O'Leary, T. J., Drake, R. B., Crump, P. P., and Allen, M. F.: The incidence of recession in young males. A further study. J. Periodont., *42*:264, 1971.
12. Schoenwetter, R. F.: Localized juvenile periodontosis. J. Dent. Child., *34*:301, 1967.
13. Stewart, D. J.: Traumatic gingival recession. Dent. Pract. Dent. Rec., *16*:64, 1965.
14. Trott, J. R., and Love, B.: An analysis of localized gingival recession in 766 Winnipeg High School students. Dent. Pract. Dent. Rec., *16*:209, 1966.
15. Woofter, C.: The prevalence and etiology of gingival recession. Periodontal Abstracts, *17*:45, 1969.

8
Orthodontic Considerations

CROWDING OF THE MANDIBULAR INCISOR TEETH

Crowding of the mandibular incisors is an extremely common finding and is not necessarily abnormal; on the contrary, a moderate degree of crowding of the mandibular incisors may even be characteristic of the human dentition.[9] In a series of 1,000 London school children it was found that by 14 years of age 62 percent had some crowding.[8] It is interesting to note that the crowding in 60 percent of the children increased between 11 and 14 years of age.

Etiology. Because crowding is often first noticed in the late teens—about the same time as the eruption of the third molars—a cause-and-effect relationship has been suggested between these two. However, the onset of crowding occurs *before* the eruption of the third molars—actually at about the time that the second molars start erupting. Present evidence suggests that crowding is probably associated with tooth size rather than with tooth eruption.[3,13,19] In fact, several studies show the lack of relationship between crowding and eruption of the third molars.[13,19] It has been found for instance that where mandibular second molars have been extracted and the third molars have erupted into good position, either with or without orthodontic help, there has been minimal effect on lower arch crowding.[8] Many investigators have also reported that crowding of the incisors has occurred where the third molars were congenitally missing,[6,19,26] or where the mandibular third molars had been removed prior to completion of orthodontic treatment.[26] In one longitudinal study of 29 adolescents (from a mean age of 15 years and 6 months to a mean age of 19 years and 5 months), some of whom had and some of whom did not have third molars, it was found that the third molars did not contribute to any irregularity in malalignment that might develop in the remainder of the arch.[28]

RELAPSE FOLLOWING ORTHODONTIC TOOTH ROTATION

Relapse following rotational movement of a tooth is a common problem in orthodontics. There appears to be little correlation between the extent of relapse and the extent to which a tooth has been orthodontically rotated.[10] The duration of retention also appears to have little effect in preventing a rotated tooth from relapsing into its former position.

Etiology. Orthodontic treatment which expands the arch into a position in which it is in an unstable relationship to the surrounding musculature may cause relapse. Another contributing factor is the strong tendency of the mandibular incisors to evidence lingual uprighting with age. Such a change in axial inclination may precipitate crowding.

During the first 1 or 2 months following termination of active therapy, the relapse may be caused by tension on the stretched principal fibers of the periodontal ligament. This phase terminates in approximately 8 weeks, at which time remodeling of the alveolar bone provides new attachment for the principal fibers.[4] After this has taken place, relapse is thought to be caused by tension in the transseptal fibers. These

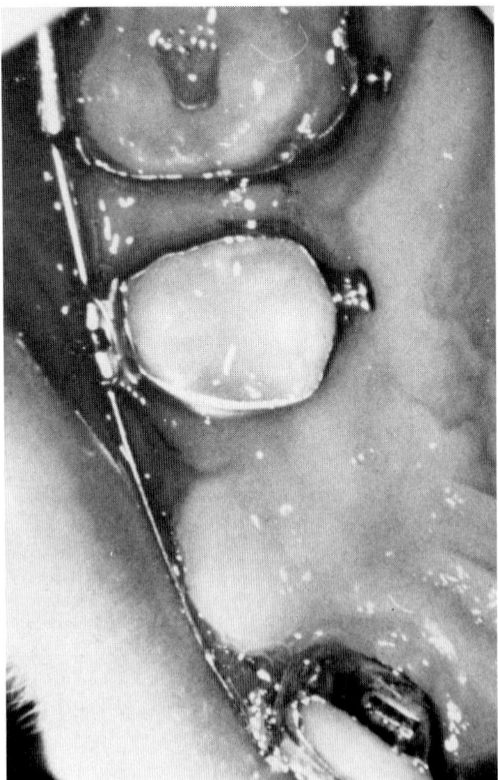

Fig. 8-1. A tooth following orthodontic rotation.

latter fibers are attached at both ends to cementum. Cementum does not remodel, so the transseptal fibers cannot readily

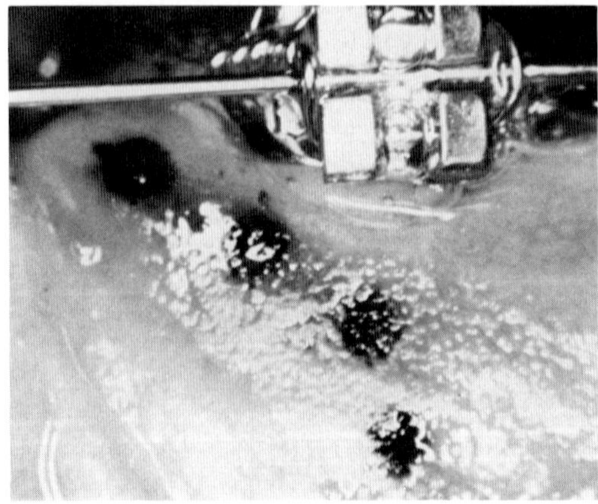

Fig. 8-2. A deviated tattoo line on the gingiva following rotation of the tooth.

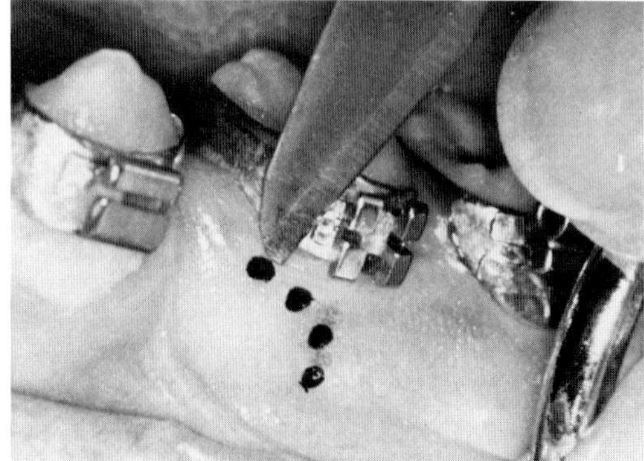

Fig. 8-3. A No. 11 Bard-Parker blade entering the gingival sulcus to sever the supracrestal fibrous attachment around the circumference of the tooth.

reorganize and find a new attachment. Therefore, even following prolonged retention, they remain compressed like a coiled spring ready to unwind and return the tooth to its original position.[5,24,27]

Overcoming Relapse. To overcome relapse, several procedures have been advocated.

1. *Prolonged retention.* As mentioned earlier, this method is ineffectual because the transseptal fibers do not reorganize following rotation.

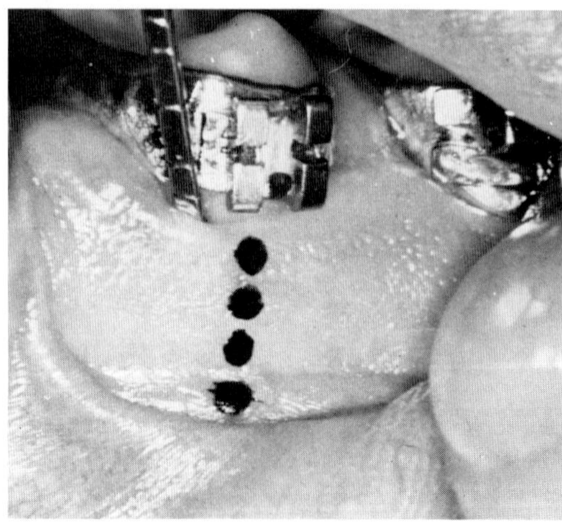

Fig. 8-4. A periodontal probe showing the normal sulcular depth one week after surgical procedure. Note that the tattoo mark has reverted to its original vertical alignment.

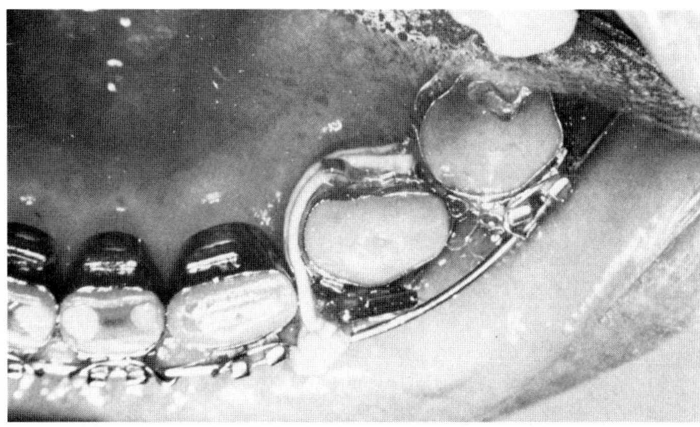

Fig. 8-5. A malaligned canine tooth under rotational force.

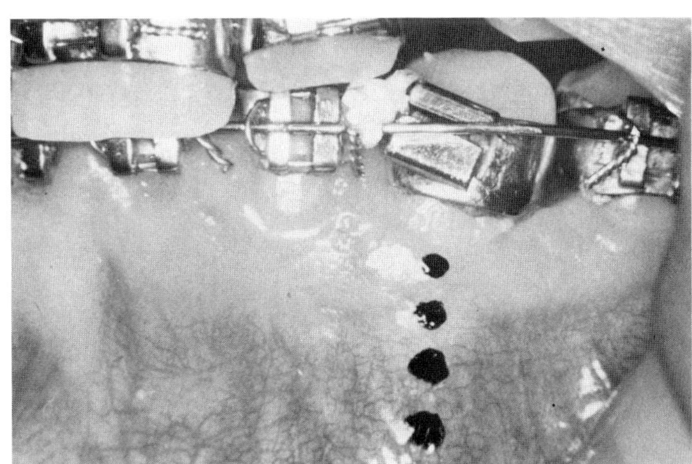

Fig. 8-6. A vertical tattoo line on the gingiva before rotational correction.

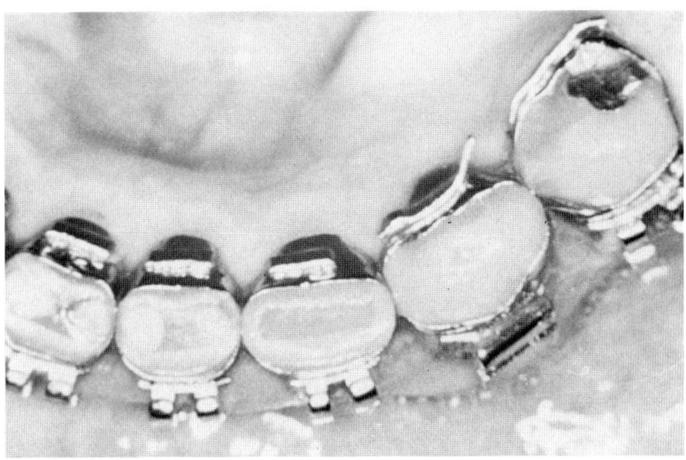

Fig. 8-7. The incisal view of a canine tooth after rotational correction.

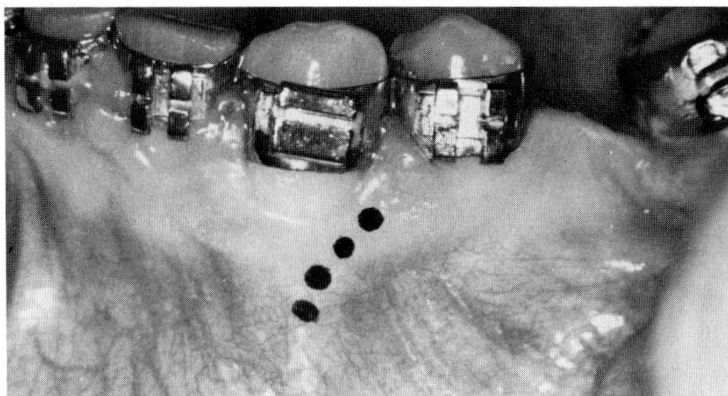

Fig. 8-8. The deviated tattoo markings in the direction of the tooth rotation. Note the accumulation of gingival tissue distal to the rotated tooth.

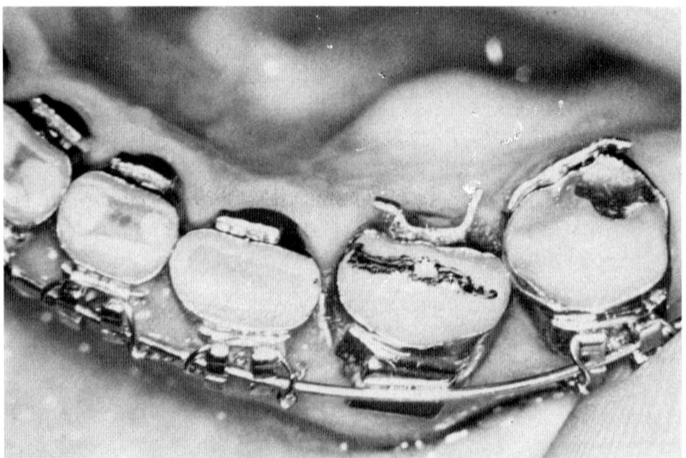

Fig. 8-9. The canine tooth has relapsed approximately 20° in two months following full rotational correction.

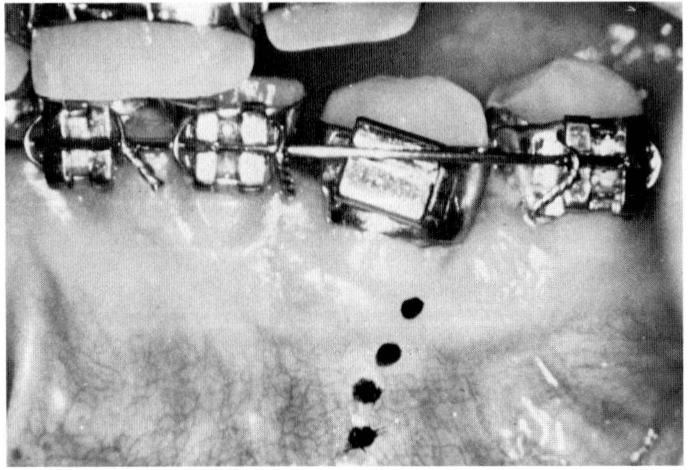

Fig. 8-10. The tattoo marking has also "relapsed" toward the vertical arrangement as the tooth relapsed. (Courtesy of Dr. John G. Edwards.)[10]

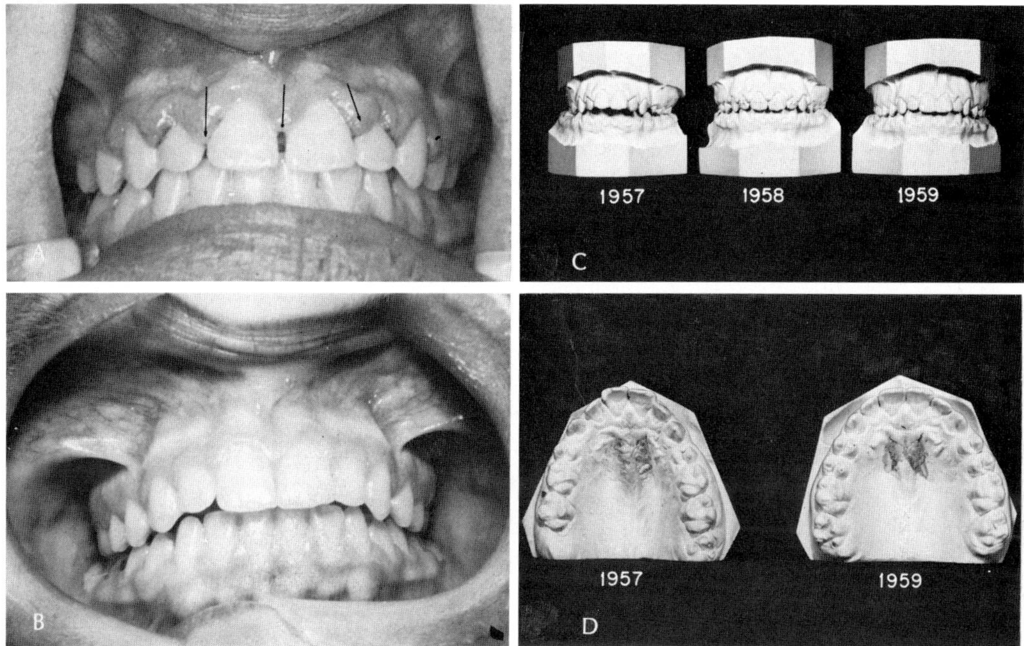

Fig. 8-11. Case 1. *A*. Note the enlarged gingival papillae (*arrows*). This photograph was taken immediately after removal of orthodontic bands.
B. Good oral hygiene was the only therapy used. Gingival architecture returned to normal in less than one year.
C. Study casts taken before, during and after completion of orthodontic therapy.
D. Note the change in the maxillary arch form following orthodontic therapy. (From Baer, and Coccaro.)[1]

2. *Over-rotation*. This method is not predictable because the extent to which an over-rotated tooth will relapse cannot be predetermined. There is no guarantee that it will relapse just the desired amount into good alignment.

3. *Rotation of teeth at an early age*. As noted earlier, relapse is not due to the principal fibers of the periodontal ligament, which reorganize as the alveolar bone remodels, but to the transseptal fibers, which do not. This method is therefore invalid.

Treatment of Relapses. Boese[4] has advocated gingivectomy to remove the transseptal fibers followed by a minimum of 8 weeks' of retention. It was found that such treatment reduces relapse by nine tenths. However, if retention is maintained for only 4 weeks following gingivectomy the principal fibers of the periodontal ligament do not have sufficient time to complete their adjustment. Under these circumstances the principal fibers are still under sufficient tension to produce relapse and nullify the effectiveness of gingivectomy. Extending the retention period to 8 weeks, however, allows the principal fibers to complete their adjustment and thereby eliminates the possibility of relapse.

Edwards,[11] in an interesting experiment using a tattooing technique, was able to demonstrate that the attached gingiva—especially the marginal gingiva—is pulled along with the tooth as it is rotated. In every instance it was observed that the amount and direction of deviation between the original vertical line of the tattoo marks coincided with the amount and direction of rotational movement of the tooth (Figs. 8-1 through 8-10). In addition, in cases of extensive rotational movements, the gingival tissue would accumulate in a "piled-up" fashion in the interdental area toward which the tooth was rotating.

Using a new surgical technique (described below), Edwards was able to show that within 20 to 40 hours the tattoo marks could be caused to realign in their original vertical position parallel to the long axis of the tooth. Following completion of the rotational movements, and before surgery, the involved tooth or teeth must be kept in mechanical retention for a period of at least 8 weeks to permit the principal fibers to readjust to their new environment. In this way the problem of relapse is minimized.

The surgical technique used is as follows:[11] The point of a No. 11 Bard-Parker blade is inserted into the depth of the gingival sulcus and moved so as to sever all fibrous attachments surrounding the tooth to a depth of approximately 3 mm. below the crest of the alveolar bone. A periodontal dressing is then placed over this area for 5 to 8 days.

During the 3 month postoperative observation when this technique was originally performed—a period in which no mechanical retention device was employed following the surgical procedure—negligible rotational relapse occurred.

THE LOOSE CONTACT IN BISCUPID EXTRACTION CASES

It has been observed[12] that in many orthodontic cases in which removal of the first bicuspids is followed by retraction of the anterior segment of the arch (so as to bring the cuspid into approximation with the second bicuspid), the contact between these teeth lacks the lively resilience to the passage of dental floss found with teeth in normal approximation.

Etiology. The cause of this type of contact is believed to be that following extraction of the first bicuspids the transseptal fibers reform to extend from the cementum on the distal of the cuspid across the extraction site to insert into the cementum on the mesial aspect of the second bicuspid. When teeth opposite such an edentulous space are brought into approximation, the elongated transseptal fibers relax, coil and become compressed. The tension resulting from the compression of these fibers explains the tendency for such contacts to reopen.

Treatment. After the teeth have been in retention for a period of 8 weeks or more, a gingivectomy on both the labial and lingual surfaces should be performed in the area of the cuspid-bicuspid to remove the old transseptal fibers.

GINGIVAL ENLARGEMENT COINCIDENT WITH ORTHODONTIC THERAPY

A gingival enlargement, particularly of the papillary area, can occur around teeth banded orthodontically. While not all patients have a gingival tissue reaction to orthodontic bands, many do have a high degree of tissue response—often severe enough to cause the gingival tissue to literally "grow" over the bands.

Etiology. The etiology of the gingival enlargement is probably multifactorial. The orthodontic bands may encroach upon the gingival papilla and act as a local irritant. The orthodontic appliance may act as an obstacle to plaque control. In such cases the accumulation of the bacterial plaque is responsible for the inflammatory gingival hyperplasia. Last, some of this enlargement is undoubtedly the result of an interproximal space that is now too small for the gingival papilla to fit into. In other words, as a result of the orthodontic therapy the diastemas originally present between the teeth were eliminated. The result is a "piling up" of the interproximal gingival tissue.

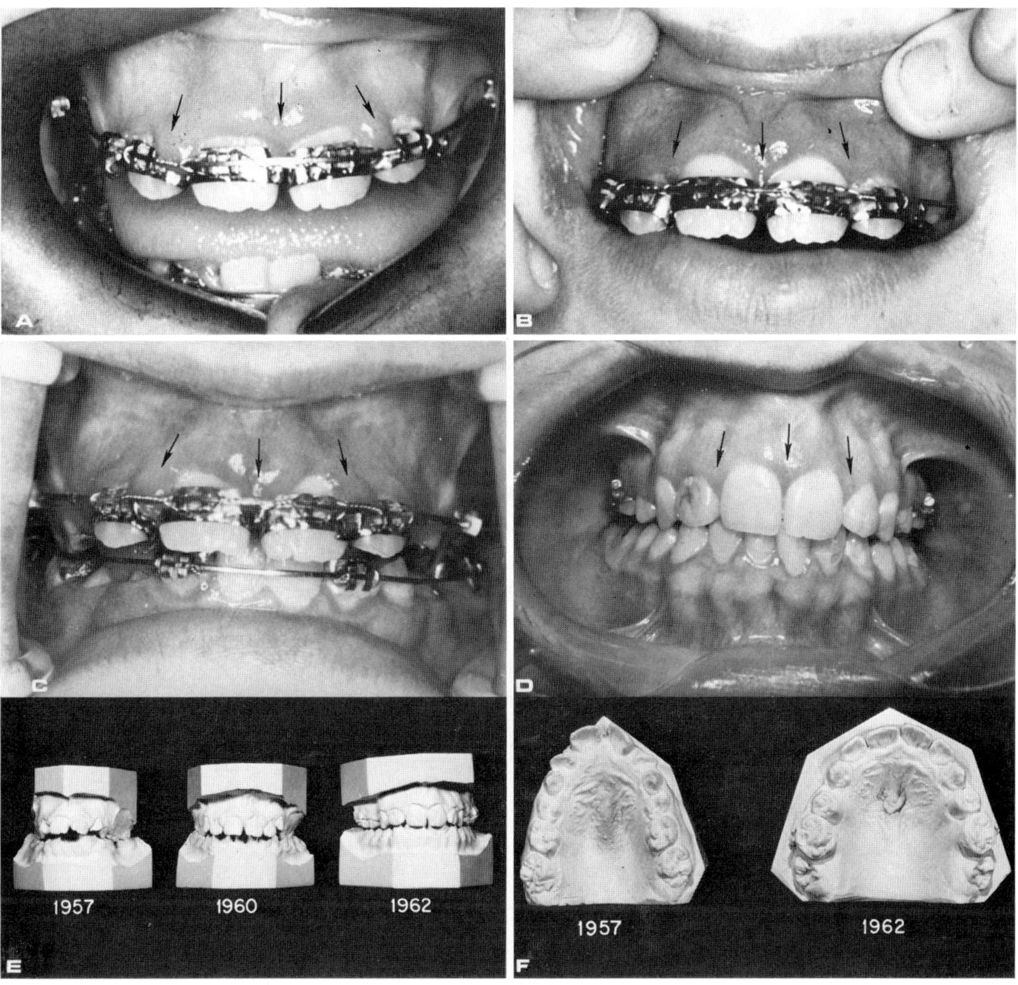

Fig. 8-12. Case 2. *A*. Enlarged gingival papillae (*arrows*).
B. Gingival papillae (*arrows*) are normal in contour after a gingivectomy.
C. Recurrence of enlarged papillae (*arrows*) within eight months.
D. Normal gingival architecture returned in less than a year following removal of the orthodontic bands. Good oral hygiene was the only periodontal therapy used.
E. Casts of the above case.
F. Note the increased maxillary width which resulted from the orthodontic treatment. (From Baer, and Coccaro.)[1]

Treatment. For those adolescents who develop marked gingival enlargement during orthodontic treatment, plaque control must be immediately instituted. Surgical removal of the enlarged gingival tissue is deferred until several months following termination of all orthodontic treatment.[1] In most instances it will then be found that surgical intervention is either unnecessary or consists at most of gingivoplasty. The results that can be obtained with good plaque control alone are usually quite gratifying. The following cases illustrate this point.

CASE HISTORY 1

An 11-year-old girl presented with a Class II division 1 malocclusion and maxillary incisor

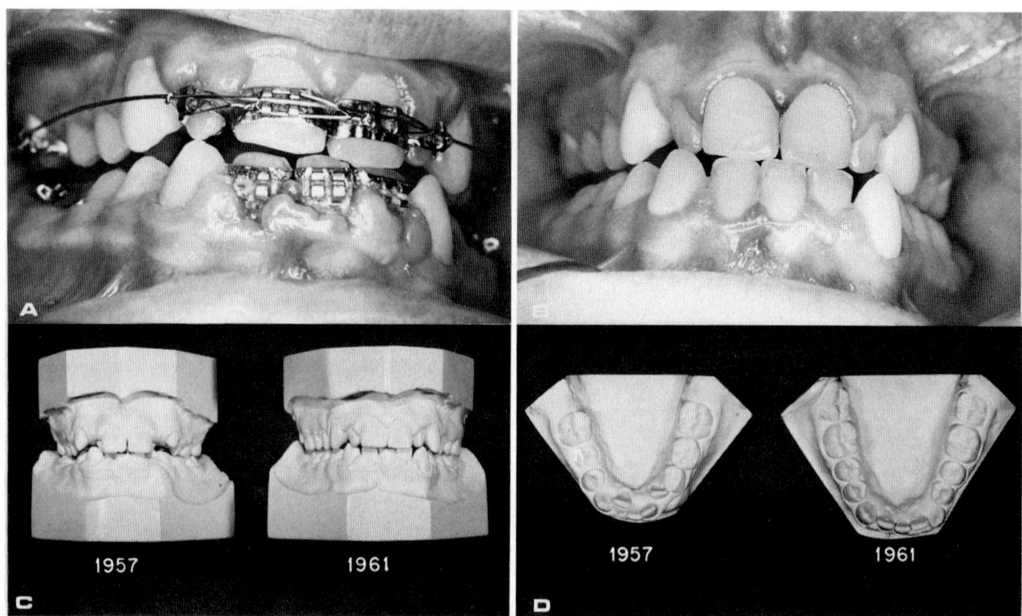

Fig. 8-13. Case 3. *A*. Note the anterior gingival enlargement.
B. Gingival improvement occurred within four months following removal of orthodontic appliances. No periodontal therapy other than oral hygiene was done.
C and *D*. These casts were taken before and after orthodontic treatment. (From Baer, and Coccaro.)[1]

protrusion. The mandibular arch was satisfactory. The right first molars were in a cross-bite relation. The gingivae were normal in appearance.

Upon completion of orthodontic treatment, and immediately after removal of her orthodontic bands, there was a moderate, generalized, gingival hyperplasia in the maxillary arch (Fig. 8-11A). The patient was instructed in proper oral hygiene but no other periodontal therapy was performed. The gingiva returned to normal in less than one year (Fig. 8-11B).

CASE HISTORY 2

An 8-year-old girl presented with a Class II division 1 malocclusion in the mixed dentition and an extreme protrusion of the maxillary incisors. During the course of treatment a marked gingival hyperplasia of the maxillary anterior (papillary) areas occurred, encroaching upon the orthodontic appliance (Fig. 8-12A). Gingivectomy was performed, restoring the gingival form to normal, (Fig. 8-12B). Within 8 months, however, the interproximal gingival tissue had returned to its previous size (Fig. 8-12C). At this time it was decided to continue orthodontic treatment without periodontal surgery. Good oral hygiene was stressed to the patient, but without apparent benefit. Upon completion of the orthodontic treatment the importance of proper oral hygiene was once again stressed. No other periodontal therapy was done. Gingival form returned to normal in less than one year (Fig. 8-12D).

CASE HISTORY 3

This 12-year-old boy had an excessive overjet and overbite, and a Class II relationship in the molar region. Before therapy was started the mandibular left central incisor was extracted, as were the remaining primary molars. During orthodontic treatment gingival hyperplasia occurred in the anterior region of both arches. It was more severe, however, in the mandibular arch (Fig. 8-13A). Within 4 months following removal of the appliances, with no periodontal therapy other than proper oral hygiene, there was marked improvement in gingival form (Fig. 8-13B).

RELATIONSHIP OF MALOCCLUSION TO CHRONIC DESTRUCTIVE PERIODONTAL DISEASE

There appears to be no statistically significant difference between the general severity of periodontal disease and various tooth and occlusal irregularities such as open-bite, crossbite, variation of the occlusal plane, anterior overlap, anterior overjet, crowding of one or more teeth, or the angle of the lower incisors. [2, 14, 15, 29] However, in patients who have periodontal disease and who also have teeth in crossbite, there is increased severity of the disease localized around the teeth that are in a crossbite relationship.

OTHER PERIODONTAL PROBLEMS CONCOMITANT WITH ORTHODONTIC THERAPY

Root Resorption

Histologically, cemental resorptions are extremely common, occurring in over 90 percent of teeth.[16] This problem, however, must not be confused with the gross root resorption that may be observed roentgenographically following orthodontic treatment (Fig. 8-14). It has been found[20] that the frequency of moderate resorption (2 to 4 mm. of the apex resolved) increased from 9.2 percent in untreated controls to 31.4 percent in a group treated orthodontically. Severe resorption (4 mm. to half the root length) increased from 0.3 percent in the untreated group to 10.8 percent after orthodontic treatment, and very severe resorption (more than half the root resolved) rose from 0.11 percent to 3.4 percent.

Severe root resorption may occasionally occur even when mechanical movement is accomplished by the most competent of orthodontists. Some patients who are otherwise completely healthy evidently possess an inherent proclivity for root resorption. There seems to be no correlation between the amount of apical root loss and the length of treatment, sex, age of the patient or the amount of movement of the tooth through bone.[22]

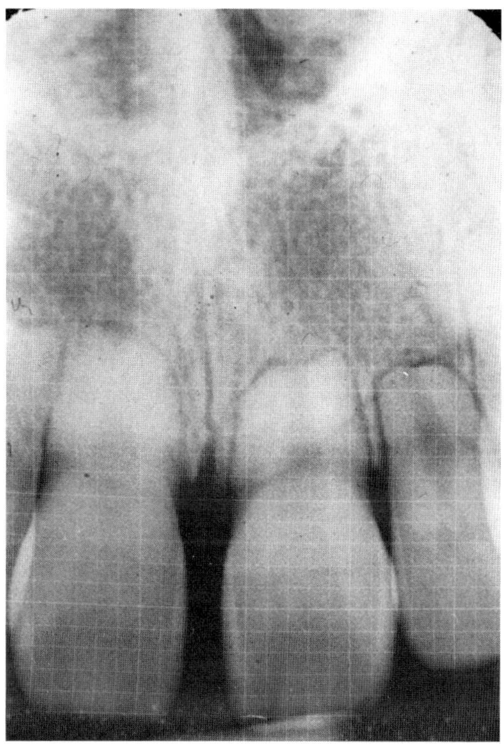

Fig. 8-14. Extreme root resorption followed orthodontic treatment.

It is felt by some that root resorption is directly related to the amount of interrupted movement experienced by a tooth.[18] If this is true the problem can be minimized clinically by using light continuous forces to move teeth directly into new positions and by avoiding interrupted movement.

Destructive Periodontal Disease

While admittedly it is impossible to indict orthodontic treatment as a primary etiologic factor in initiating destructive periodontal disease,[25] there is sufficient circumstantial evidence to incriminate it in certain cases. The following examples illustrate this point.

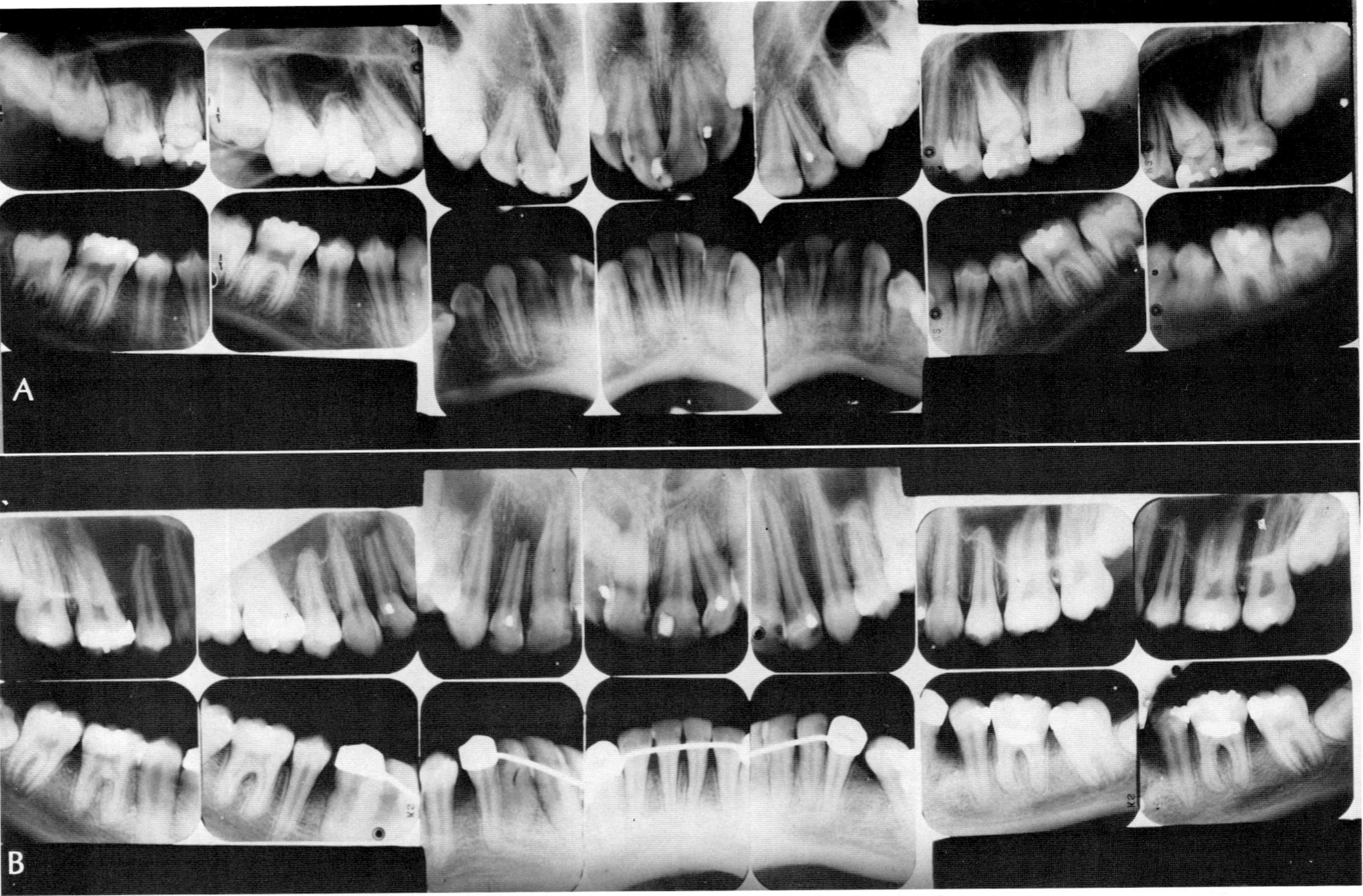

Fig. 8-15. *A*. Roentgenographs were taken before orthodontic treatment. *B*. Upon completion of the treatment, note there is alveolar bone loss and apical root resorption about the maxillary lateral incisor. *C*. The disease had further progressed one year later. *D*. The response following periodontal and endodontic therapy.

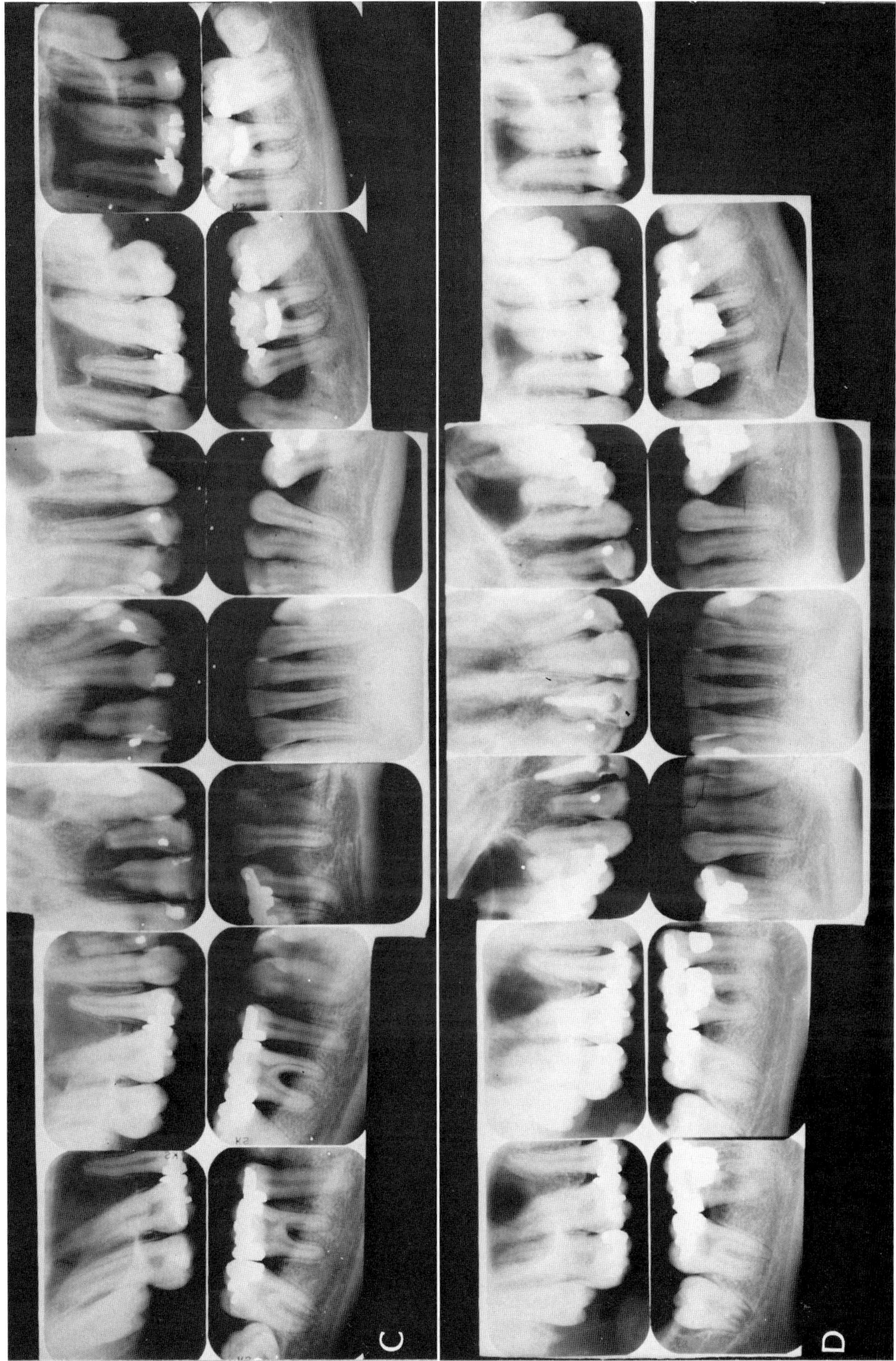
C
D

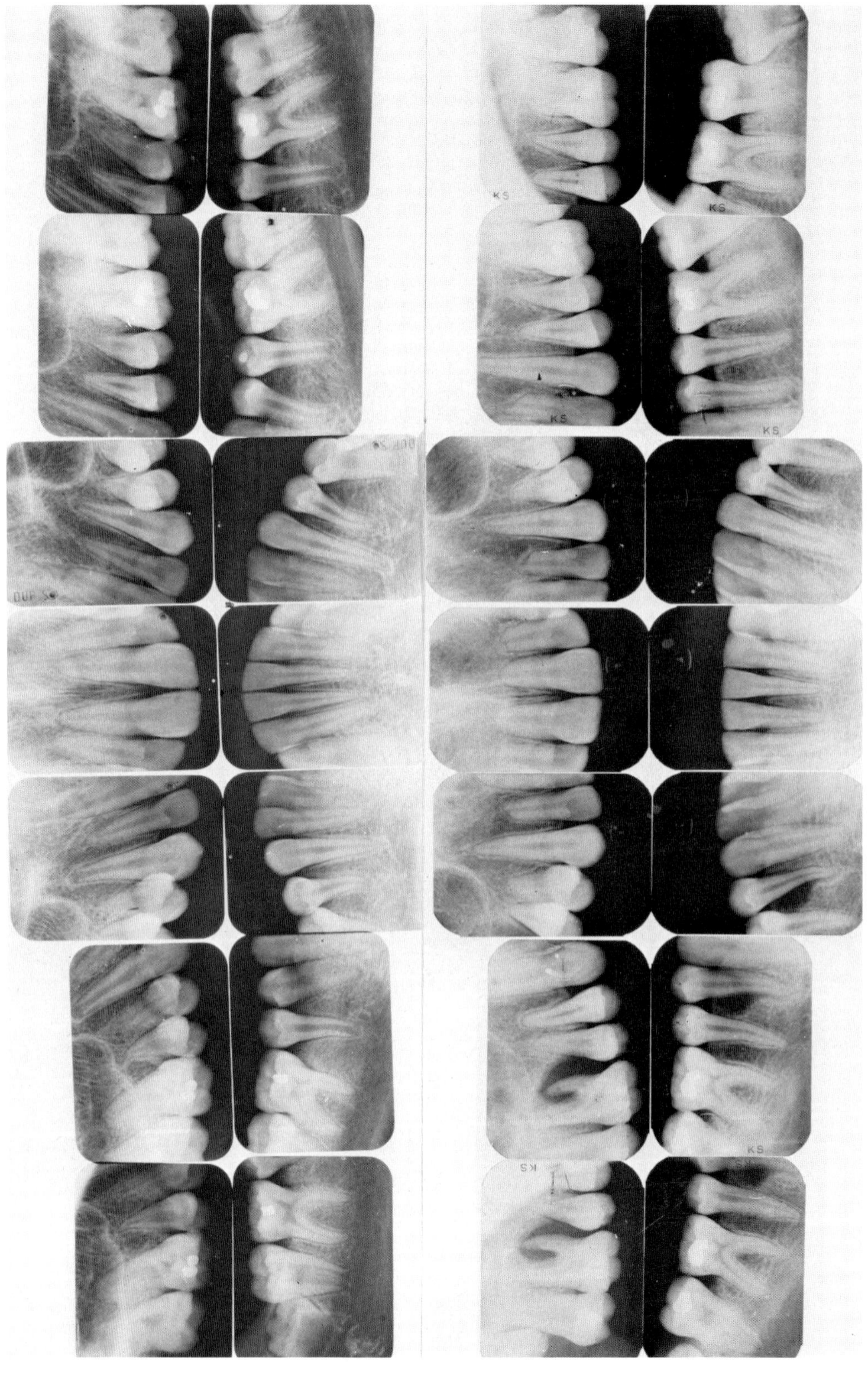

Fig. 8-16. *Top*. Roentgenographs were taken before orthodontic treatment.
Bottom. Note the alveolar resorption in the maxillary left first molar and mandibular first bicuspid region following completion of the orthodontic treatment.

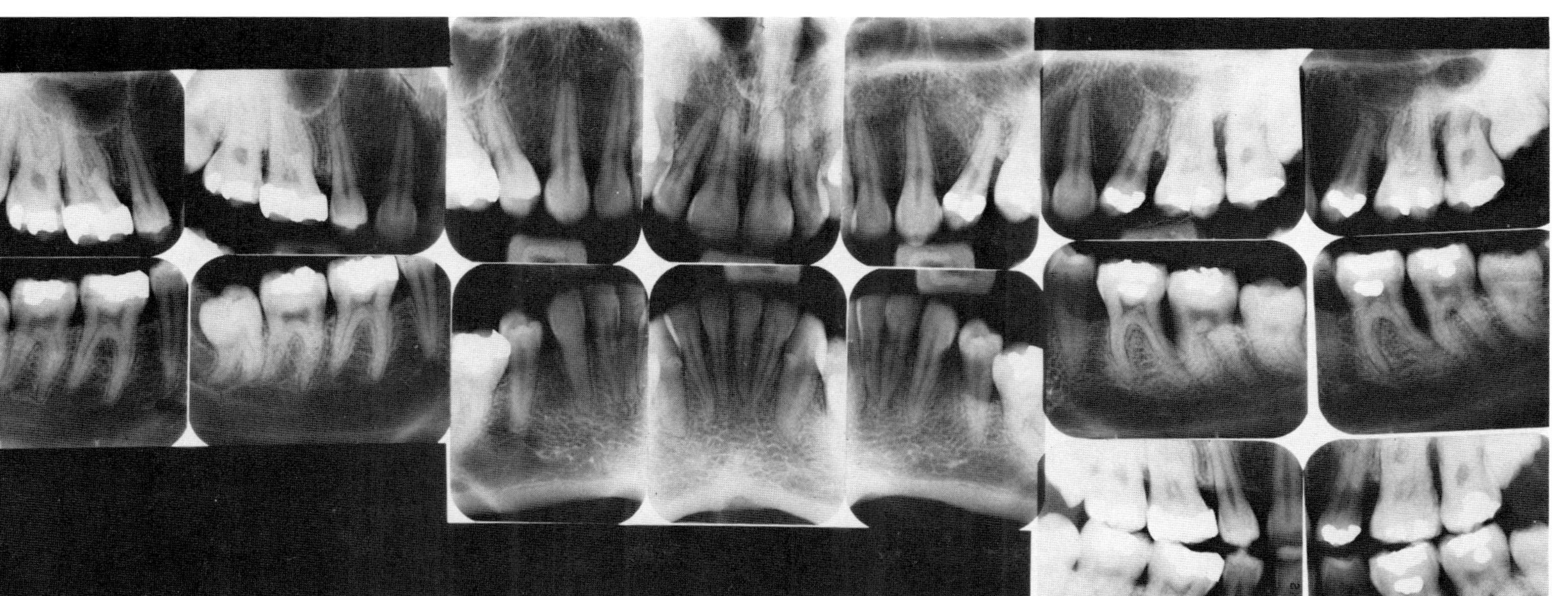

Fig. 8-17. Alveolar bone resorption present on the distal of the mandibular right first molar. The patient previously had orthodontic therapy.

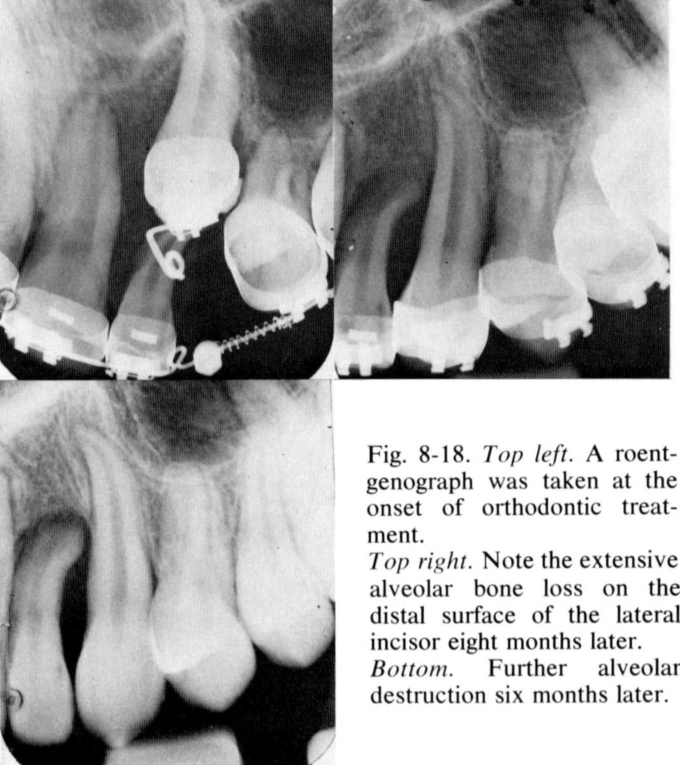

Fig. 8-18. *Top left.* A roentgenograph was taken at the onset of orthodontic treatment.
Top right. Note the extensive alveolar bone loss on the distal surface of the lateral incisor eight months later.
Bottom. Further alveolar destruction six months later.

CASE HISTORY 1[21]

Roentgenographs obtained before orthodontic treatment was instituted in this 16-year-old patient revealed a periodontium within normal limits (Fig. 8-15A). Roentgenographs were taken immediately upon completion of treatment (Fig. 8-15B). Alveolar bone loss can be seen in the mandibular incisor region, interproximally between the mandibular left and right bicuspids, and in the bifurcation area of the mandibular left first molar. Apical root resorption was also noted about the maxillary right lateral incisor. Roentgenographs taken one year later (Fig. 8-15C) revealed further progression of bone loss and root resorption about this tooth. Following periodontal and endodontic therapy (Fig. 8-15D) there was a favorable response.

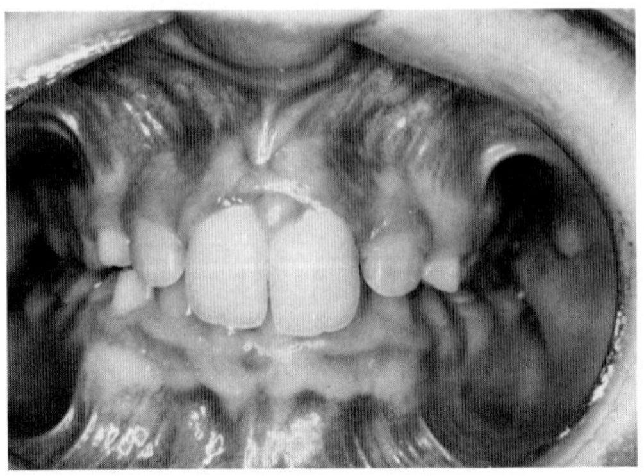

Fig. 8-19. A 9-year-old female patient with 10 mm. periodontal pockets on the distal of both maxillary central incisors.

Diagnosis. The diagnosis of the above case was periodontitis associated with orthodontic tooth movement. This was based on the following diagnostic criteria:

1. The pattern of bone loss did not correspond to that seen in periodontosis.
2. All the teeth that were periodontally involved had been banded.
3. The interproximal mandibular bicuspid areas, which showed extensive loss of

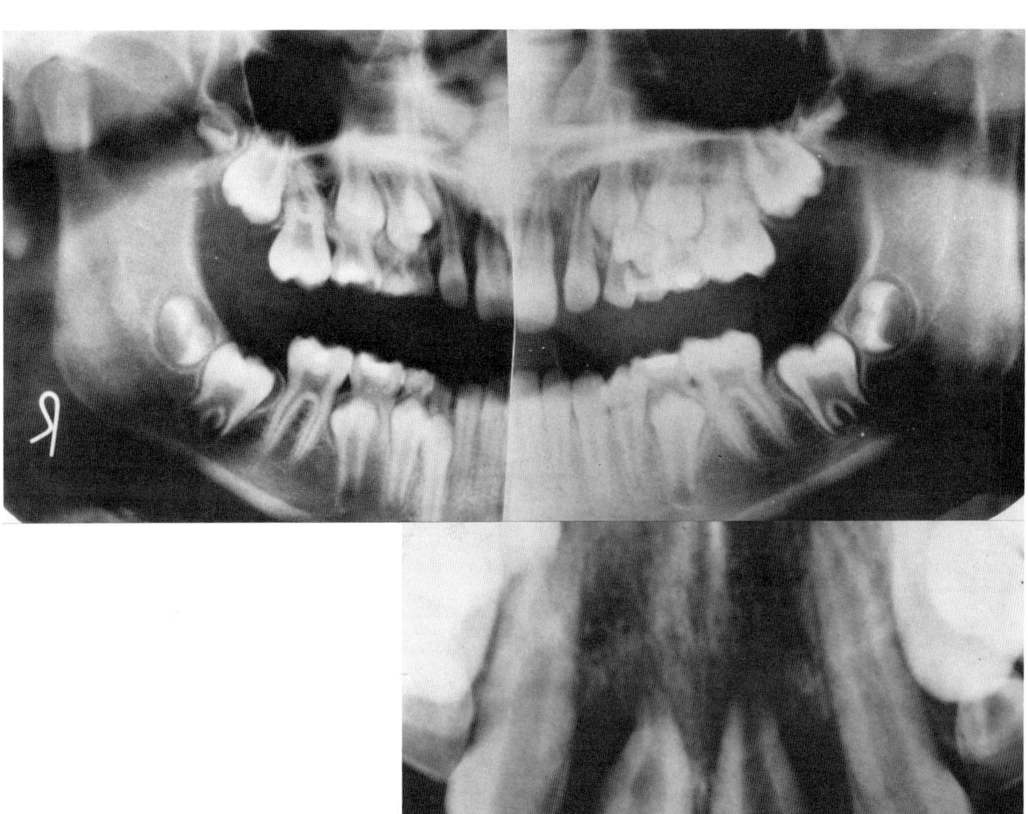

Fig. 8-20. *Top* and *bottom*. Roentgenographs made when the patient was first seen. Note the destruction on the distal of both maxillary central incisors.

alveolar bone, were not in proximal contact. This would encourage impaction of food.

4. In teeth with two roots, such as the mandibular first molars, the area which would be most severely injured during mechanical movement of the tooth would be in the region of the bifurcation. This could explain the periodontal involvement in the area of the bifurcation in these teeth in the absence of alveolar bone loss on the proximal surfaces.

In several other cases, advanced periodontal disease was found to be present in only a few localized areas in an otherwise healthy mouth (Figs. 8-16, and 8-17). In all instances these patients had recently completed orthodontic treatment. Since this severe localized loss of alveolar bone could not be explained by any other local factors it is felt that the orthodontic treatment probably was most responsible for these lesions. The following case report is an example of another inherent danger in orthodontic therapy.

CASE HISTORY 2

As part of the treatment plan it was decided to properly realign an impacted maxillary cuspid (Fig. 8-18 *Top left*). A roentgenograph taken of

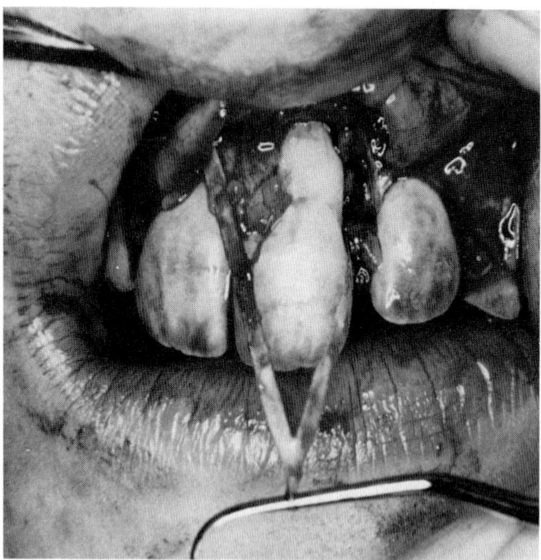

Fig. 8-21. A rubber band was found at the time of operation.

this area 8 months later revealed extensive loss of alveolar bone on the distal proximal surface of the lateral incisor (Fig. 8-18 *Top right*). Six months later the bone loss extended down to and around the apex of the lateral incisor (Fig. 8-18 *Bottom*). Clinical examination revealed deep periodontal pockets and bone loss on the distal and lingual surfaces of the lateral incisor extending down to and around the apex of the root. Subsequently, the tooth had to be extracted.

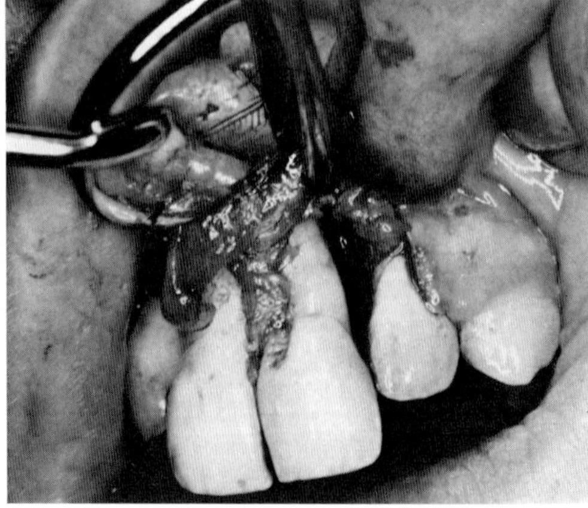

Fig. 8-22. Appearance of the bony lesion after granulations were removed by curettage.

Improperly Used Rubber Bands

As mentioned previously (Chap. 6), the diastema between the maxillary central incisor generally begins to close upon the eruption of the lateral incisors. Proximal contact of the central incisor is usually reached when the cuspids have completed eruption. Thus, what may appear to be an abnormality at an early age develops into an arch with proper alignment as the patient becomes older. The use of rubber bands to close a diastema between the maxillary central incisors in children is, therefore, contraindicated for two reasons: First, it is superfluous, secondly, there is always danger that the patient may forget to remove the rubber band—as a result it may gradually work its way toward the apices of the teeth. The ultimate result is severe destruction of alveolar bone and occasionally tooth exfoliation.

CASE HISTORY 1

The patient was 9 years old when first seen (Fig. 8-19). She had been referred because radiographs had revealed severe localized destruction of alveolar bone on the distal surfaces of both maxillary central incisors (Fig. 8-20). A clinical examination revealed deep 10 mm. pockets on the distal of both incisors and the presence of a purulent exudate. All other areas in the mouth were within normal limits.

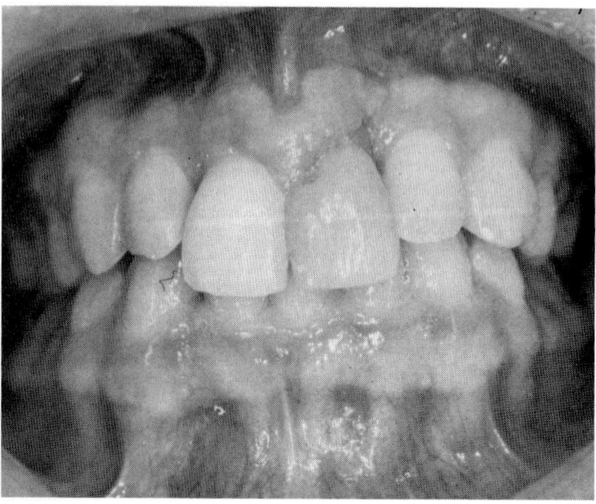

Fig. 8-23. The same patient seven years postoperative.

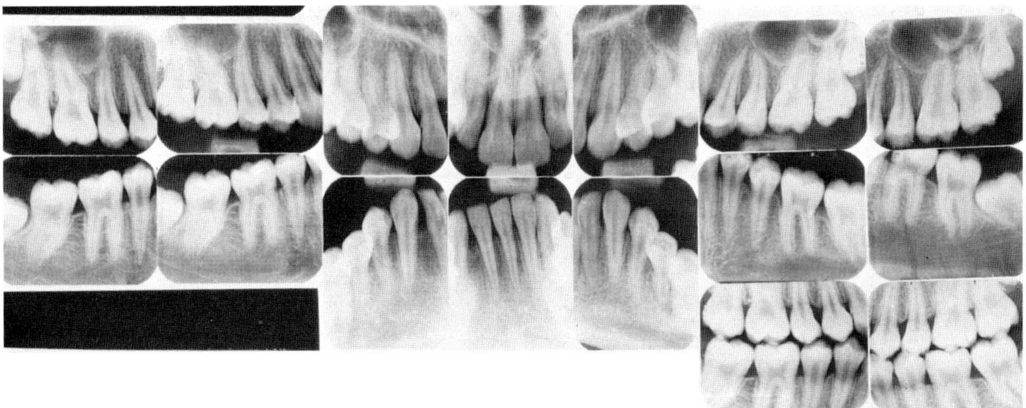

Fig. 8-24. Roentgenographs eight years postoperative.

The medical history was noncontributing and the laboratory tests and physical findings were within normal limits. Roentgenographs revealed lesions not usually seen in either periodontosis or juvenile periodontitis. There was insufficient clinical evidence of local factors to explain the extreme amount of localized destruction revealed. The patient was carefully questioned. After much effort she finally remembered that at one time her dentist had prescribed rubber bands to close the diastema between her maxillary central incisors.

At the time of operation, a rubber band was found about the roots of the maxillary incisors (Fig. 8-21). This was removed and the area thoroughly curetted (Fig. 8-22). Healing appeared to progress uneventfully. However, one year later deep pockets were again found on the distal of the incisor. The area was reoperated upon, this time successfully. A 7-year postoperative roentgenograph shows the healing of the alveolar lesion (Figs. 8-23, and 8-24).

Three other reports of cases involving the maxillary incisors have appeared in the literature.[7,17,23]

The same type of periodontal destruction resulting from the improper use of rubber bands can occur on any tooth. Figure 8-25 shows the severe destruction of alveolar bone which occurred in a biscuspid. Fortunately, since in most of these cases the reaction is an acute one with severe destruction of alveolar bone occurring within

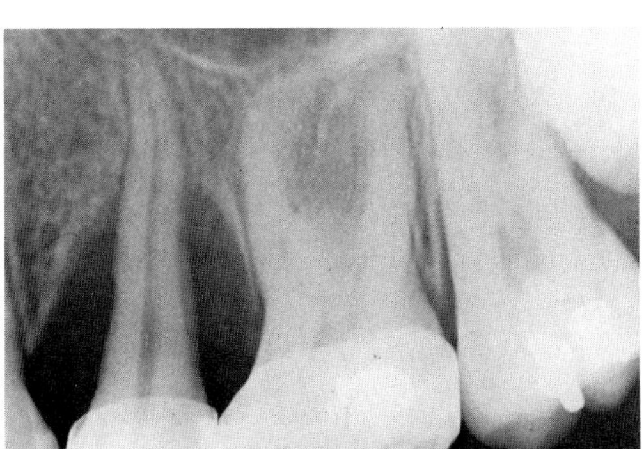

Fig. 8-25. Destruction about the maxillary bicuspid was due to a rubber band. (Courtesy of Dr. Sheldon Holen.)

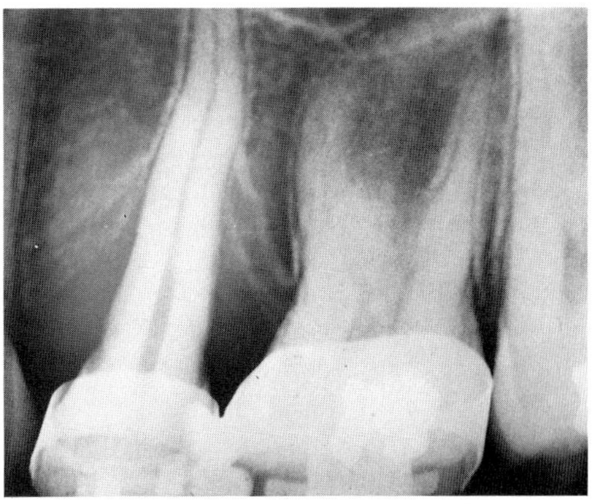

Fig. 8-26. Postoperative healing. (Courtesy of Dr. Sheldon Holen.)

a relatively short period of time, the response to the removal of the imbedded rubber band is usually gratifying (Fig. 8-26).

Periodontal Abscess. On occasion a periodontal abscess may develop on a tooth that is banded. The treatment for this is discussed in Chapter 3.

REFERENCES

1. Baer, P. N., and Coccaro, P. J.: Gingival enlargement coincident with orthodontic therapy. J. Periodont., *35:*436, 1964.
2. Beagrie, G. S., and James, G. A.: The association of posterior tooth irregularity and periodontal disease. Br. Dent. J., *113:* 239, 1962.
3. Begg, P. R.: The evolutionary reduction and degeneration of man's jaws and teeth. Proc. Tenth Congress Austral. Dent. Assoc., pp. 542-564, 1939.
4. Boese, L. R.: Increased stability of orthodontically rotated teeth following gingivectomy in macaca nemestrina. Am. J. Orthod., *56:*273, 1969.
5. Brain, W. E.: The effect of surgical transsection of free gingival fibers on the regression of orthodontically rotated teeth in the dog. Am. J. Orthod., *55:*50, 1969.
6. Broadbent, B. H.: The influence of the third molars on the alignment of the teeth. Am. J. Orthod., *29:*312, 1943.
7. Burstone, C. J.: Distinguishing developing malocclusion from normal occlusion. Dent. Clin. North Am. *8:*484, 1964.
8. Cryer, B. S.: Third molar eruption and the effect of extraction of adjacent teeth. Dent. Pract., *17:*405, 1967.
9. Dewel, B. F.: Serial extraction in orthodontics: indication, objective and treatment procedure. Am. J. Ortho., *40:*906, 1954.
10. Edwards, J. G.: A study of the periodontium during orthodontic rotation of teeth. Am. J. Orthod., *54:*441, 1968.
11. Edwards, J. G.: A surgical procedure to eliminate rotational relapse. Am. J. Orthod., 57:35, 1970.
12. Erikson, B. E., Kaplan, H., and Aisenberg, M. S.: Orthodontics and transseptal fibers. Am. J. Orthod. Oral Surg., *31:*1, 1945.
13. Fastlicht, J.: Crowding of mandibular incisors. Am. J. Orthod., *58:*156, 1970.
14. Geiger, A. M.: Occlusal studies in 188 consecutive cases of periodontal disease. Am. J. Orthod., *48:*330, 1962.
15. Grewe, J. M., Chadha, J. M., Hagen, D., and Zermeno, J. A.: Oral hygiene and occlusal disharmony in Mexican-American children. J. Periodont. Res., *4:*189, 1969.
16. Henry, J. L., and Weinman, J. P.: Pattern of resorption and repair of human cementum. J.A.D.A., *42:*270, 1951.
17. Hogeboom, F. E., and Stephens, K. A.: The dangerous rubber band. J. Dent. Child., *32:*199, 1965.
18. Horowitz, S. L., and Hixon, E. H.: The Nature of Orthodontic Diagnosis, p. 67. St. Louis, C. V. Mosby, 1966.
19. Keene, H. J.: Third molars agenesis, spacing and crowding of teeth, and tooth size in caries resistant naval recruits. Am. J. Orthod., *50:*445, 1964.
20. Massler, M., and Malone, A. J.: Root resorption in human permanent teeth. Am. J. Orthod., *40:*619, 1954.
21. Moskow, B. S., and Baden, E.: Unusual gingival characteristics having a familial tendency: A case report. Periodontics, *5:*259, 1967.
22. Phillips, J. P.: Apical root resorption under orthodontic therapy. Angle Orthod., *25:* 1, 1955.
23. Prichard, J. F.: Advanced Periodontal Disease: Surgical and Prosthetic Management, pp. 363-365. Philadelphia, W. B. Saunders, 1965.
24. Reitan, K.: Tissue rearrangement during the retention of orthodontically rotated teeth. Angle Orthod., *29:*105, 1959.
25. Ruben, M. P., Frankl, S. N., and Wallace, S.: The histopathology of periodontal disease in children. J. Periodont., *42:*473, 1971.
26. Selmer-Olsen, R.: The normal movement of the mandibular teeth and the crowding of the incisors as a result of growth and function. Dent. Rec., *57:*465, 1937.
27. Thompson, H. E., Myers, H. P., Waterman, J. M., and Flanagen, V. D.: Preliminary macroscopic observations concerning the potentiality of supre-alveolar collagenous fibers in orthodontics. Am. J. Orthod., *44:*485, 1958.

28. Weinstein, S.: Third molar implications in orthodontics. J.A.D.A., *82*:819, 1971.
29. Winter, B. A.: The relationship between anterior tooth irregularities and periodontal disease. Thesis. Indiana Univ.-Purdue Univ. School of Dentistry, 1971.

9

The Third Molar

CONGENITAL ABSENCE OF THIRD MOLARS

Prevalence. In a study of congenitally missing teeth in skeletal material from museums it was found that there were some persons in all racial groups who have completely missing third molars. The range was from 2.6 percent among West Africans to 49 percent among certain Europeans.[7] In a more recent investigation it was found that 25 percent of 195 men studied had one or more third molars congenitally missing.[8] On the other hand the prevalence of agenesis of permanent third molar teeth in an adolescent group aged 14 through 16 years was reported to be about 13 percent. [11]

As can be seen from Table 9-1, some studies show that congenitally missing third molars are more numerous among females (35%) than among males (27%), while other studies have reported no sex differences.[11] The distribution of congenitally missing third molars is shown in Table 9-2.

Concomitant with congenitally missing third molars is an increased incidence of agenesis of other teeth, delay in posterior tooth formation and a reduction in size of all remaining teeth in the arch—with the result that the teeth in both arches are more frequently spaced and less frequently crowded.[3,6,8] This effect is most pronounced when all 4 third molars are congenitally missing (Table 9-3).

THIRD MOLARS AS POTENTIAL PERIODONTAL PROBLEMS

Patially erupted or impacted third molar teeth, even when asymptomatic, have to be carefully evaluated, since they may be important etiologic factors in recurrent pericoronal infections and destructive periodontal disease in that area.[1,2] The following are indications for extraction of overerupted third molars.

1. An impacted or congenitally missing third molar in one arch that enables the opposing third molar to continue erupting until it reaches the opposing edentulous saddle area (Fig. 9-1) or is stopped by the intervention of the tongue or cheek. Overeruption of a third molar may lead to occlusal problems, caries and periodontal pathology as a result of food impaction and plaque formation. Therefore, if it is deemed desirable to preserve an unapposed third molar tooth, it must be splinted to an adjacent tooth to prevent its overeruption.

2. Recurrent pericoronal infections that are impossible to prevent or to treat successfully because of the anatomical posi-

TABLE 9-1. INCIDENCE OF CONGENITALLY MISSING THIRD MOLARS

	Males		Females	
Total No. of Specimens	735		314	
Incidence of Missing Third Molars	No.	%	No.	%
	201	27.35	110	35.04

After Hellman[7]

TABLE 9-2. DISTRIBUTION OF CONGENITALLY MISSING THIRD MOLARS

No. of Third Molars Missing	Males		Females	
	No.	%	No.	%
1	64	31.84	30	27.27
2	74	36.82	31	28.19
3	28	13.93	18	16.36
4	35	17.41	37	28.19

After Hellman[7]

tion of the third molar. For example, a manidbular third molar that cannot fully erupt because it is situated so far distally in the arch that it invades the ramus cannot be successfully treated.

Another inoperable situation occurs when the pterygomandibular raphe inserts into the distal portion of the gingival operculum. To retain such a tooth following surgical removal of the gingival operculum, a short distal saddle area should be obtainable. If it is not, the tooth should be extracted.

3. Roentgenographic evidence that the crown of the third molar is in close approximation to the distal cervical area of the second molar (Fig. 9-2). This might prevent complete development of the supporting structures on the distal of the second molar. In such cases the third molars should be extracted to prevent periodontal destruction interproximally between the second and third molars.

Once destruction has occurred in such a situation, extraction of the third molar will not restore the supporting structure lost on the distal of the second molar. In an investigation of this problem,[1] impacted molars were sorted into the following 3 groups on the basis of radiographic ap-

TABLE 9-3. RELATIONSHIP BETWEEN AGENESIS OF THIRD MOLARS AND SPACING OF TEETH

Arrangement of Teeth	No Third Molar Agenesis		Agenesis of One or More Third Molars		Agenesis of Four Third Molars	
	Men	%	Men	%	Men	%
Maxilla						
Spacing	66	45.2	28	57.2	11	91.6
No Spacing, No Crowding	57	39.0	13	26.5	1	8.3
Crowding	23	15.7	8	16.3	0	0
Totals	146	99.9	49	100.0	12	99.9
Mandible						
Spacing	22	15.0	23	47.0	8	66.6
No Spacing, No Crowding	54	37.0	11	22.4	1	8.3
Crowding	70	47.9	15	30.6	3	25.0
Totals	146	99.9	49	100.0	12	99.9

After Keene[8]

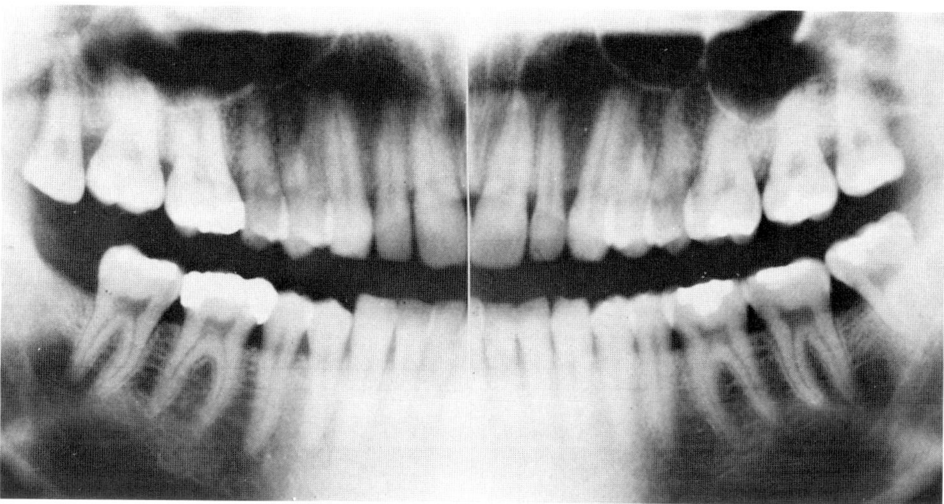

Fig. 9-1. The maxillary left third molar has overerupted because of the absence of its antagonist.

proximation of the third molar to the second: broad separation, thin separation and no apparent separation. It was found that of the 58 broadly separated molars, 15 developed pockets and/or root exposure one year after the extraction. In the group in which the second and third molars were thinly separated, there was a total of 79 teeth, of which 34 developed pockets and/or root exposure. In the group without apparent separation, 65 pockets and/or root exposures were found in a total of 88 teeth one year after extraction of the third molars. It is apparent therefore that the possibility for loss of periodontal structure is considerable when the third molar is in close contact with the distal aspect of the second molar (Table 9-4).

4. Deeply or horizontally impacted third molars (Fig. 9-3) that might cause future problems. Such teeth should be extracted at an early age since their removal in the late twenties or after frequently requires extensive surgical procedures, which may lead to a permanent loss of supporting structures on the distal and buccal aspects of the second molar. This might ultimately lead to progressive destruction of the supporting structure and loss of this tooth.

5. The position of the ascending ramus, buccal fat pad and almost total absence of a

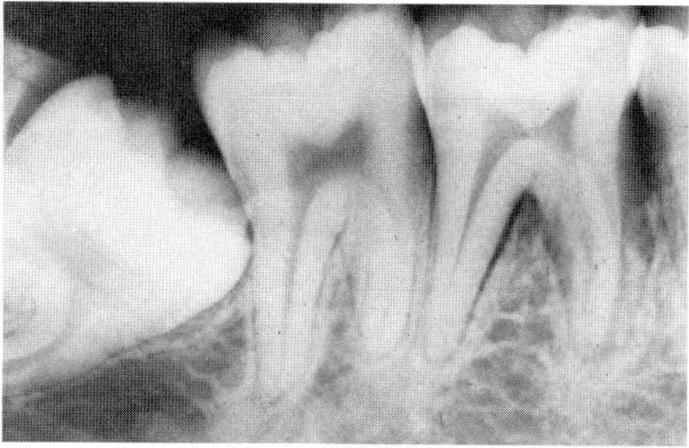

Fig. 9-2. Third molars in close approximation to the distal cervical area of the second molar should be extracted.

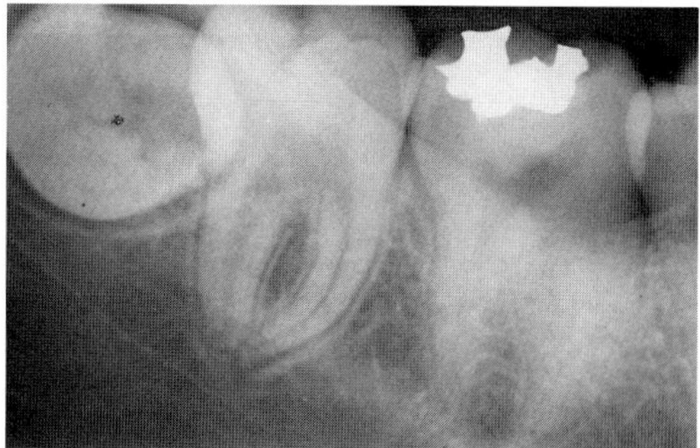

Fig. 9-3. Deeply or horizontally impacted third molars should be extracted at an early age.

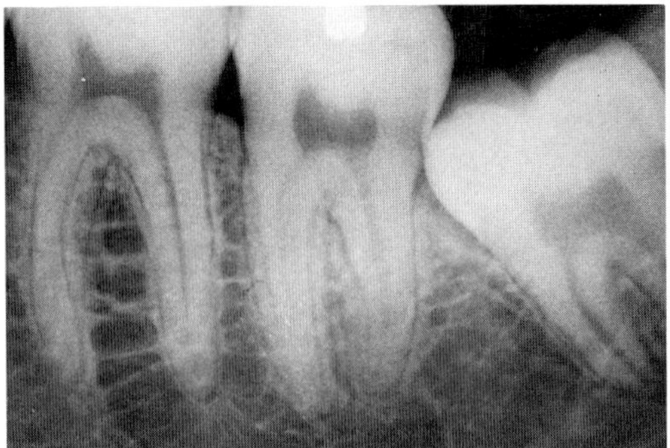

Fig. 9-4. The third molar in this 18-year-old girl should be extracted.

mucobuccal fold area has caused the gingival margin on the distobuccal aspect of the second molar to be continuous with the buccal mucosa. If extraction of a third molar is delayed until adult life, particularly in these cases, deep periodontal pockets will tend to occur on the distal of the mandibular second molar.

Age to extract third molars. Periodontal hazards, such as faulty development of the supporting tissues on the distal of the second molar and/or loss of supporting tissues on the distal of the second molar following extraction of the third molar, can be prevented by extraction at any early age. Present evidence indicates that repair of the supporting structures on the distal of the second molar is better in younger than in older persons (Figs. 9-4, 9-5, 9-6

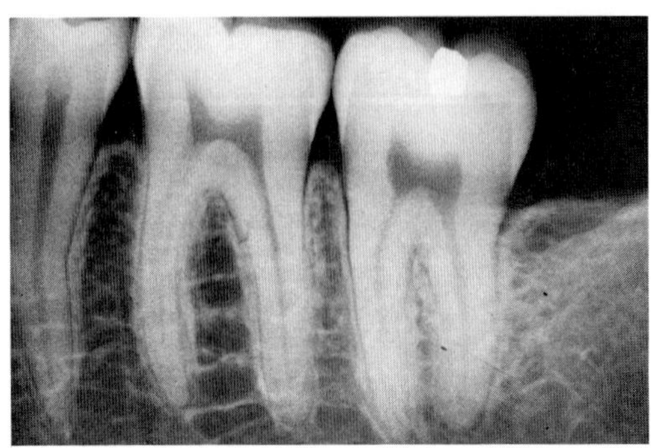

Fig. 9-5 Following extraction, healing is excellent. Compare with Fig. 9-4.

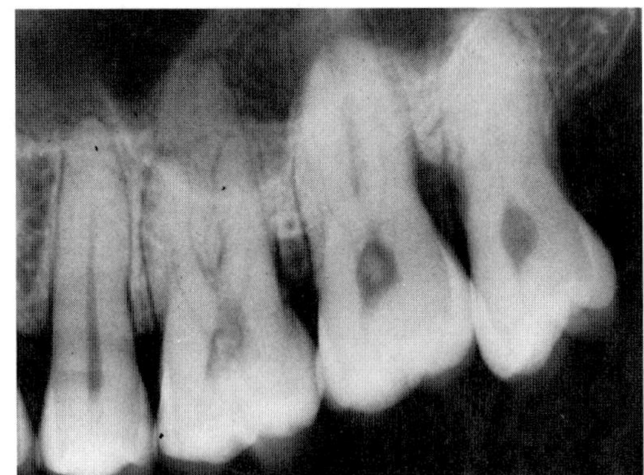

Fig. 9-6. An overerupted third molar in an adult.

TABLE 9-4. POCKET FORMATION AND/OR ROOT EXPOSURE ACCORDING TO PROXIMITY OF THIRD MOLARS TO SECOND MOLARS

Proximity of Third Molars to Second Molars	No. in Each Group	No. of Pockets 1 yr. After Extraction
Broad Separation	68	15
Thin Separation	69	34
No Separation	88	65

After Ash, Costich, Hayward[2]

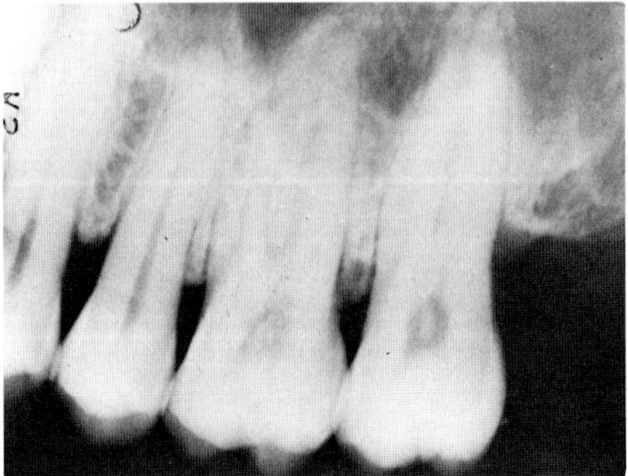

Fig. 9-7. A distal periodontal defect remained following extraction of the third molar shown in Fig. 9-6.

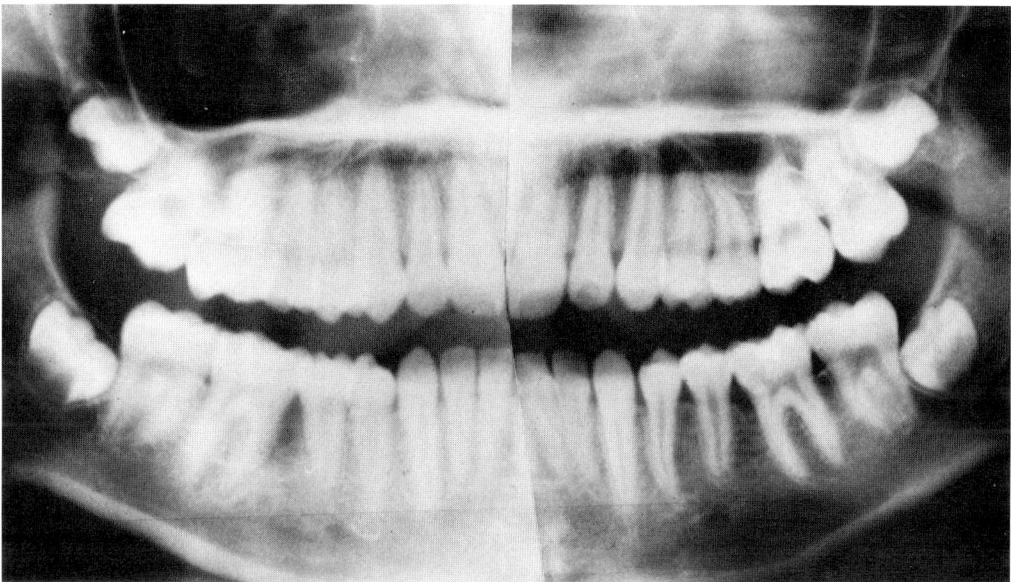

Fig. 9-8. Note the position of the mandibular third molar in this 12-year-old girl.

and 9-7). A favorable time for extraction of the third molar is prior to the full development of the roots of the third molar,[1] since permanent loss of bone does not occur if teeth are extracted at a time when the supporting bone on the distal of the second

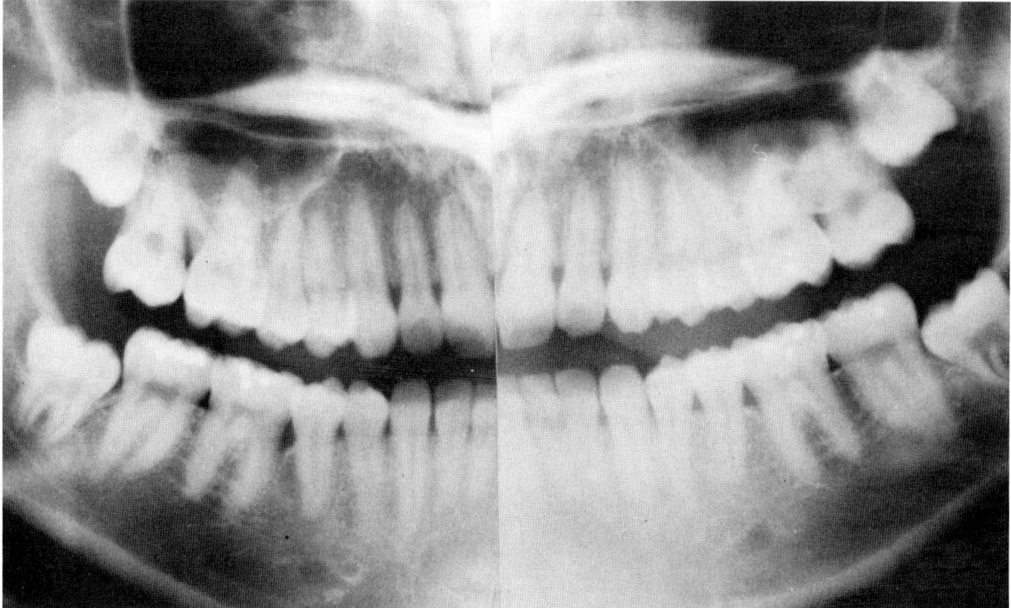

Fig. 9-9 Note the position of the mandibular third molars when the patient was 16 years of age. (Same patient as Fig. 9-8.) There is no doubt now but that the mandibular third molars will not be able to erupt in a good position and therefore should be extracted.

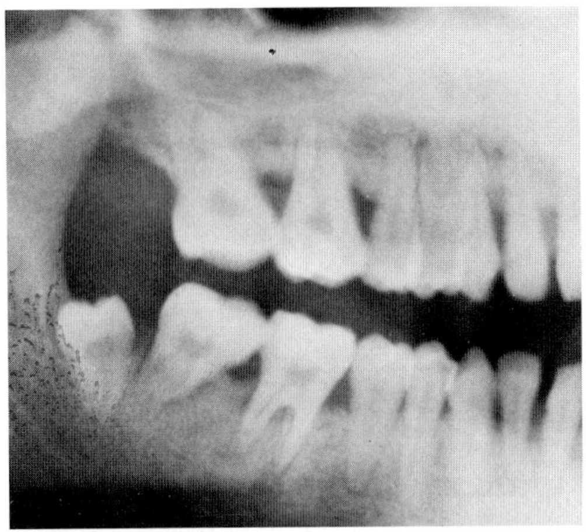

Fig. 9-10. Prediction as to whether or not a third molar will erupt properly is difficult to make. Note the position of the third molar in 1967.

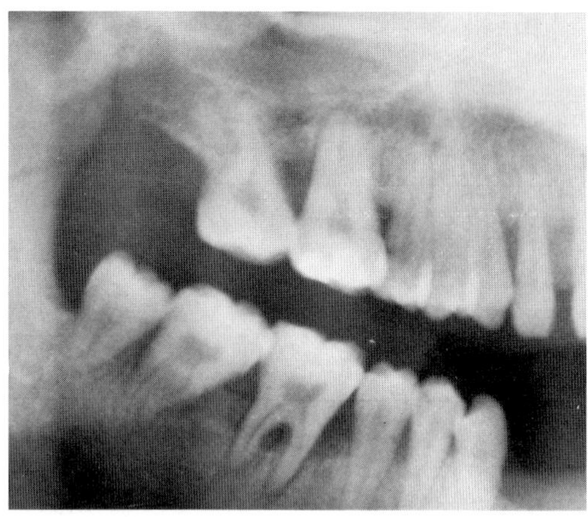

Fig. 9-11. Same case as Figure 9-10 five years later. Note the new position of the third molar (patient has Down's syndrome).

molar is developing. Because growth of the mandible with accompanying resorption of the anterior border of the ramus is also essentially completed about this same time, the ideal age for extraction of the third molar would be between 16 and 20 years of age.[9, 10, 12]

Contraindication for extraction. In orthodontics it has become increasingly popular to extract 4 bicuspids to facilitate

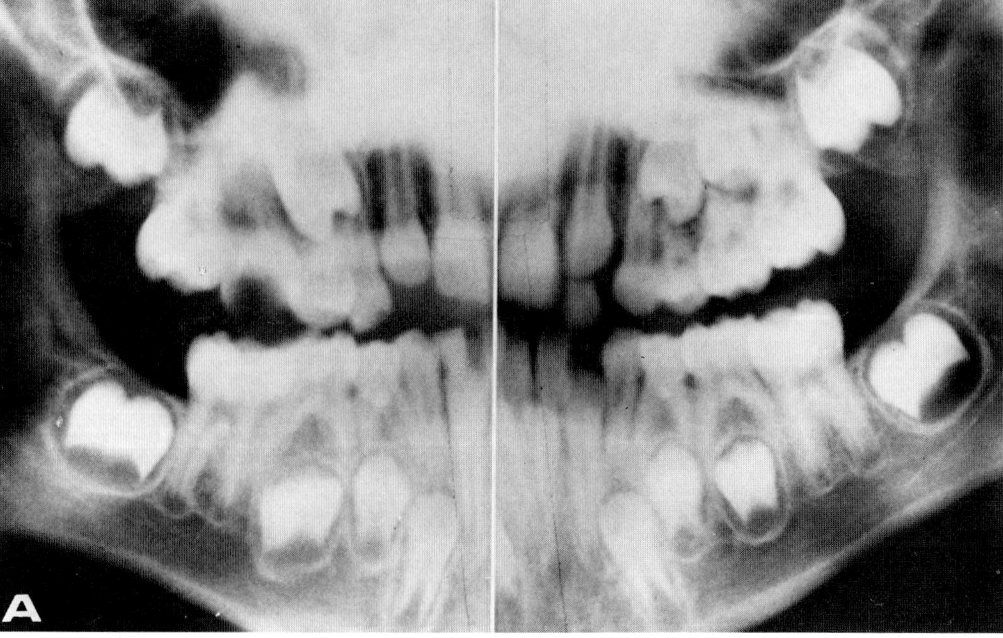

Fig. 9-12. A. There was no roentgenographic evidence of third molars in this patient at 7 years of age.

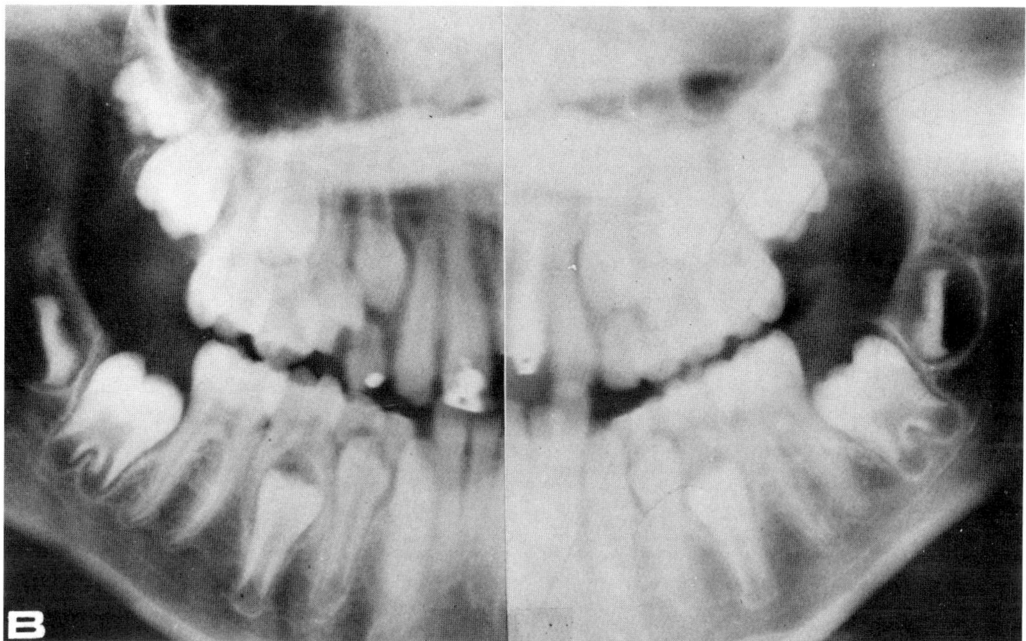

Fig. 9-12. B. Third molar tooth buds were present when the patient was 10 years of age.

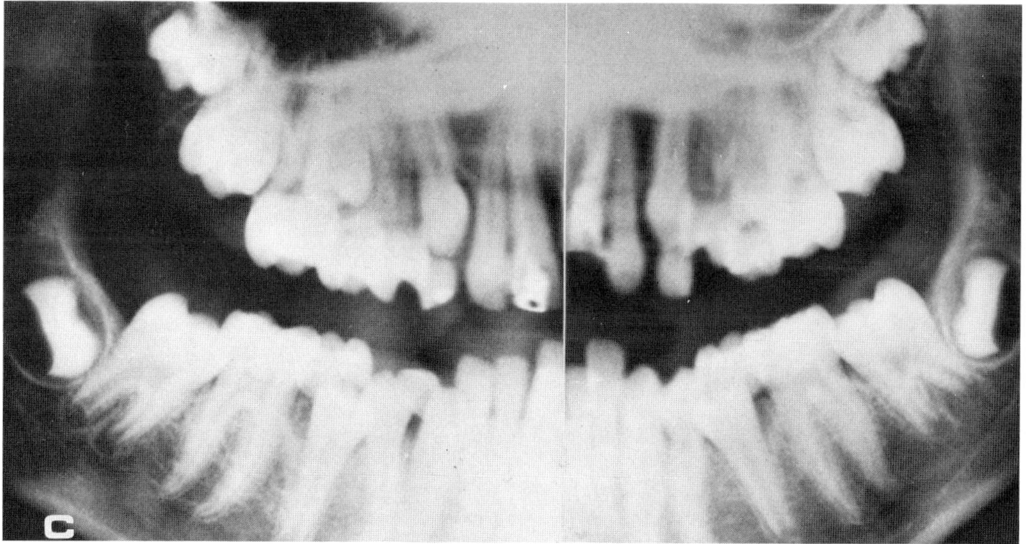

Fig. 9-12. C. Same patient at age 11 years.

treatment. This often permits all the molars to move forward.[5, 13] However, in a study in which the lower second permanent molars were extracted for orthodontic purposes (in lieu of the bicuspids), it was found that a high proportion of third molars in such cases erupted in good position.[4] Similarly, when first molars are lost the third molars may contribute to an acceptable occlusion.

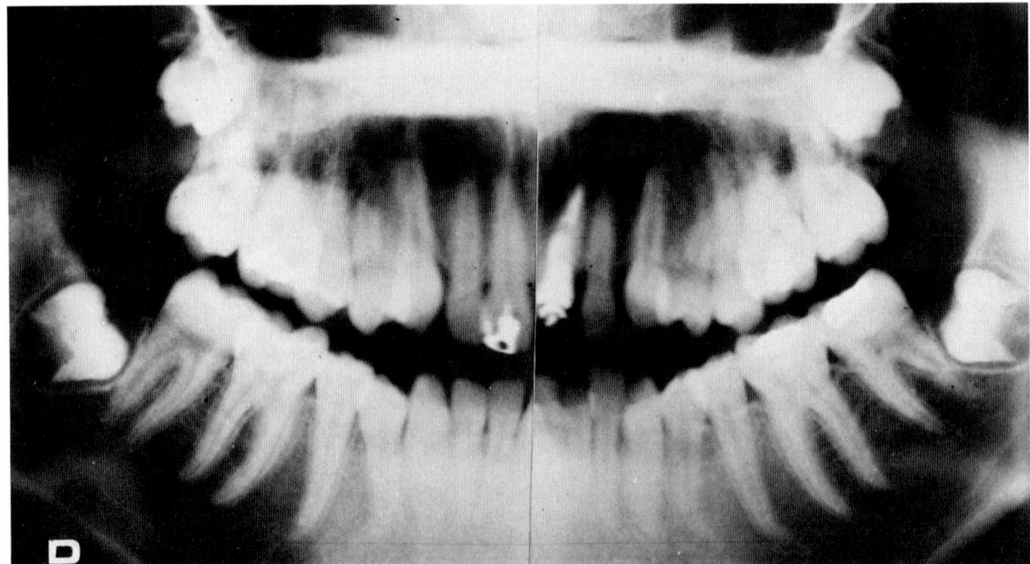

Fig. 9-12. D. Note the position of the third molars at age 14 years.

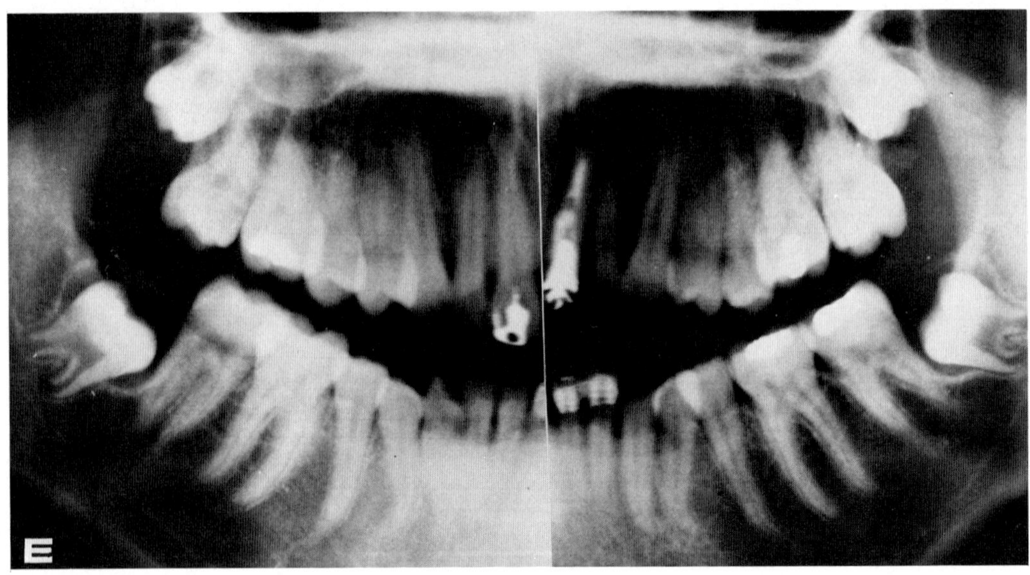

Fig. 9-12. E. When the patient was 16 years of age the third molars were ready to be extracted.

A deeply impacted third molar which has no roentgenographic or subjective symptoms should not be extracted because the hazard of losing extensive supporting periodontal structures, which may accompany the surgical removal of such a tooth, may far outweigh the hazards of retaining it.[1] Another indication for retaining the third molars is if it is likely that the second molars might be lost because of extensive caries.

The third molars should also be retained in young patients with periodontosis. They might be needed for autotransplantation to replace first molars that might become lost because of extensive periodontal involvement. The third molars may also prove to be useful as terminal abutments in adults who might in the future lose their first and second molars from periodontal disease. Finally, since it cannot generally be predicted whether or not a third molar will erupt properly before its roots have started to develop, the third molars should not as a rule be extracted before 16 years of age. (Figs. 9-8–9-12).

REFERENCES

1. Ash, M. M., Jr.: Third molars as periodontal problems. Dent. Clin. North Am., *8:*51061, 1964.
2. Ash, M. M., Costich, E.R., and Hayward, J. P.: A study of periodontal hazards of third molars. J. Periodont., *33:*209, 1962.
3. Baum, B. J., and Cohen, M. M.: Agenesis and tooth size in permanent dentition. Angle Ortho., *41:*100, 1971.
4. Cryer, B. S.: Third molars eruption and the effect of extraction of adjacent teeth. Dent. Pract., *17:*405, 1967.
5. Faubion, B. H.: Effect of extraction of premolars on eruption of mandibular third molars. J.A.D.A., *76:*316, 1968.
6. Garn, S. M., Lewis, A. B., and Kerewsky, R. S.: Third molar agenesis and size reduction of the remaining teeth. Nature, *200:*488, 1963.
7. Hellman, M.: Our third molar teeth, their eruption, presence and absence. Dent. Cosmos, *78:*750, 1936.
8. Keene, H. J.: Third molar agenesis, spacing crowding of teeth, and tooth size in caries-resistant naval recruits. Am. J. Orthod., *50:*445, 1964.
9. Laskin, D. M.: Evaluation of the third molar problem. J.A.D.A., *82:*824, 1971.
10. Laskin, D. M.: Indication and contraindications for removal of impacted third molars. Dent. Clin. North Am., *13:*919, Oct. 1969.
11. Rantanen, A. V.: The age of eruption of the third molar teeth. Acta. Odont. Scand. Suppl. *25:*48, Helsinki, 1967.
12. Waite, D. E.: Evaluation and determination of the proper time to remove third molars. J.A.D.A., *75:*1170, 1967.
13. Weinstein, S.: Third molar implication in orthodontics. J.A.D.A., *82:*819, 1971.

10

Resorptive Lesions of the Alveolar Bone

PERIODONTOSIS

Since its first suggestion as a clinical entity by Gottlieb,[12] periodontosis has been an enigma to the dental profession. The term itself is a controversial one, and there are many who do not believe it exists as a clinical entity. Even among those who agree that the disease does exist, there is considerable variation in opinion as to its frequency and as to how it should be defined.

In 1949[18] the Committee on Nomenclature of the American Academy of Periodontology defined periodontosis as a "degenerative noninflammatory destruction of the periodontium originating in one or more of the periodontal structures, characterized by migration and loosening of the teeth in the presence or absence of secondary epithelial proliferation and pocket formation or secondary gingival disease." There are several reservations to be made to this definition.

1. Nothing is stated about the general health of the individual. A distinction should be made as to whether the changes noted in the alveolar bone occurred in an otherwise healthy individual or were really an oral manifestation of a systemic disease.

2. It is unclear as to whether the disease affects the primary or permanent dentitions or both.

3. The degenerative nature of the disease has not been documented.

4. Migration and loosening of the teeth is never observed as an early manifestation. It is one of the late clinical signs of its more advanced stage.

In a recent workshop in periodontics,[26] it was recognized that while the term periodontosis was ambiguous, there was, nevertheless some evidence to indicate that a clinical entity different from adult periodontitis may occur in the adolescent and young adult.

We prefer to define periodontosis as a disease of the periodontium occurring in an otherwise healthy adolescent and is characterized by a rapid loss of alveolar bone around more than one tooth of the permanent dentition.[2] There are two basic forms: In one, only the first molars and incisors are affected (Fig. 10-1 *Top*). In the other more generalized form most of the dentition is affected (Fig. 10-1 *Bottom*). The amount of destruction manifested is not commensurate with the amount of local irritants present. Single tooth involvement should not be considered as a case of periodontosis, since too many local factors may produce isolated osseous defects (Fig. 10-2 *Top*).

Prevalence. The prevalence of the disease is difficult to ascertain, since its very existence depends upon the investigator's own personal bias and prejudices. Those who do not believe in the existence of such an entity report a prevalence of zero.[25] However, even for those who do believe in the existence of periodontosis, there is a wide variation in its reported incidence. This may be due in part to real geographic differences, to differences in examination procedures or to differences of opinion as to what actually does constitute periodontosis. Several examples from the field of epidemiology illustrate the confusion that presently exists in this field. Miglani and Sharmi[16] reported periodon-

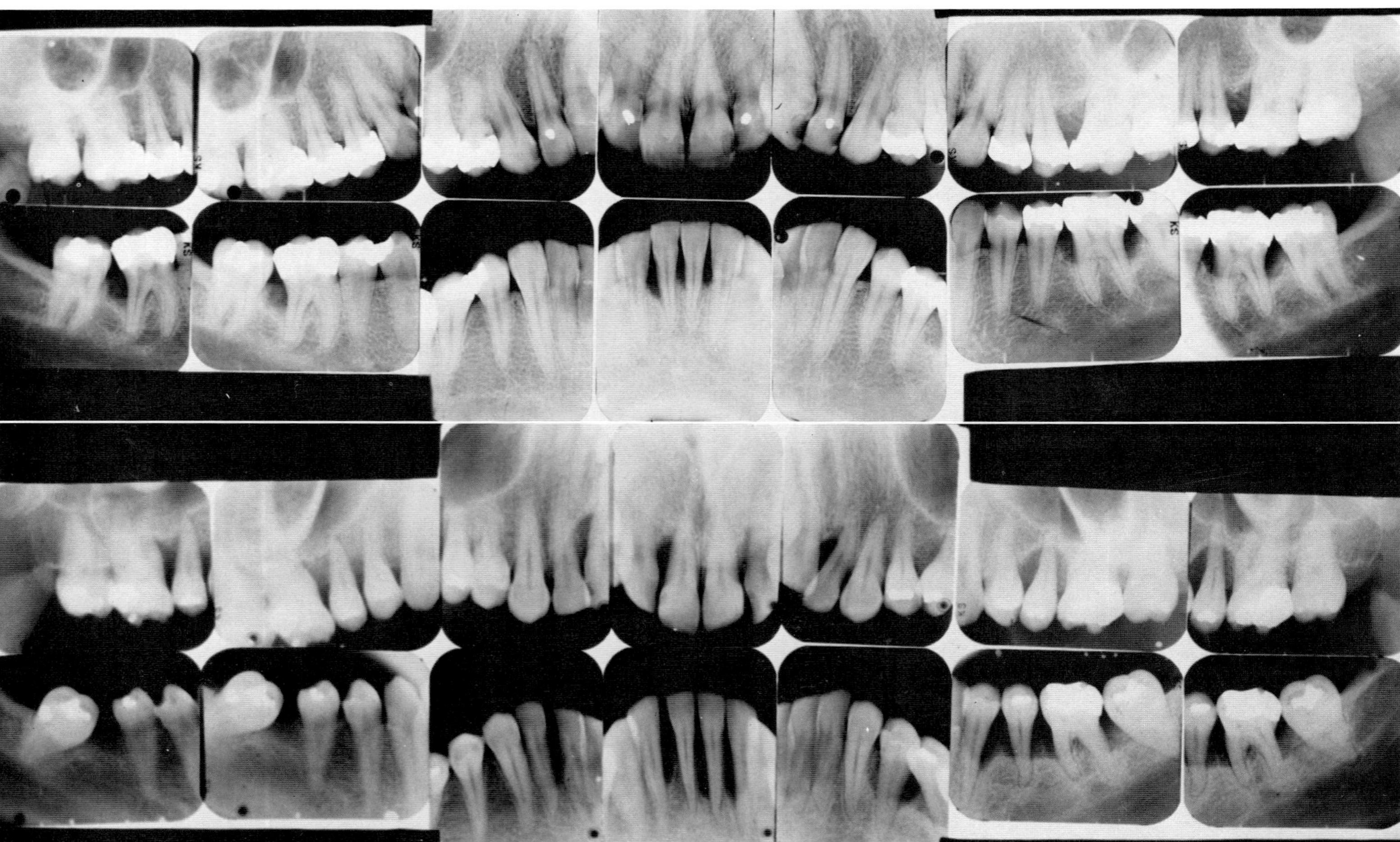

Fig. 10-1. *Top.* A localized form of periodontosis. The disease remains limited to the incisors and first molars. *Bottom.* The sister of the above patient with a generalized form of periodontosis.

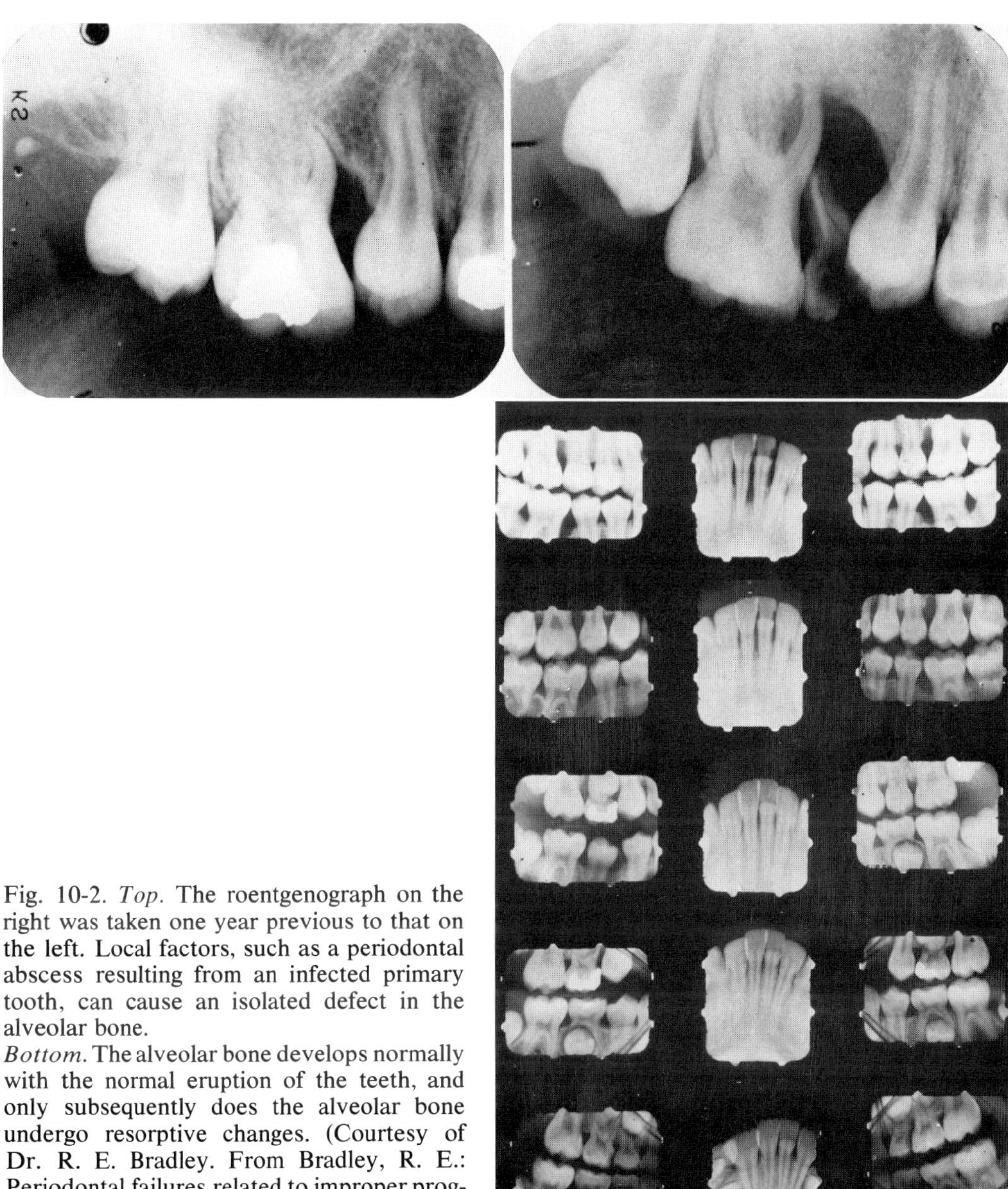

Fig. 10-2. *Top.* The roentgenograph on the right was taken one year previous to that on the left. Local factors, such as a periodontal abscess resulting from an infected primary tooth, can cause an isolated defect in the alveolar bone.
Bottom. The alveolar bone develops normally with the normal eruption of the teeth, and only subsequently does the alveolar bone undergo resorptive changes. (Courtesy of Dr. R. E. Bradley. From Bradley, R. E.: Periodontal failures related to improper prognosis and treatment planning. Dent. Clin. N. Am., *16*:33, 72.)

tosis in 0.1 percent of the patients they examined in Madras, India, while Rao and Tewani[20] reported 6.8 percent in Bombay, and Basu and Dutta[5] found 28.4 percent of 12- to 17-year-old Indians living in Calcutta had periodontal pockets. It is unknown what percentage of these latter cases might have been considered periodontosis by other investigators. Russell[22] stated the problem well when he said that if the term periodontosis is used to describe a condition seen in adolescents and young adults in which the rapidity and severity of tissue destruction seem out of proportion to local irritating factors, then this condition is consistently seen by

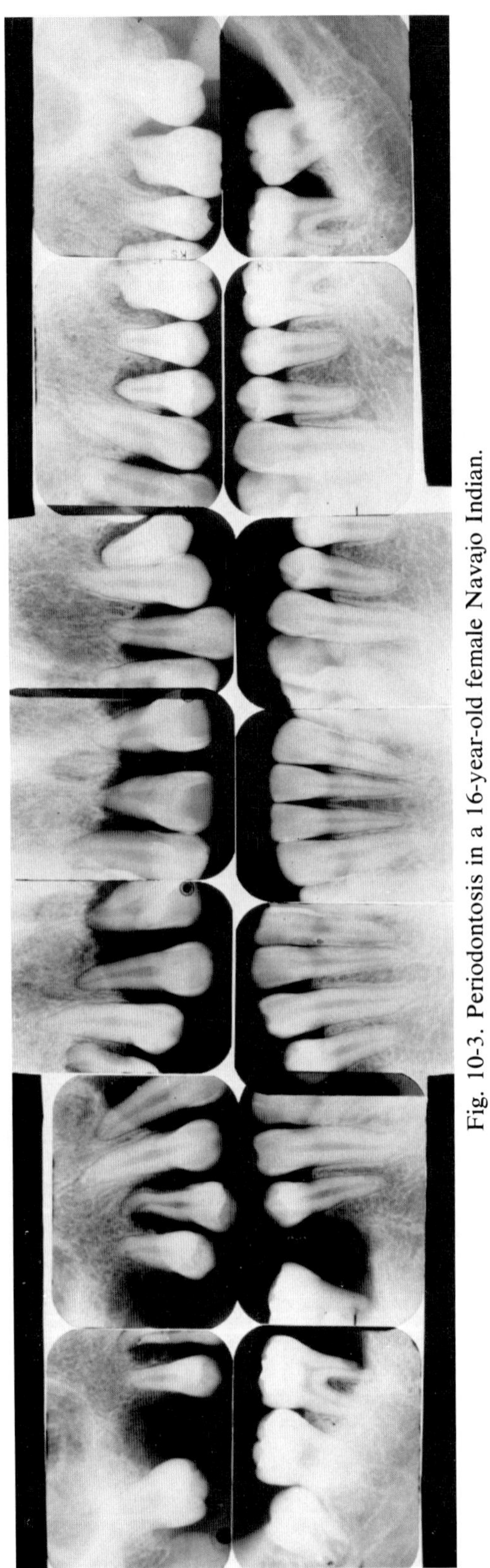

Fig. 10-3. Periodontosis in a 16-year-old female Navajo Indian.

epidemiologists. Advanced disease was seen in 5 percent of Lebanese children aged 10 to 14 years, and in 10 percent of Palestinian children in refugee camps in Lebanon. Refugee girls in Lebanon as young as 12 years of age were found with extensive loss of alveolar bone. Russell[21] has also reported finding advanced periodontal disease in about 3.0 percent of white and 3.2 percent of black children in the United States. In Nigeria, on the other hand, the prevalence was so extremely high that by age 20 to 29 years most of the villagers were already approaching the terminal stages of periodontal destruction.[22] In a study[11] at a Navajo Indian School, in which the student body ranged from 12 to 18 years of age, 14 cases were found out of a total student body of 2,050. Orban[19] stated that this group of diseases comprised about 15 percent of all periodontal disorders. This extremely high figure was probably the result of his interpretation of what constituted periodontosis. For instance, adults were included in his cases but excluded from most other reports.

There are several distinctive features of this disease that we think justifies its classification as a distinct clinical entity different from periodontitis. These features are:

1. Age of onset
2. Sex ratio
3. Familial background
4. Lack of relationship between local etiologic factors and severity of response (deep periodontal pockets).
5. Distinctive roentgenographic pattern of alveolar bone loss.
6. Rate of progression.
7. Lack of involvement of the primary teeth.

Onset. The onset of the disease is insidious and occurs during the circumpubertal period, that is, between the ages of 11 and 13. Available evidence indicates that the alveolar bone loss is not due to a developmental or congenital absence

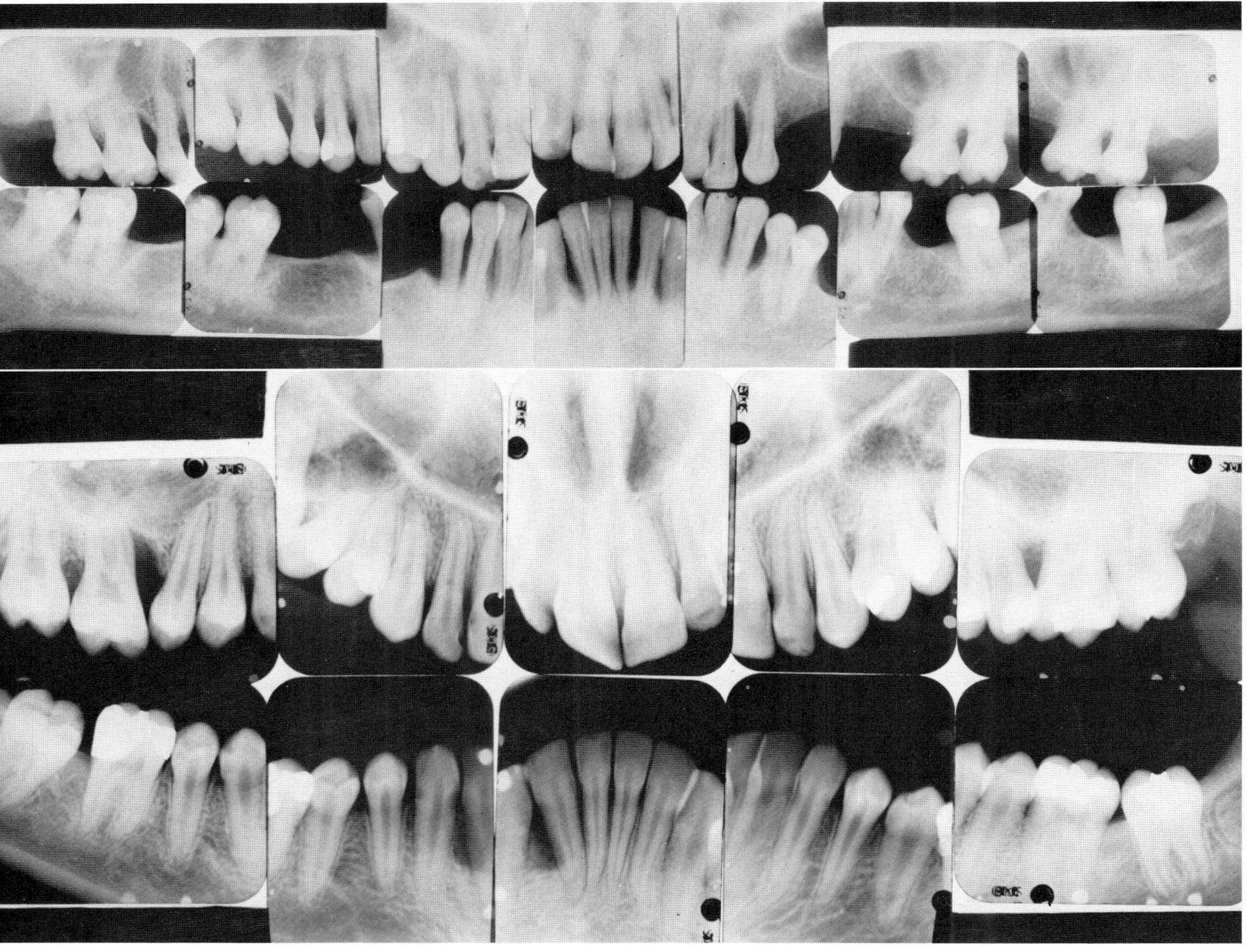

Fig. 10-4. *Top.* Periodontitis in mother, 31 years of age. *Bottom.* In daughter, 13 years old.

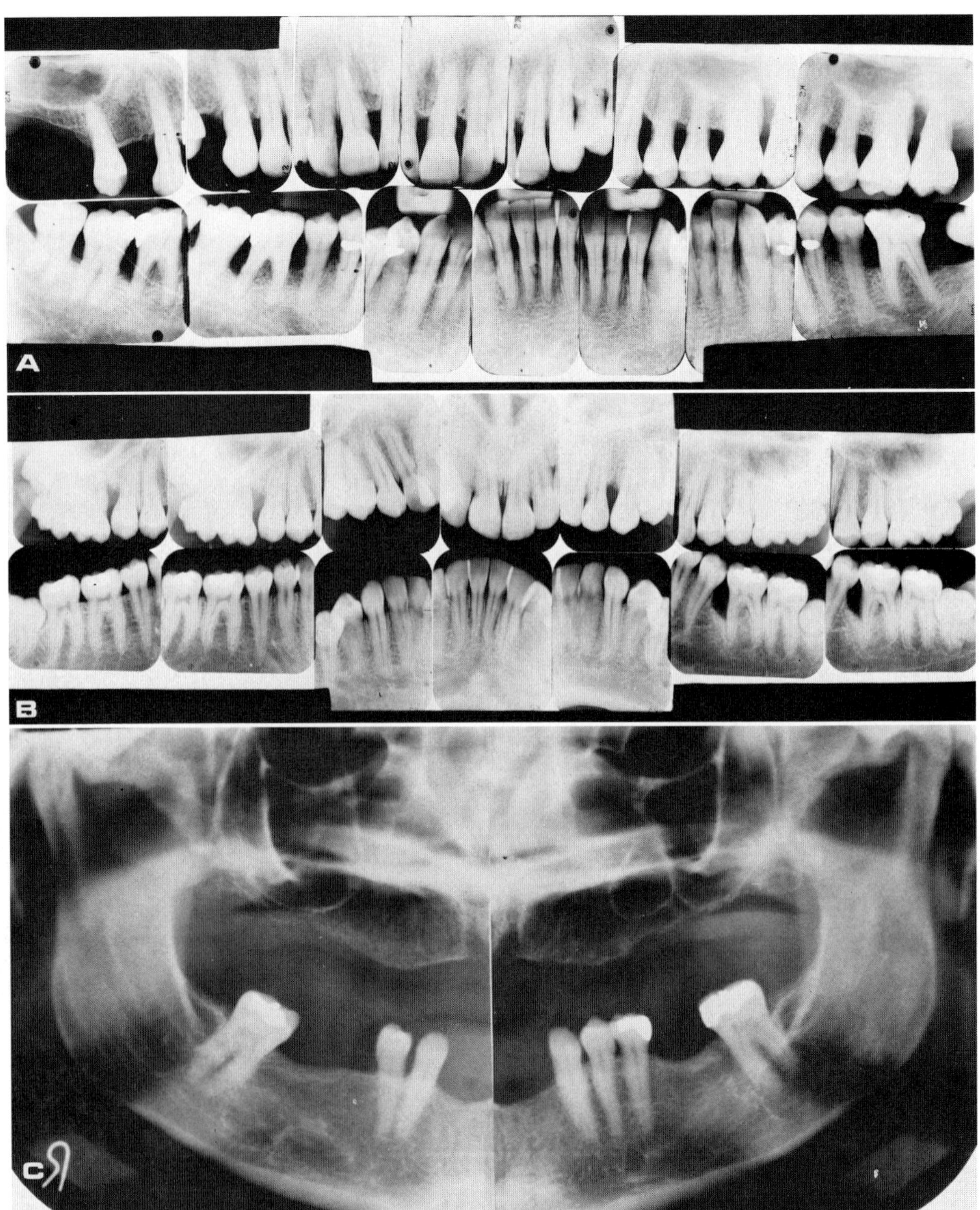

Fig. 10-5. *A*. A father, 41 years old, with adult type periodontitis.
B. The daughter, 14 years old, showed roentgenographic evidence of bone loss confined to the maxillary left first molar and the maxillary right lateral incisor and mandibular right first molar.
C. The mother, 32 years of age, had a history of early tooth loss as a result of periodontal disease. The pattern of remaining teeth is consistent with that found in periodontosis.

or defect. The alveolar bone is present and does appear to develop normally with the normal eruption of the teeth, and only subsequently does the alveolar bone undergo resorptive changes (see Fig. 10-2 *Bottom*).

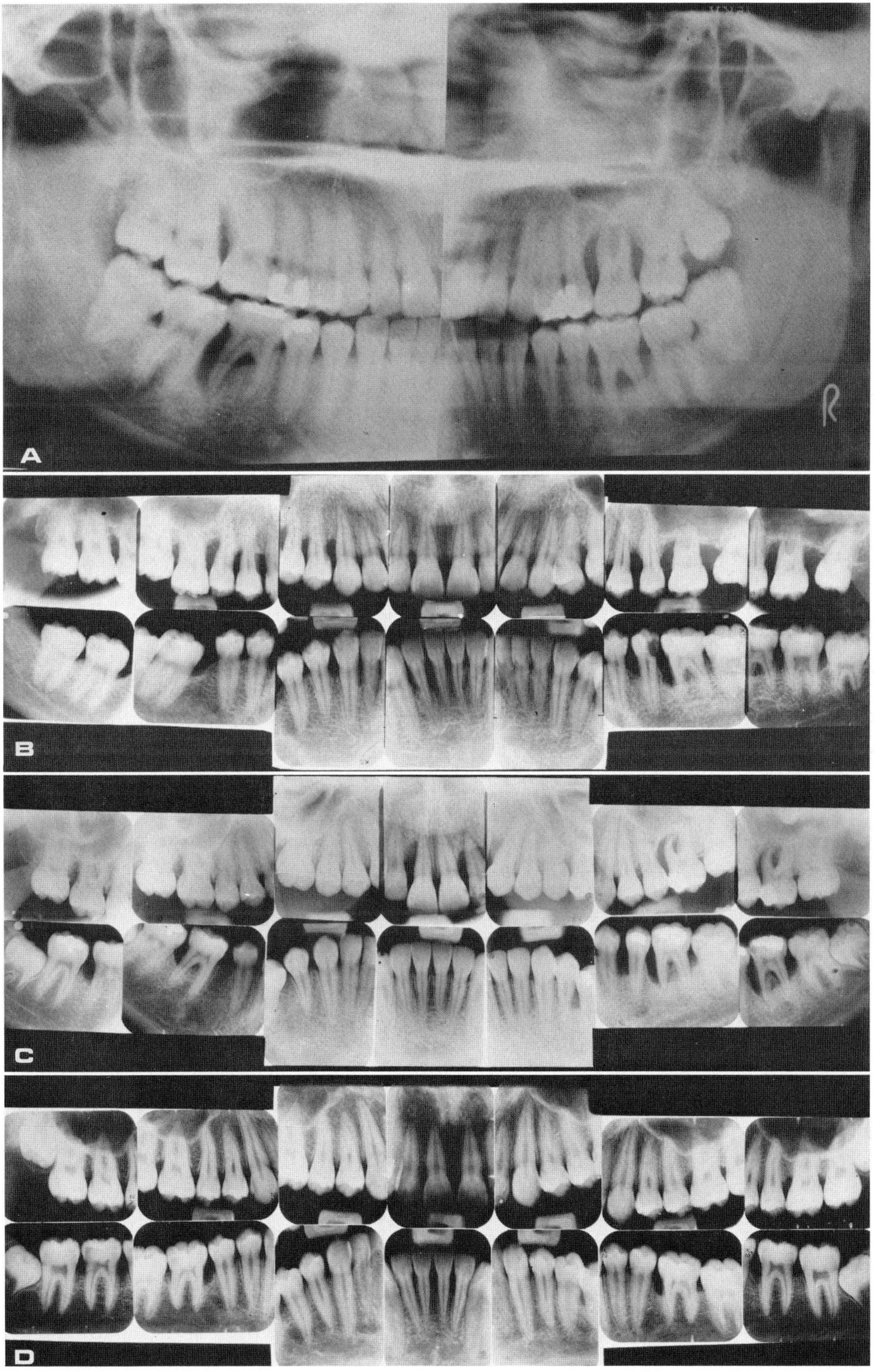

Fig. 10-6. Periodontosis in siblings. *A*. A 22-year-old female. *B*. A 21-year-old female. *C*. A 16-year-old female. *D*. A 15-year-old male.

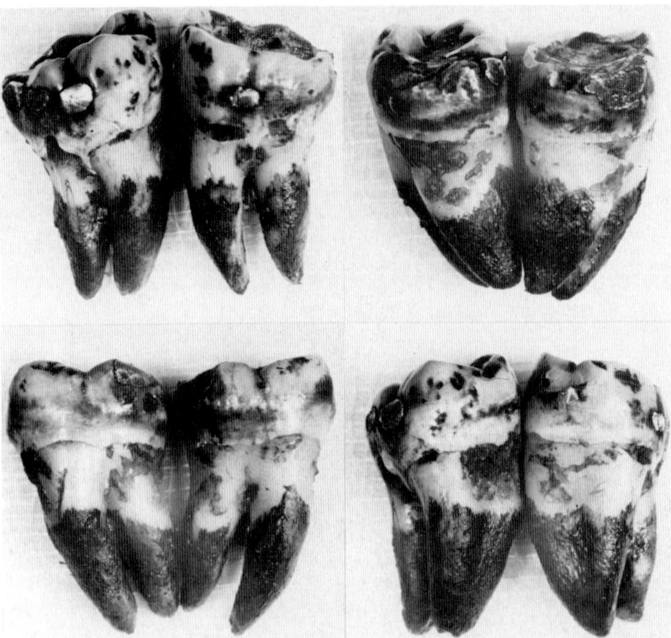

Fig. 10-7. Stained extracted molars exhibiting a three-dimensional "mirror image" pattern of connective tissue loss. (Courtesy of Dr. Ralph S. Kaslick.)

In the generalized form of this disease the age of onset varies with different teeth in the same individual. For instance, while all the first molars and mandibular incisors may be involved at 13 years of age, the maxillary lateral incisors or bicuspids may not show roentgenographic evidence of alveolar bone loss until 3 to 5 years later.

Sex ratio. It has been consistently reported that this disease affects more females than males. In our own studies of over 85 cases, the sex ratio has been approximately 3:1 females to males affected.

Race. This disease has been found in all racial groups studied to date. It has been seen in the Caucasian, Negro, Chinese, American Indian (Fig. 10-3) and in patients from India.

Familial background. In more than half the cases in our studies the disease has been found to have a familial background.[6,7,8] We have found it in 3 sets of identical twins, in numerous parent-offsprings (Figs. 10-4 and 10-5), siblings (Fig. 10-6), first cousins and uncles and nephews. It has also been found to have a tendency to follow the maternal side of the line.

Kaslick and Chasens[15] have shown that in many instances the lesions produce a bilateral mirror image pattern of loss of periodontal ligament attachment on the roots of the teeth (Fig. 10-7) when they are stained. This evidence further supports the role of genetic factors in the etiology of periodontosis.[1]

In two cases, other problems of an unusual nature occurred in a sibling. In one

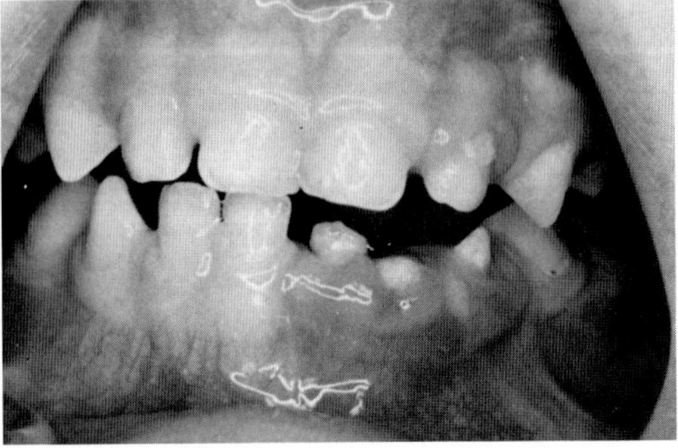

Fig. 10-8. Odontodysplasia in the 3-year-old brother of patient shown in Figure 10-10.

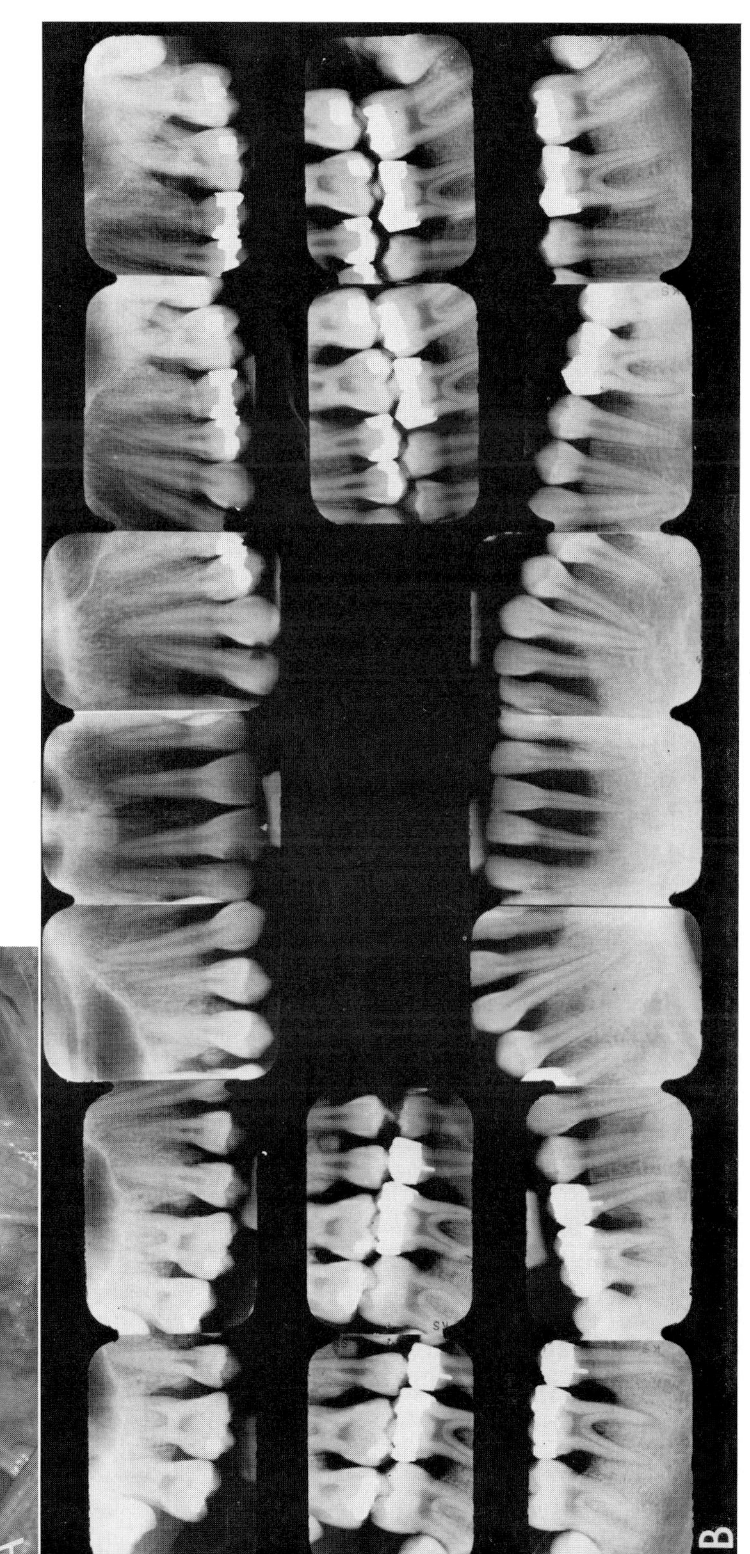

Fig. 10-9. *A*. Periodontosis in a 14-year-old female. Clinically, the inflammation is minimal, although the periodontal pockets are deep.
B. Roentgenographs of the above patient. All areas demonstrating bone loss can be probed.

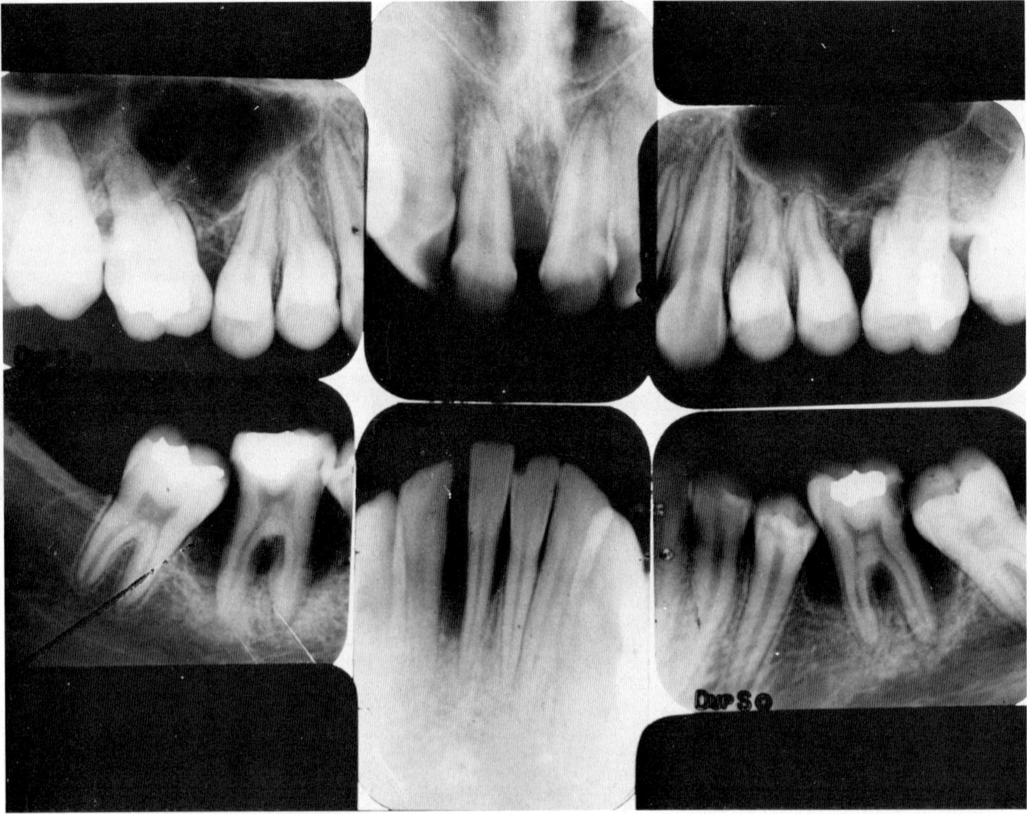

Fig. 10-10. Note the malalignment of the mandibular posterior teeth in this 14-year-old female. Improperly contoured jackets are present in maxillary central incisors, placing these teeth in occlusal trauma.

instance the 3-year-old brother of a periodontosis patient was found to have odontodysplasia of the mandibular left cuspid, and lateral and central incisors (Fig. 10-8). In the other case, the sister of a periodontosis patient developed glaucoma at 25 years of age.

Etiology and Clinical Characteristics. During puberty the most common form of periodontal disease is an inflammatory hyperplastic gingivitis associated with poor oral hygiene, plaque and supragingival calculus. Untreated, the disease usually progresses into a periodontitis. In periodontosis, on the other hand, the gingiva, at least in the early stages, is most frequently normal in appearance, having a normal color and physiologic contour. In the very early stages of this disease, therefore, the diagnosis is most often made as a result of a routine dental examination in which roentgenographs are used. However, even where the gingiva does have a normal clinical appearance, if bone loss is evident roentgenographically an examination with the aid of a periodontal probe will reveal a true periodontal pocket. Gross deposits of subgingival calculus are uncommon, even in pockets that extend almost down to the apices of the roots (Fig. 10-9). This is true whether the teeth are examined clinically with the aid of an explorer, roentgenographically, or visually after the affected teeth have had to be extracted. If these teeth are decalcified and studied microscopically, plaque

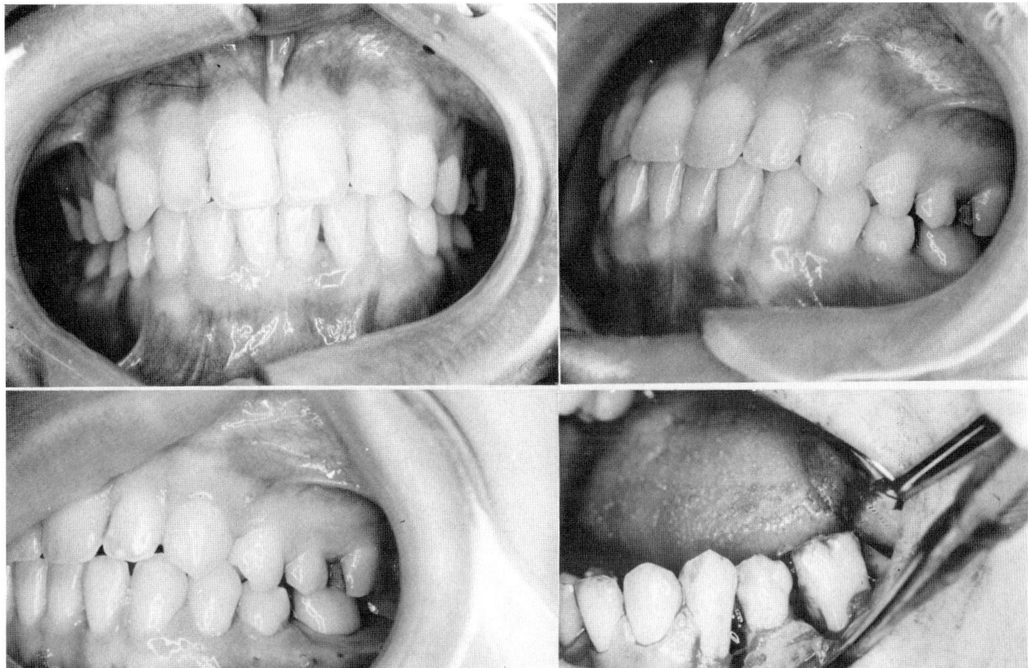

Fig. 10-11. *Top left.* A 19-year-old female with advanced periodontosis, anterior view. The gingiva is within normal limits.
Top right. The same patient, lateral view.
Bottom left. Probe has marked the depths of the periodontal pockets in the mandibular posterior region.
Bottom right. The flap is retracted and granulation is removed to demonstrate the extent of bony involvement.

will be seen adhering to the root surfaces. There are of course patients whose oral hygiene is poor and who do have obvious plaque and supragingival calculus. In these instances gingival inflammation is present. Gingival inflammation is also commonly observed in the very advanced cases.

In some patients with periodontosis one can elicit a history of their having injured (actually fractured) a crown of one or more of their incisor teeth as a result of an accident. Subsequently in these cases the affected tooth or teeth were restored improperly and thus placed in occlusal trauma. In a few instances other occlusal problems, such as a malalignment of the posterior teeth (Fig. 10-10) or some obvious centric or balancing side prematurity in the first molar region, can also be found. However, even after such a premature contact has been established, it is impossible to tell whether it is a cause for the disease, or as Gottlieb[13] assumed, a consequence of it.

In the majority of cases of periodontosis the amount of periodontal destruction observed is not commensurate with the amount of local irritants that can be found. The alveolar bone loss is vastly out of proportion to what one would expect from the local etiologic factors present in a patient of that age (Fig. 10-11).

Bacteriologic findings. Preliminary findings at the Forsyth Dental Center indicate that there is an unusual bacterial flora in the periodontal pockets of patients with periodontosis.[17A] The microbiota of their periodontal pockets is dominated by gram–anaerobic rods. Two clearly distinguishable types were found: a motile, curved, fermentative rod, and a nonmotile pleo-

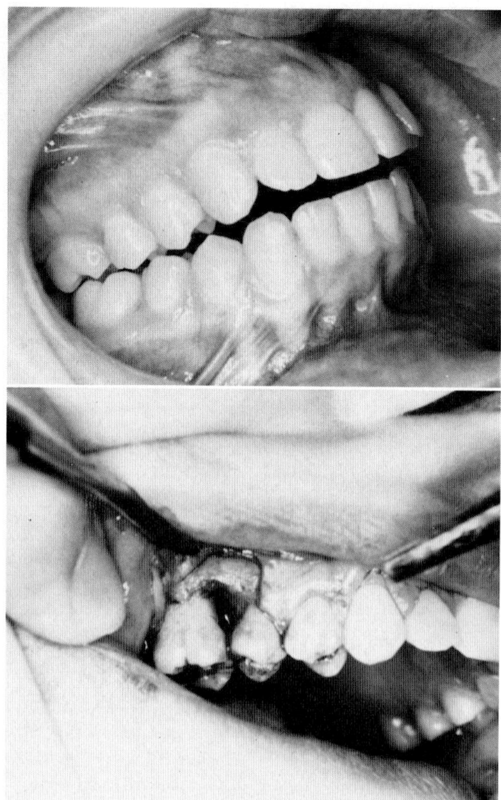

Fig. 10-12. *Top.* In the early lesion the gingival color and contour may be within normal limits.
Bottom. Type of bony defect found in the above patient (i.e., a 3-walled infrabony pocket).

morphic, small rod. This group of microorganisms presents a strong contrast to the organisms usually found in the periodontal pockets of patients with periodontitis.

Medical histories, examinations and laboratory tests. The medical histories by and large are noncontributory. This assessment is based on the fact that every patient in our study received the following minimal laboratory tests: a urinalysis, complete and differential white blood counts, sedimentation rates, hemoglobin, hematocrit, serology and chest plate; in addition, every patient received a physical examination. In selected cases the following laboratory tests and/or roentgenograms were also done: glucose tolerance, serum calcium, phosphorus and alkaline phosphatase, C-reactive protein, capillary fragility, chromosome study, calcium metabolism studies utilizing calcium-47;[19] skeletal surveys that included the thoracic spine, lumbosacral spine, cervical spine, both hands and wrists, right arm, right femur and right lower leg; and hemoglobin electrophoresis studies. It was not possible to demonstrate any generalized metabolic defect in any of these patients with any of the techniques used.

Psychiatric component. In the absence of a familial history the one outstanding feature which has occurred with marked regularity has been the presence of emotional or psychiatric problems. The following case histories illustrates this point.

CASE HISTORY 1

The patient was an 18-year-old female who admitted a fingernail and lip-biting habit. She was aware also that she clenched her incisor teeth when under emotional tension.

The past medical history included the usual childhood illnesses without sequellae. Her father had died of accidental causes. Because she did not feel welcome in the home of her stepfather she had been living with an aunt, several hundred miles away from her home.

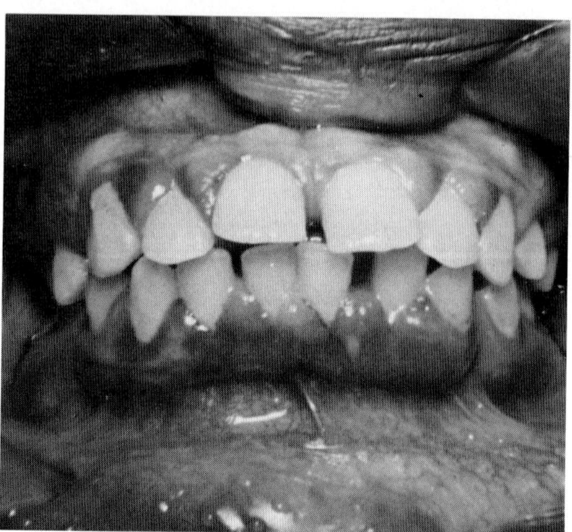

Fig. 10-13. An 18-year-old female with advanced periodontosis. Diastema formation and inflammation are common in the very advanced stage.

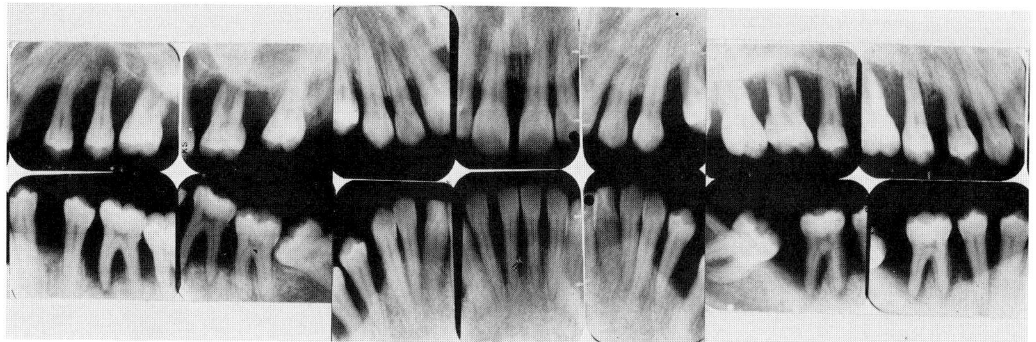

Fig. 10-14. The same patient shown in Figure 10-13. Note generalized form of the disease.

She had a poor school record and had not received a high school diploma. She was hospitalized overnight on one occasion, at age 17, for taking an overdose of sleeping pills. She had little or no interest in working at the jobs available to her. She had received some psychiatric care on a temporary basis. Her only physical complaints had been intermittent headaches and an episode of temporary blindness at age 17 which was treated at Massachusetts General Hospital as an emotional disorder.

CASE HISTORY 2

A 13-year-old female with a 2-year history of periodontosis was referred for psychiatric evaluation. During a stress interview, she was able to localize some of her sources of anxiety:

1. Her grandmother has been taken to the hospital on several occasions and the patient is concerned that she will die.
2. The patient is also concerned that she will lose her teeth as her parents did. Both parents had all their teeth extracted, the mother in her thirties and the father just recently.
3. The patient's father drinks excessively on the weekends and when drunk becomes sexually abusive to the patient, which she reacts to by fleeing from the house and running off to her friends.
4. She is excessively concerned over her weight. She is slightly obese, but not fat, and feels that she is unattractive and will be unable to date.

On testing, her IQ was found to be in the above normal range, 110 to 120. There are no organic signs or symptoms present, neither are there any symptoms suggesting a psychosis. The patient does exhibit numerous signs of excessive anxiety. She has been a nail-biter all her life and during the interviews constantly twirled her hair with her fingers. The mother stated that she is constantly doing something with her hands at home, moving objects from one place to another, picking things up, putting things down. It is also of note that according to her mother the patient grinds her teeth in her sleep at night.

The family setting is somewhat less than ideal, the patient being the only child. Her father, aged 50, had been married previously, was divorced secondary to infidelity on his wife's part, and had married the patient's mother, who is 51, who also had been married previously and whose husband had died overseas. The patient's father holds two jobs, is away from home from 6:00 in the morning until 4:00 in the afternoon, then leaves at 4:30 to return at 11:00 p.m. On Saturdays he is away from home from 7:00 a.m. to 3:00 p.m. The patient is a good student in school, getting A's and B's. It is of note that her extracurricular activities consist of baton twirling, which her mother forced upon her as "a good source of income in her later life." The patient, I believe, is not really enjoying this activity, and is using passive-aggressive defense by just not practicing at it.

Diagnosis: Anxiety reaction in an adolescent with secondary excessive grinding and clenching of the teeth.

CASE HISTORY 3

A 21-year-old female, married since last November, was referred to psychiatry because of extreme sensitivity to dental examination

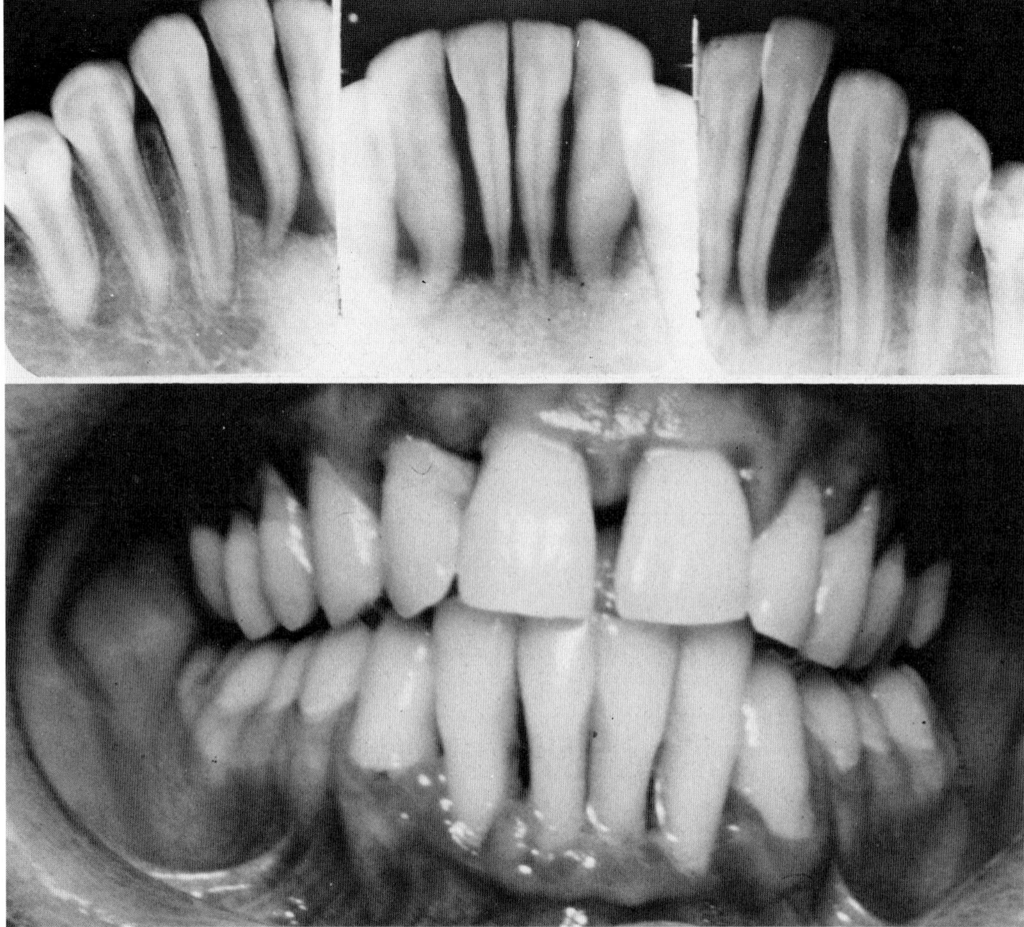

Fig. 10-15. *Top.* Circumferential loss of alveolar bone in a 16-year-old male. *Bottom.* The same patient shows extensive gingival recession. This is an unusual form of periodontosis.

as well as some bizarre features and an admission that she sometimes feels she is "going crazy."

The patient easily revealed that for the past two or three years she had suffered repeated hallucinatory experiences. Most commonly she sees a man in her bedroom or wakes up after a nightmare and hears people laughing at her. She also has "headaches" which turn out not to be really painful but are sensations of "something wrong" in the head, concentrated at both temples and the occiput. During these episodes, which may last as long as two days, she feels as though her head is filled with hair. The episodes are precipitated by upsetting events, either arguments or visual or auditory experiences which seem to have particular meaning for her. For example, she was looking at a psychedelic record album cover and suddenly thought that it had hair coming out of it, and she quickly went on to have a headache. She did not report olfactory hallucinations, "unreality" feelings or any evidence that she goes into automatic activities or has long amnesic spells.

The patient grew up in a large family, first in Alabama, then in Chicago and the Washington area. Several siblings have "emotional problems" of probably considerable severity. She had been living with her brother until she married. She said that marriage had been a disappointment. She works as a secretary, enjoys the job, and is successful at it.

Diagnosis. She appears to be a psychotic person who has managed to live a reasonably stable life by limiting her activities to relatively conflict-free areas, particularly work. I believe that marriage has been a stress on her and has increased the frequency and intensity of her hallucinatory episodes, which seem clearly related to unconscious sexual fantasies. Her dynamics are probably of the hysterical type, but the severity of the symptoms, particularly the hallucinations and the flattening of affect, point to a psychotic disturbance, probably schizophrenia. The sensations of something being wrong in her head, which take a very concrete form clearly related to unconscious fantasies, are very characteristic of schizophrenia.

Clinical Characteristics. *Early lesion.* There are neither subjective symptoms, tooth mobilities, nor obvious defects in gingival color, tone or contour early in the disease. The diagnosis is usually made fortuitously as a result of a routine dental examination, which includes a full mouth series of roentgenographs. Gingivitis, however, may be present if local irritational factors, such as calculus, or poor restorative dentistry, is present. Examination with a periodontal probe, nevertheless, will always reveal the presence of a periodontal pocket on one or more proximal surfaces of two or more first molar teeth and, also frequently, one or more incisor teeth. The initial lesions are generally confined to the first molar and incisor teeth. When a buccal flap is retracted about the involved teeth, invariably a 3-walled infrabony defect is present (Fig. 10-12). It is usually confined to one proximal tooth surface of two or more of the first

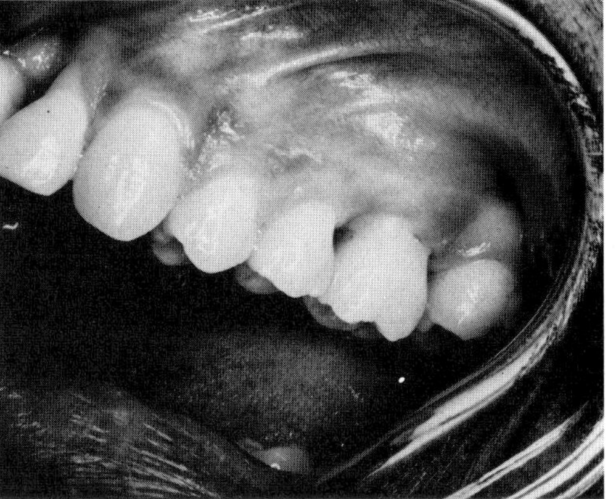

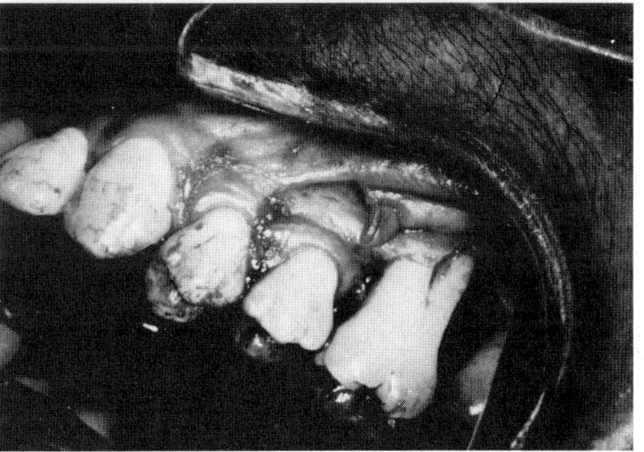

Fig. 10-17. *Top.* The clinical appearance of the gingiva in an advanced case in a 16-year-old male.
Bottom. Note the extent of bone loss in the above patient.

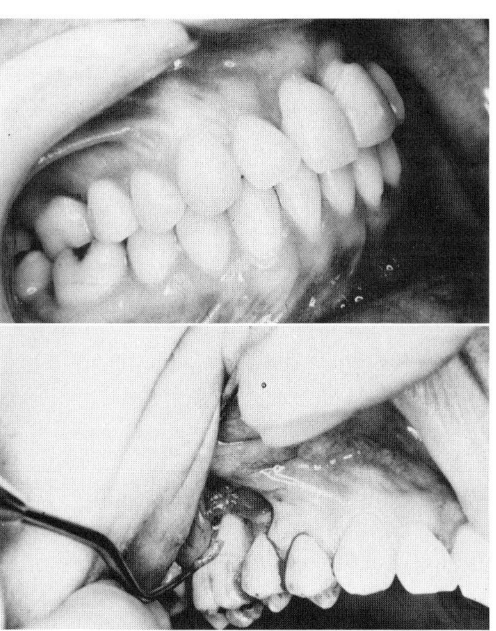

Fig. 10-16. *Top.* The clinical appearance of the maxillary posterior teeth in a moderately advanced case in a 16-year-old female.
Bottom. The flap is retracted to show bone loss extending around the proximal surface and involving the buccal aspect of the molar.

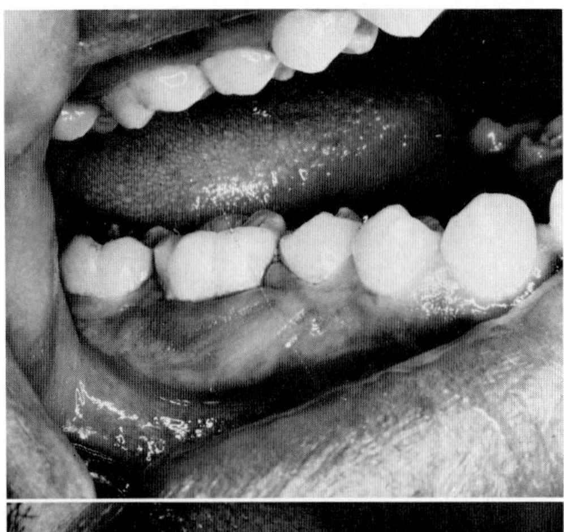

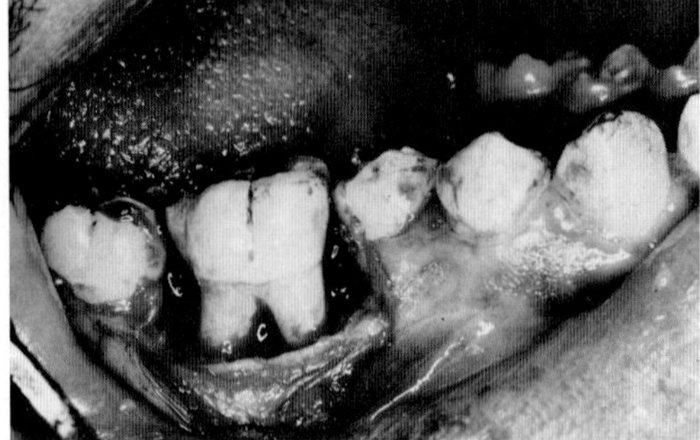

Fig. 10-18. *Top.* The clinical appearance of the gingiva in an advanced case.
Bottom. Note the extent of bone loss in the above patient.

molars. The straight buccal and lingual plates of cortical bone, in all cases examined to date, have always been intact early in the disease. This explains the lack of clinically detectable tooth mobility.

Advanced lesion. Pathological tooth mobility, wandering and diastema formation are prominent features of the advanced disease. The presence of gingival inflammation is variable, but more common as the disease increases in severity (Fig. 10-13). The increased tooth mobility and tooth migration encourage food impactions and retention. In some patients the disease remains limited to the first molars and one or more incisors, while in others it affects almost the entire maxillary dentition (Fig. 10-14) and, to a lesser degree, most, but not all of the mandibular arch. Periodontal pockets measuring 8 to 10 mm. and furcation involvements of the molar and first bicuspid teeth are common findings. In a few patients the loss of bone is circumferential in nature (Fig. 10-15 *Top*) and severe gingival recessions occur concomitant with the alveolar bone loss. (Fig. 10-15 *Bottom*). Most frequently in the advanced molar-incisor case, the bone loss about the molar teeth extends from the proximal surface around the mesio- and/or distobuccal line angles (Fig. 10-16) until it involves the bifurcation (Figs. 10-17 and 10-18). The buccal cortical plate is more often involved to a greater degree than the lingual or palatal cortical plate, although there are exceptions to this. Excluding the terminal cases in which no bone is present about one or more of the molar roots, the apical portion of the deep infrabony defect is invariably a 3-walled pocket. The more cervical portions, on the other hand, are usually one or 2-walled infrabony pockets. While calculus is frequently present on the more cervical portion of the root, it is rarely seen further apically on the root surface.

When the incisor teeth are involved, the labial plate as well as both proximal walls of alveolar bone are frequently found to be missing.

In cases in which the disease has progressed to the point that extractions of all the maxillary teeth are indicated, it has been our observation that these patients experience little difficulty in adjusting to a full maxillary denture (Fig. 10-19).

Roentgenographic Findings. Vertical loss of alveolar bone about the first molars and one or more incisor teeth in an otherwise healthy adolescent is a diagnostic sign of periodontosis. The pattern of bone loss in the well-established so-called "classical" case is usually described as an arc-shaped loss of alveolar bone extending from the distal surface of the second bicuspid to the mesial surface of the second molar. The bone loss in the posterior regions occurs bilaterally, and the right and left sides are generally mirror images of each

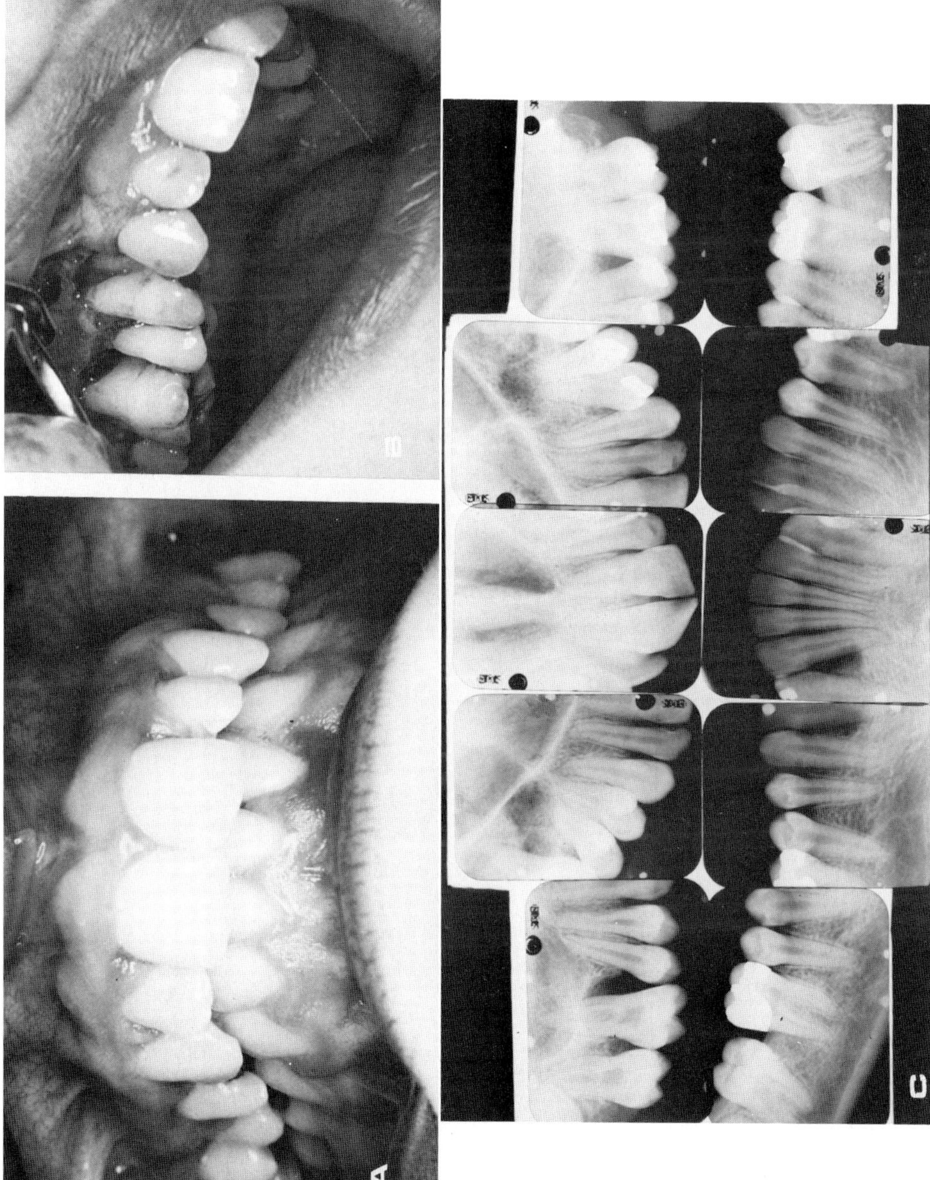

Fig. 10-19. *A*. A female patient, 13 years old.
B. The flap is retracted to demonstrate extent of bone loss in first bicuspid and first molar area in this 13-year-old patient.
C. Roentgenographs taken at 13 years of age did not reveal bicuspid involvement even though it was actually present as shown in *B* above.

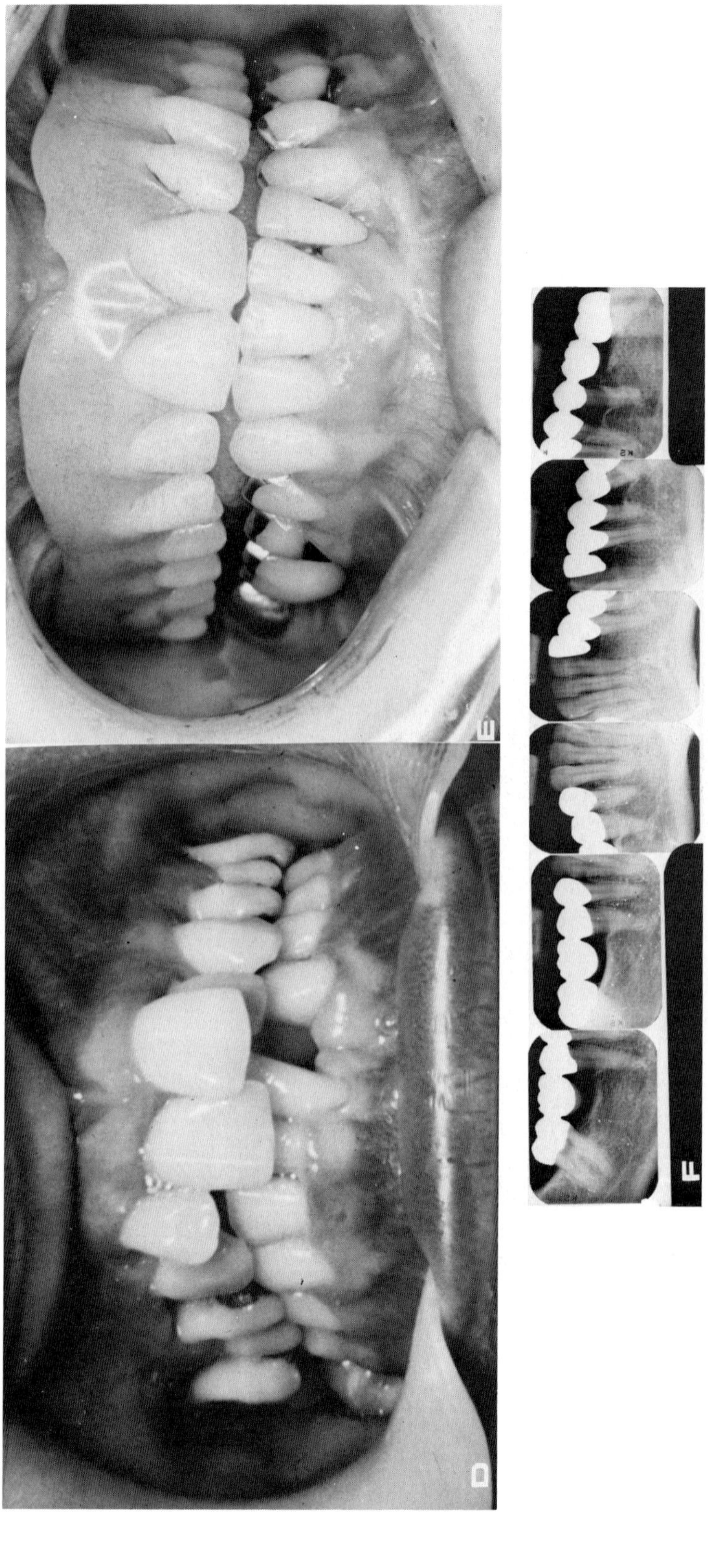

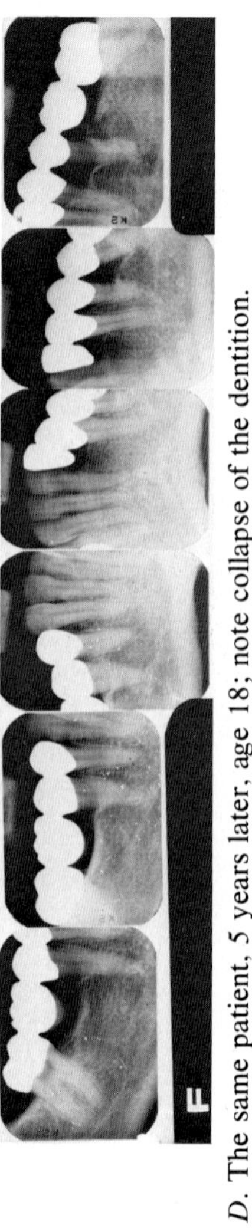

Fig. 10-19. *D*. The same patient, 5 years later, age 18; note collapse of the dentition. *E*. The same patient, age 29; full maxillary denture and mandibular fixed prosthesis. *F*. Roentgenographs, at age 29, that is 16 years postoperative result. The patient has been stabilized with full maxillary denture and mandibular fixed prosthesis since age 18.

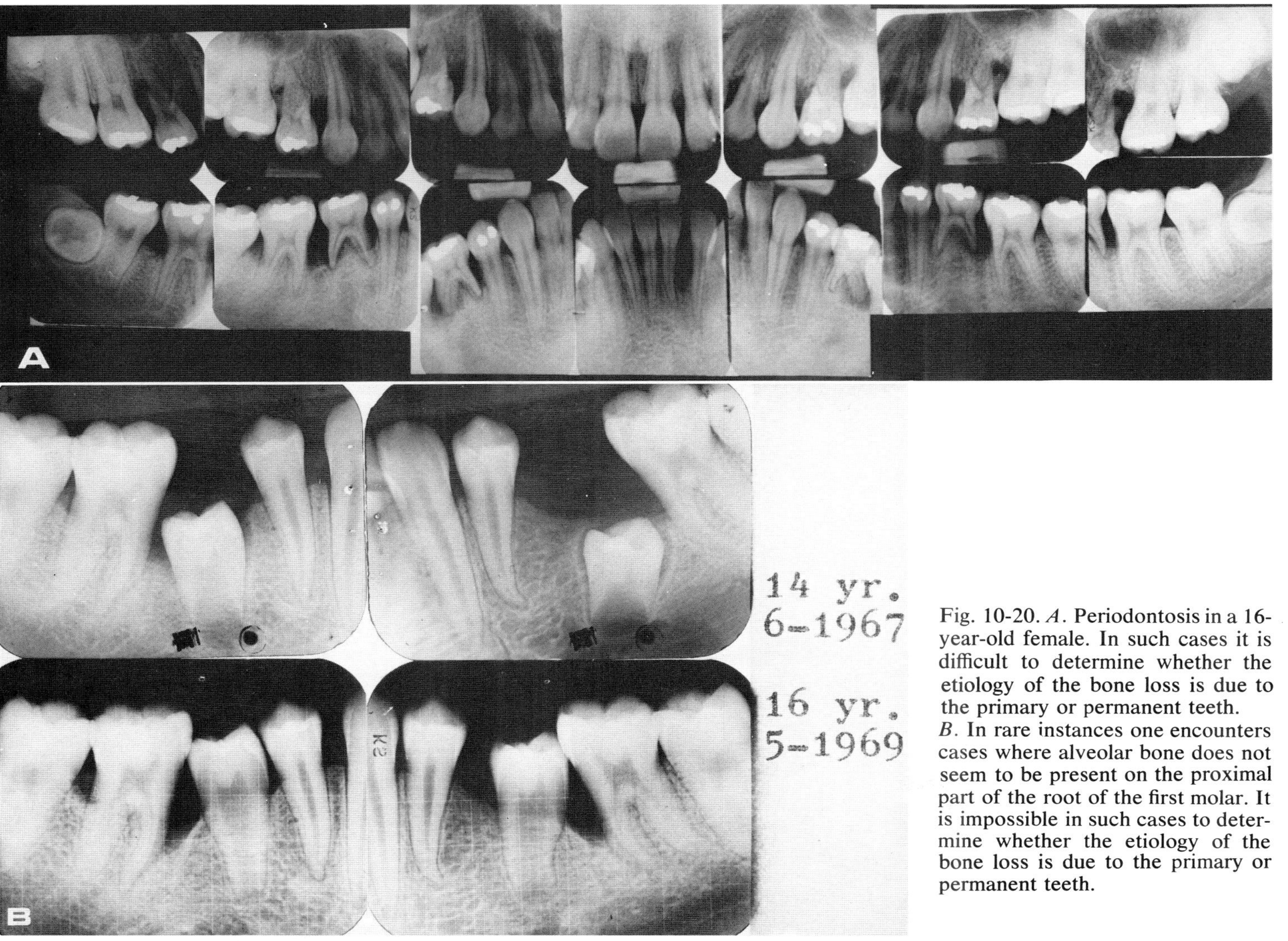

Fig. 10-20. *A*. Periodontosis in a 16-year-old female. In such cases it is difficult to determine whether the etiology of the bone loss is due to the primary or permanent teeth. *B*. In rare instances one encounters cases where alveolar bone does not seem to be present on the proximal part of the root of the first molar. It is impossible in such cases to determine whether the etiology of the bone loss is due to the primary or permanent teeth.

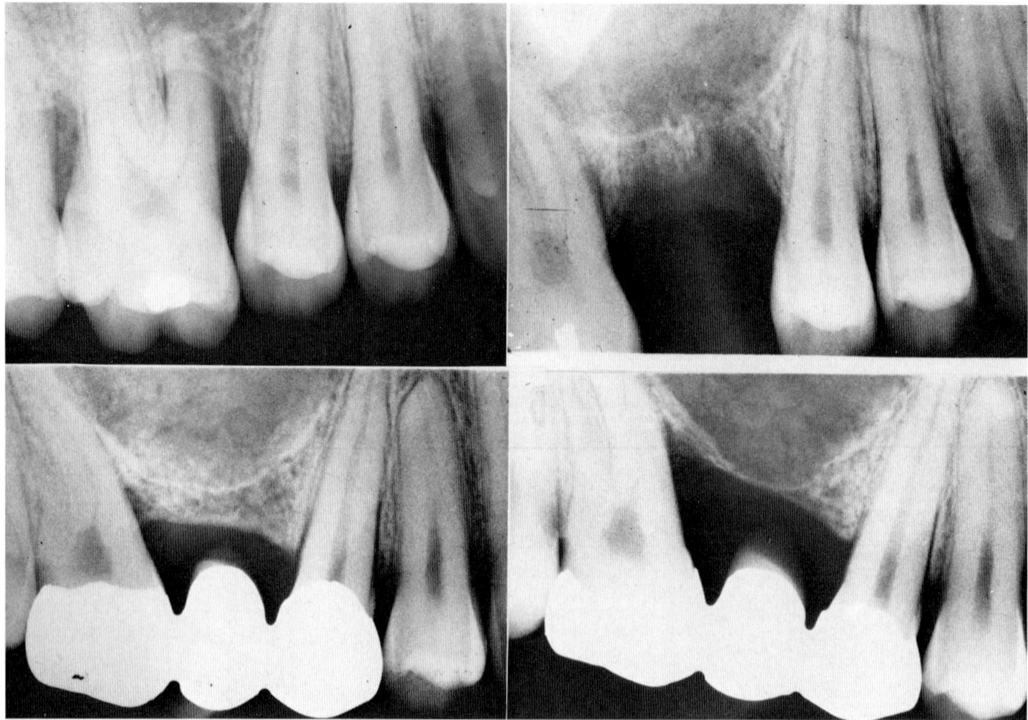

Fig. 10-21. *Top left.* Twenty-year-old male had periodontosis. The maxillary molar has severe periodontal involvement.
Top right. The maxillary first molar area following extraction.
Bottom left. The healed extraction site one year later.
Bottom right. Note the change in the position of the maxillary sinus in this three-year post-operative photograph. Compare with above. (Baer, and Everett.)[4]

other. While this is the so-called classical description, the patterns of bone loss are actually much more protean in nature. For instance, in rare instances the incisors are not involved, only the 4 first molars are (see Fig. 10-6 *A*). In other cases, only one proximal surface of the first molars may show loss of alveolar bone, and the disease may never progress to involve any of the other surfaces. In this latter instance it is the mesial surface which is most often affected. There are cases, however, where it is the distal surface. The extent and morphology of the bone loss generally depends upon whether the lesion is diagnosed in an early or advanced stage of the disease and whether the patient has the localized or generalized form. In the patient with the incipient localized disease the pattern of bone loss is not, as a rule, bilaterally similar. Most frequently, only one proximal surface of the first molar in each arch is initially involved (see Fig. 10-6*D*, p. 145). As the disease progresses, the contralateral proximal surfaces usually become affected until all 4 first molars assume their so-called classical mirror-image appearance. Since the buccal and lingual plates of alveolar bone are the last to resorb, the furcation areas of the molar teeth generally show radiolucencies only as a late manifestation of the disease. Also, as the disease progresses, the affected teeth tend to develop open proximal contacts. In the generalized form, all the teeth roentgenographically may approximate the same degree of alveolar bone loss (see Fig.

10-14). Therefore, as the terminal stage of the disease is reached, the bone loss is no longer vertical in nature but assumes a horizontal shape. The maxillary teeth are generally more severely affected. The molar teeth in both arches tend to have spindly roots, which results in a poor crown-root ratio. Histologic examination of the roots of the teeth has failed to reveal the presence of accessory root canals.

Progression. Unlike periodontitis, which progresses at a slow rate, periodontosis progresses rapidly. The present available roentgenographic evidence indicates that an affected tooth can have approximately three-fourths of its alveolar bone lost about one or more of its involved root surfaces within a period of 5 years or less from the time its inception is noted roentgenographically. This would be about 3 to 4 times the rate of progression for periodontitis.

In a few patients, the loss of alveolar bone may progress only to a certain point and then may remain stationary for many years. It is not known at this time whether this represents a "burnt-out" lesion, or whether it is merely one in which the disease process is progressing at an extremely slow rate. This phenomena is most often seen in a patient over 21 years of age.

Lack of Involvement of the Primary Teeth. In contradistinction to certain oral manifestations of systemic diseases, such as Down's syndrome, cyclic neutropenia, hypophosphatasia and Papillon-Lefèvre syndrome, the primary teeth in periodontosis are not affected and are not prematurely exfoliated because of destructive periodontal disease. It is true that in certain patients in whom the onset of the disease occurs during the period of the mixed dentition, it is sometimes difficult, if not impossible, to determine by roentgenographic examination alone whether the bone loss is associated with the normal exfoliation of the primary second molar or with the the onset of a destructive type

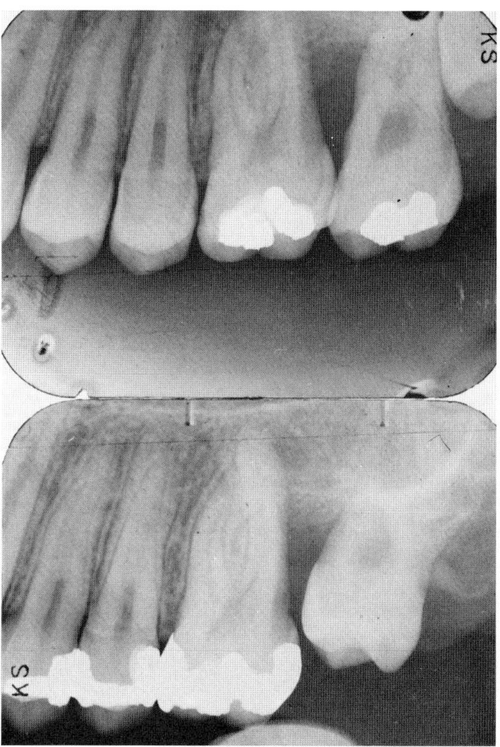

Fig. 10-22. *Top.* Horizontal bone loss between maxillary first and second molar. *Bottom.* The maxillary second molar was extracted but this did not solve the problem on the distal of the first molar.

of periodontal disease on the mesial aspect of the first permanent molar tooth (Fig. 10-20; see also Fig. 10-2 *Top* and Chap. 20). A careful evaluation of our own cases and those in the literature have led us to the conclusion that in periodontosis the primary teeth are not affected. It is a disease entirely of the permanent dentition. It should be remembered, however, that in a study on the prevalence of periodontal disease of the deciduous teeth[14] 25.2 percent of the 159 children examined had destructive periodontal disease of their primary teeth. It was also found that proportionately more boys than girls had the disease—just the reverse of periodontosis—but that the difference was not statistically significant. This type of destructive periodontal disease was thought to be related to the process of exfoliation that occurs

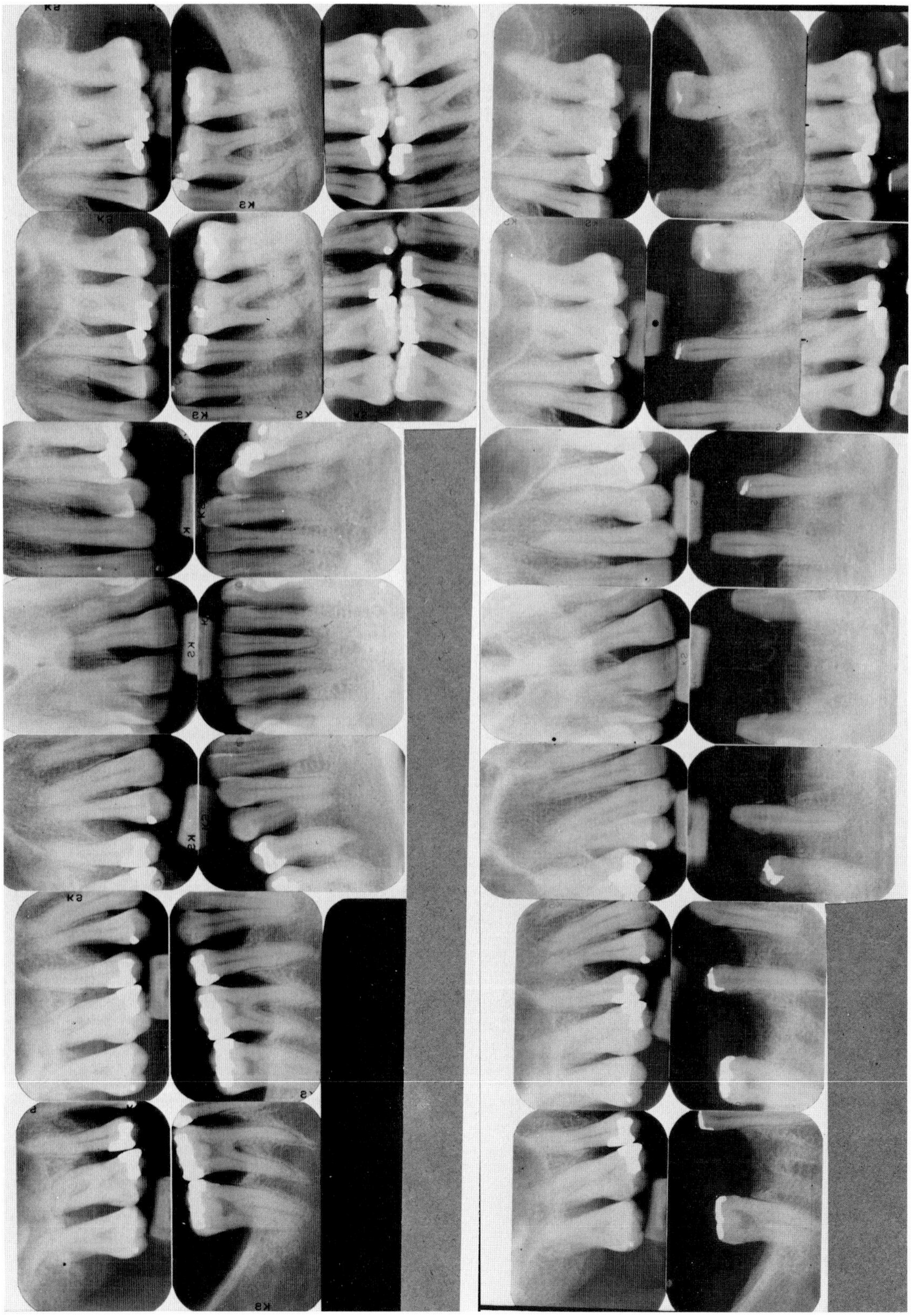

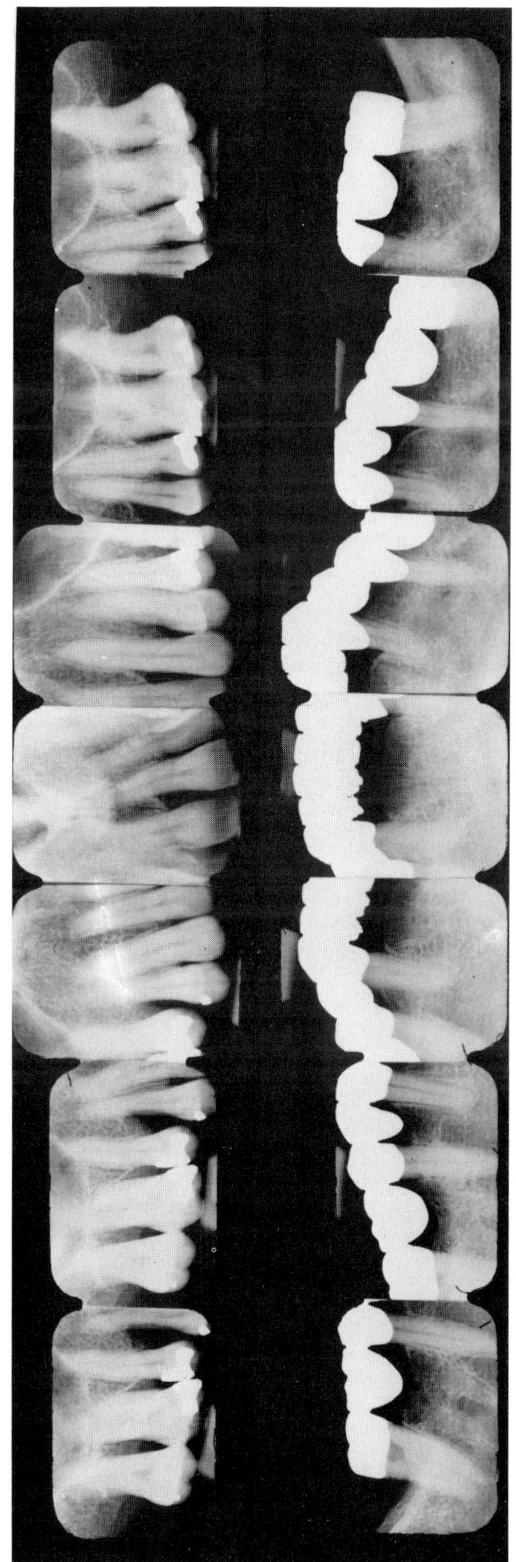

Fig. 10-23. *Top*. Extraction can be an excellent form of therapy when alternate teeth in the arch are affected. *Central*. A patient in a provisional mandibular splint, three years postoperative. *Bottom*. A patient in permanent mandibular splints, one year postoperative.

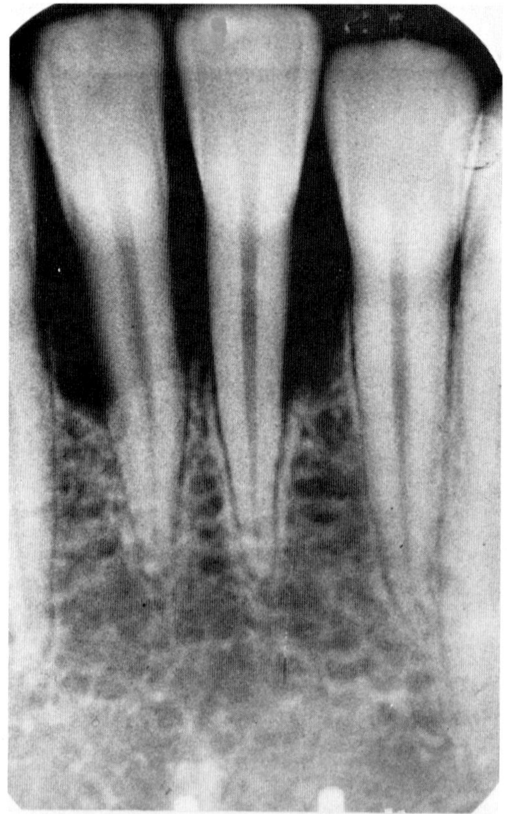

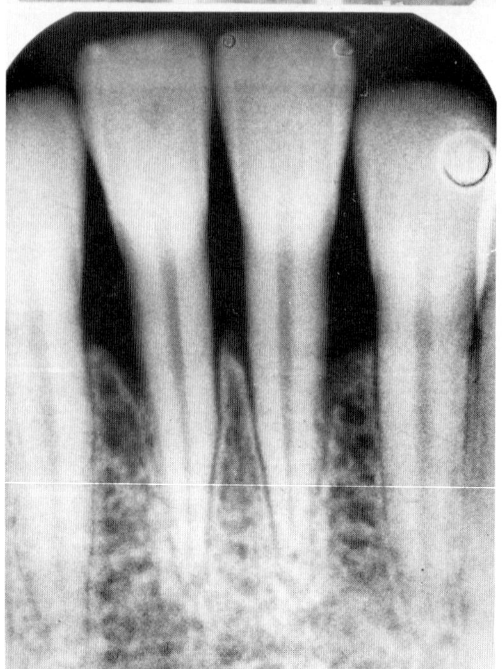

Fig. 10-24. *Top.* Note the bony defects and diastemas in this preoperative roentgenograph.
Bottom. This roentgenograph was taken two years postoperatively. Note the improvement in the bony contour and spontaneous closure of the diastema.

concomitantly with the normal eruption of the permanent teeth and should not be confused for periodontosis.

Caries and Periodontosis. We have not found that patients with periodontosis are any more immune to dental caries than other patients of their age and socioeconomical level. Occasionally one does see a patient with periodontosis who is caries free. This finding, however, may be fortuitous—particularly in areas of the country where the water supply is fluoridated. In fact, in our patients, caries has been a real problem in the maintenance of teeth with severe periodontal involvement.

Morphologic Dental Findings. The occurrence of short, slender roots, with a crown-root ratio of 1:1, instead of the normal ratio of 1:1½, is another frequent finding.

Treatment of Localized form of Periodontosis. *Selective tooth extraction.* Following extraction of the maxillary molar teeth, the maxillary sinus invariably enlarges [4,9,24,27] by resorbing the alveolar bone that formerly served to support the missing molar teeth. This can lead to the sinus occupying almost the entire edentulous area, leaving only a very thin cortical plate of bone over the alveolar ridge. If this condition occurs, periodontal therapy may be difficult or impossible for any of the remaining teeth in the area. This is the justification for employing sophisticated methods for the retention of the maxillary molar teeth which are involved with advanced disease. In carrying out these periodontal procedures, care must be taken to avoid violating the integrity of the maxillary sinus. The following example will illustrate this point.[4]

CASE HISTORY 4

The patient was a 20-year-old male with a diagnosis of periodontosis. The maxillary first molar had such severe periodontal involvement that it was extracted (Figs. 10-21 *Top left* and *right*). A roentgenograph taken one year later (Fig. 10-21 *Bottom left*) showed the extraction site completely healed. However, roentgenographs of this same area taken 2 years later revealed that the sinus was now located practically at the level of the alveolar crest (Fig. 10-21 *Bottom right*).

Another problem that may be encountered occurs when the loss of alveolar bone is horizontal and occurs between the maxillary first and second molars (Fig. 10-22 *Top*). In this type of situation the problem is whether to extract the first or second molar. In the case cited, the maxillary second molar was extracted in the hope that in the healing process, the bony defect on the distal of the first molar would be eliminated, but unfortunately this did not occur. By the time the patient was referred to us, not only was the periodontal lesion still present on the distal of the first molar, but the maxillary third molar had partially erupted, tilted and drifted mesially into the space formally occupied by the second molar (Fig. 10-22 *Bottom*). This situation caused food impaction interproximally between the maxillary first and third molar and led to the formation of a carious lesion on the distal of the first molar.

In the mandibular arch the extraction of a first molar may prove to be an easy solution for solving a difficult periodontal problem (see Fig. 10-19*F*).

Extractions also appear to be an excellent form of therapy in cases where al-

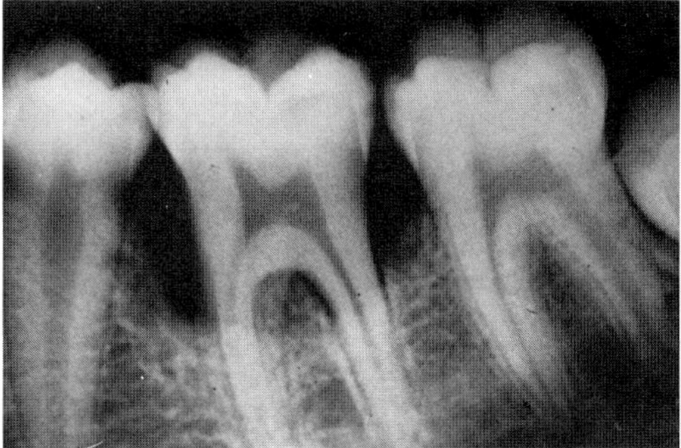

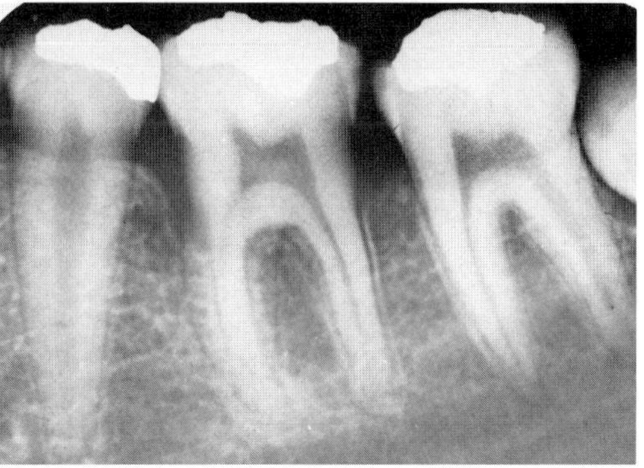

Fig. 10-26. *Top*. Preoperative roentgenograph.
Bottom. Two-year postoperative roentgenograph.

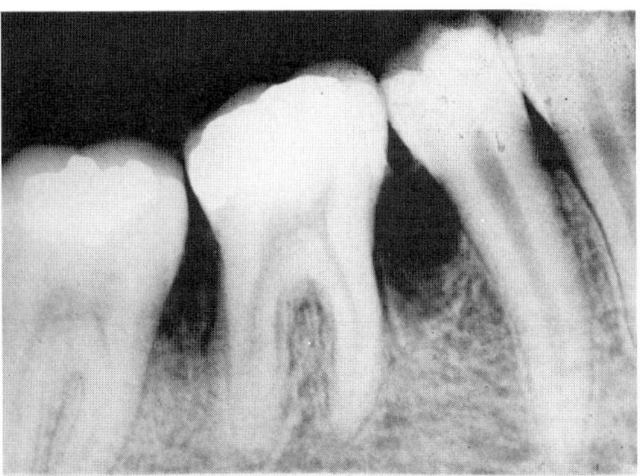

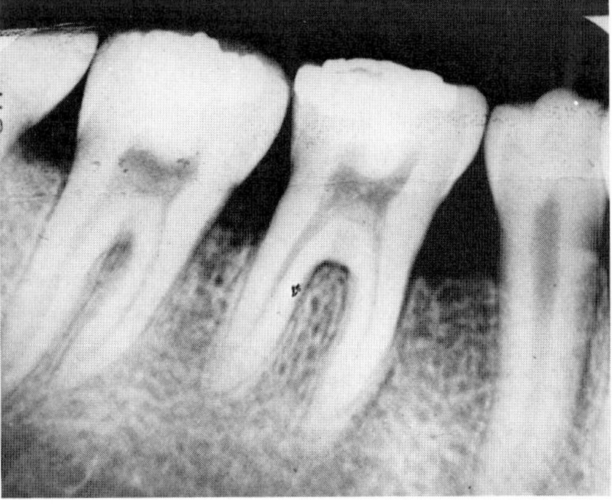

Fig. 10-25. *Top*. Note the proximal defect in the first molar area preoperative.
Bottom. Five-year postoperative results.

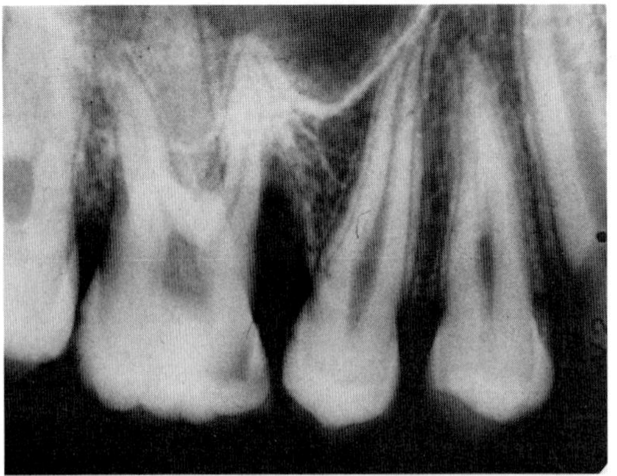

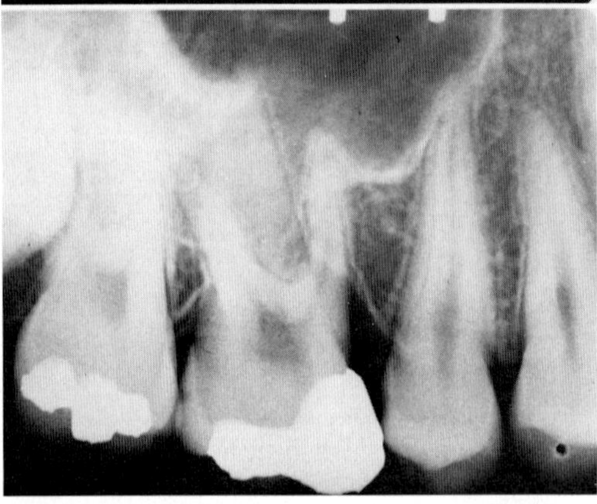

Fig. 10-27. *Top.* Preoperative roentgenograph.
Bottom. Postoperative result obtained.

ternate teeth in the arch are affected by the disease process. (Fig. 10-23).

Pedicle flap and grinding tooth. An excellent method of treating the tooth with an isolated infrabony defect is to use a full thickness mucoperiosteal pedicle flap to insure complete removal of all granulomatous tissue, and grinding the morsal surface of the tooth, at the same visit, until it is taken just slightly out of occlusion.[10] Grinding of the morsal surface to encourage eruption of the affected tooth should be repeated at weekly intervals during the first 4 to 6 weeks. The success encountered with this method of therapy may in part be explained by the rather unusual method of tooth grinding procedure used. If one believes that the etiology of periodontosis is cementopathia, as Gottlieb has stated, then the results obtained could be explained by the fact that grinding a tooth out of occlusion stimulates cementum formation.

It has been proven[23] experimentally, that cementum formation can be stimulated by taking a tooth out of occlusion and enabling it to erupt in a vertical direction (Figs. 10-24 through 10-30). This is another explanation for the results obtained. Of course, taking a tooth out of occlusion also eliminates occlusal trauma as an etiologic factor.

Root amputation. This technique is especially recommended for those cases where the periodontal lesion affects only one proximal surface of a maxillary first molar. Endodontic therapy, followed by amputation of the affected buccal root (Fig. 10-31) is an excellent means of eliminating the bony defect and creating an environment conducive to periodontal health in such situations.

Autotransplantation. Where other methods of periodontal therapy have been tried and have failed, or where the lesion is too advanced to be treated by the above methods, autotransplantation of the developing third molar into the extraction site of the periodontally involved first molar may prove to be a most effective method of therapy.[3] In the use of autotransplants it is recommended that the following rules be observed.

1. The developing donor third molar should have roots which are no less than 1/4 or more than 3/4 their completed length. Once root formation has been completed and the apices have closed the chances of success are minimal.

2. Check to see that the mesiodistal width of the donor third molar crown will fit into the first molar extraction site, and that the roots of the donor third molar are not so divergent that the tooth cannot be seated in the space available in the extraction site.

3. All granulation tissue should be left in situ following the extraction of the first molar.

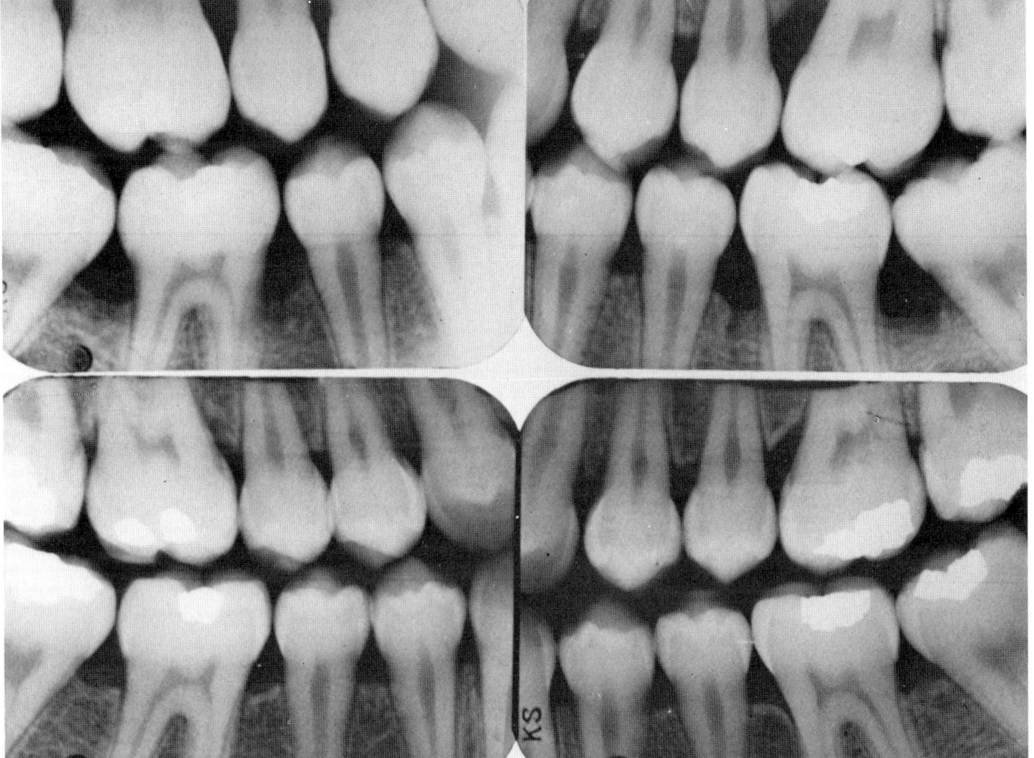

Fig. 10-28. Note the improved bone contours adjoining both lower and left upper first molars in the bottom pictures taken five months after the top two pictures.

4. The transplant should be seated so that it is in infra occlusion. To accomplish this it may be necessary to remove some of the alveolar bone from the bifurcation area of the extraction site. It is essential that the third molar be placed in a position below the occlusal plane of the adjacent teeth, thus preventing occlusal trauma. This will also encourage eruption of the transplant. The tooth must be carefully examined during the first 2 months to insure that it is not in traumatic occlusion, and is in fact kept just slightly out of occlusion during this critical period.

5. Do not use a rigid splint to hold the transplant in place. Crisscross sutures placed over the occlusal surface, plus the placement of a noneugenol periodontal dressing, should be sufficient to secure the transplant in place initially.

6. Extreme mobility of the transplant during the first 3 weeks is no cause for alarm. The transplantation procedure is shown in Figure 10-32. Results obtained are shown in Figures 10-33 through 10-40.

Prognosis. In the molar-incisor type of periodontosis the prognosis of the dentition as a whole is favorable. The prognosis of the individually involved teeth varies with the extent and type of bony lesion, tooth mobility, anatomy of the roots and cooperation of the patient. The earlier the diagnosis is made and treatment started the more favorable the prognosis becomes. In the final analysis the choice of treatment depends upon the clinical judgment of the therapist.

Treatment. *Generalized form of periodontosis.* In approximately 25 percent of the periodontosis cases in our study, the disease

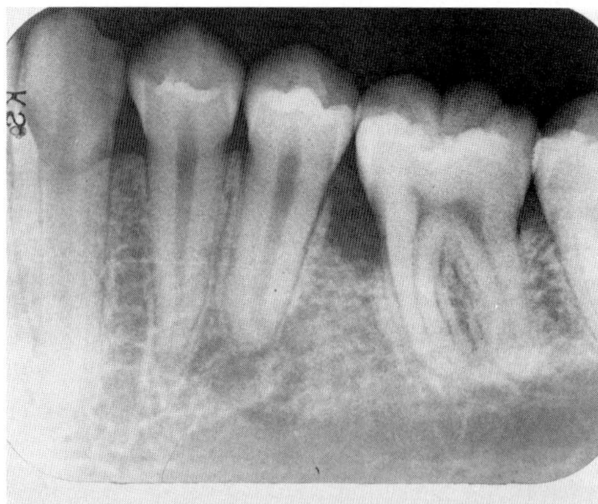

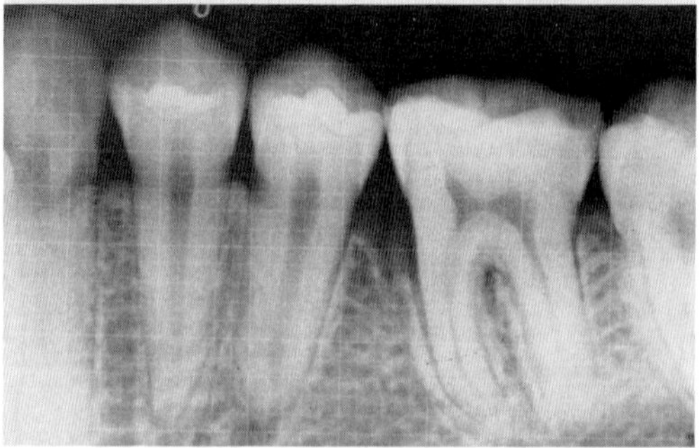

Fig. 10-29. *Top.* Preoperative roentgenograph showing bone loss on the mesial aspect of the mandibular first molar.
Bottom. Postoperative result.

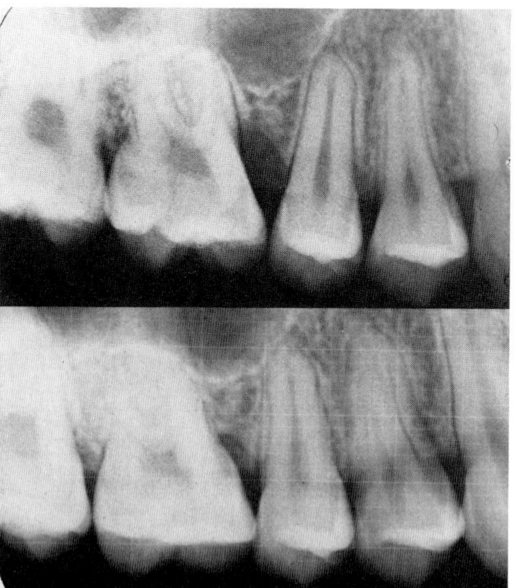

Fig. 10-30. *Top.* This preoperative roentgenograph shows bone loss on the mesial aspect of the maxillary first molar.
Bottom. Postoperative result.

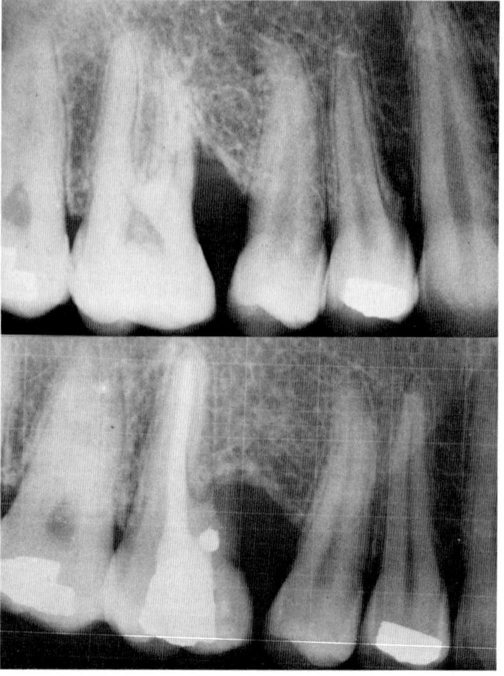

Fig. 10-31. *Top.* The periodontal pocket about the mesiobuccal root of the maxillary first molar extends down, resulting in a mesial furca involvement.
Bottom. A five-year postoperative result following endodontic therapy and root amputation.

was not limited to the molars and incisors but involved, or progressed to involve, other teeth in the dentition. The maxillary teeth in this form of disease are usually more severely involved than the mandibular ones. The prognosis, for the dentition as a whole, is guarded to poor. Treatment can be quite discouraging, since the disease may progress rapidly despite all efforts at therapy. Loss of the entire maxillary dentition while the patient is still in his teens or early twenties is not uncommon. Fortunately, a sufficient number of mandibular teeth are spared, or sufficiently resistant to the disease, so that a full mandibular denture can, as a rule, be avoided (see Fig. 10-19).

It is also common in these cases to observe that the crown-root ratio is poor. The teeth have small spindly roots and rela-

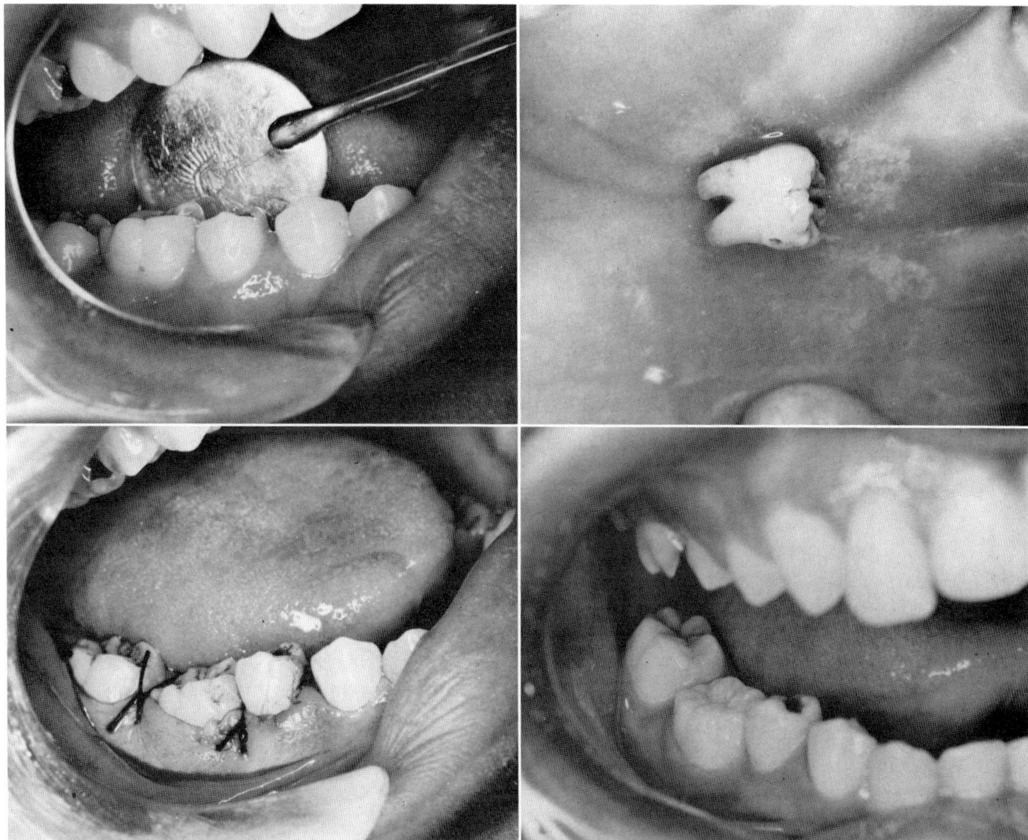

Fig. 10-32. *Top left.* The mandibular first molar is to be extracted because of severe periodontal disease.
Top right. The third molar tooth is to be used as a transplant.
Bottom left. The transplant in place.
Bottom right. Within four to six weeks the implant became firm.

tively large crowns. While this unfavorable crown-root ratio probably does not play a role in the etiology of the disease, it does have an adverse effect on the prognosis.

Once a tooth in this form of periodontosis becomes involved, it invariably takes a downhill course, regardless of the type of therapy used. However, with periodontal treatment, including splinting of the very mobile teeth, the patient can usually be kept comfortable and the rate of progression of the disease retarded.

In devising a definitive treatment plan for the mandibular arch, it is recommended that only those mandibular teeth that have not been affected by the disease be considered as abutments in the permanent restoration. This will permit the treatment plan to be completed more rapidly and will generally prove to have a beneficial effect on the patient's mental attitude.

General Comment on Treatment. *Patient with a poor prognosis.* Most often, by the time the patient is referred to a periodontist, the case is so far advanced that it is usually impossible to arrest the disease. It must be remembered, however, that it is a traumatic experience for an adolescent to be faced with the realization that he has a form of periodontal disease that cannot be cured

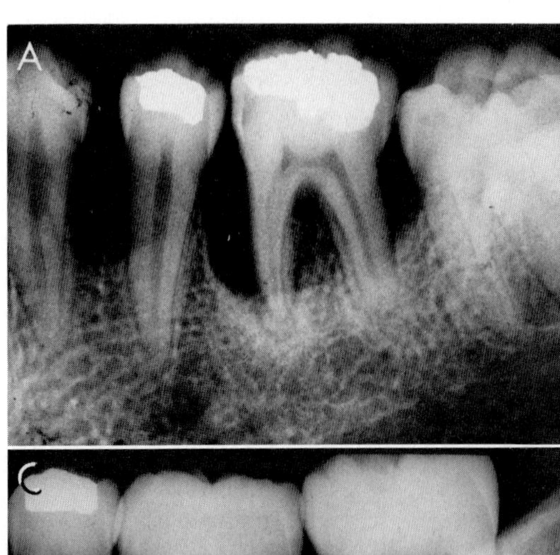

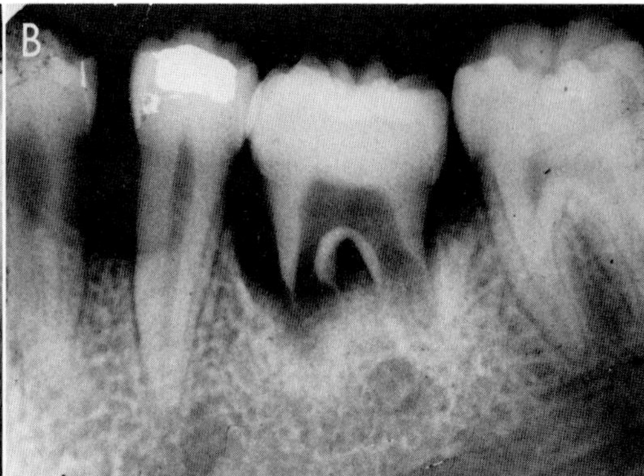

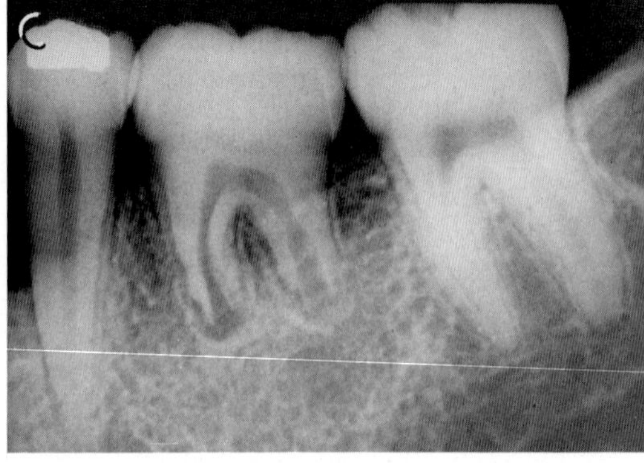

Fig. 10-33. *A*. Preoperative view of this tooth shows the transplant procedure in Figure 10-32.
B. The third molar is autotransplanted into the first molar site.
C. Eighteen months after the transplant. (Baer, and Gamble.)[3]

and that he may lose many if not all of his teeth. At the time the case is presented, the patient is desperately in need of comforting and reassurance that although the disease cannot be cured a great deal can be done to maintain the teeth for a good many years. With therapy most of the teeth in the natural dentition can be maintained to tide the patient through the teenage period and into his twenties. This length of time permits the adolescent time for psychological adjustment to the condition. It also permits him to get through an important social and cultural phase of his life. It has been our experience that those who have accepted therapy have been most grateful for all that was accomplished.

JUVENILE PERIODONTITIS

Chronic gingival inflammation may spread into the deeper supporting tissues of the periodontium where it then becomes periodontitis. It is the most common form of chronic destructive periodontal disease. Periodontitis is invariably associated with obvious local etiologic factors (Fig. 10-41) such as plaque, calculus, food impaction and faulty dental restorations. Roentgenographically, a cupping effect is seen at the crest of the interseptal bone in the posterior regions in the early stages of the disease (Fig. 10-42).

Treatment. Plaque control, root planing, curettage and various surgical procedures to correct bony and soft-tissue deformities are appropriate treatment. Plastic procedures for the correction of various gingivomucosal problems may also be required in selected cases. In addition, adjustment of the occlusion may be necessary to correct problems of occlusal trauma and splinting where tooth mobilities do not respond to occlusal correction. In those cases in which the periodontally involved teeth are in poor relationship to the sur-

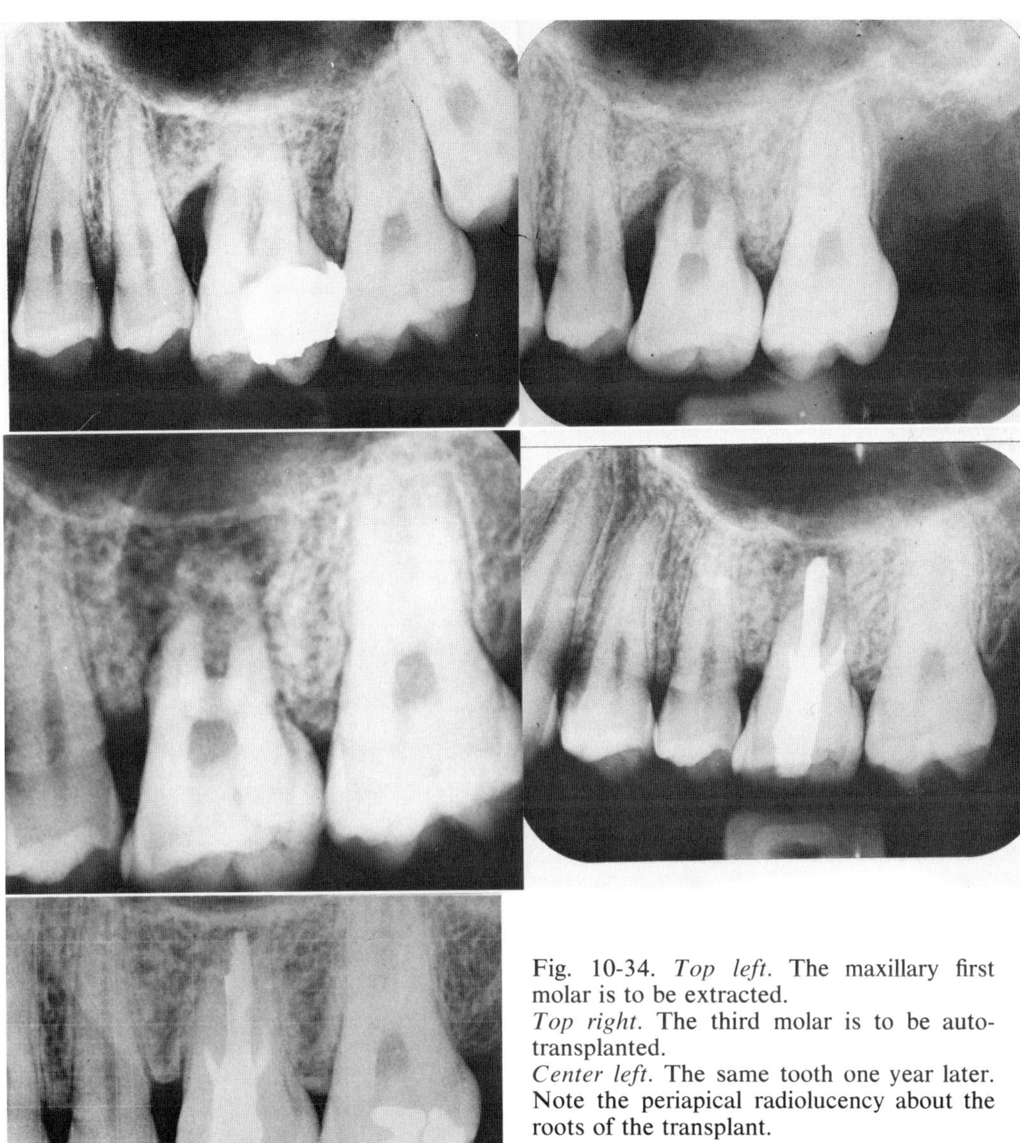

Fig. 10-34. *Top left.* The maxillary first molar is to be extracted.
Top right. The third molar is to be autotransplanted.
Center left. The same tooth one year later. Note the periapical radiolucency about the roots of the transplant.
Center right. Endodontic therapy was completed six months previously.
Bottom. Eight-year postoperative results. (Baer, and Gamble.)[3]

rounding alveolar bone, orthodontic therapy may be required to place the teeth in an environment more conducive to periodontal health. This disease is preventable by plaque control, removal of calculus at periodic intervals, elimination of food impaction areas and the placement of properly contoured and designed dental restorations.

ACUTE LOCALIZED DESTRUCTION OF ALVEOLAR BONE

This uncommon phenomenon affects only one permanent mandibular first molar tooth of children.

Etiology. Unknown. Food impaction does not appear to play a significant role.

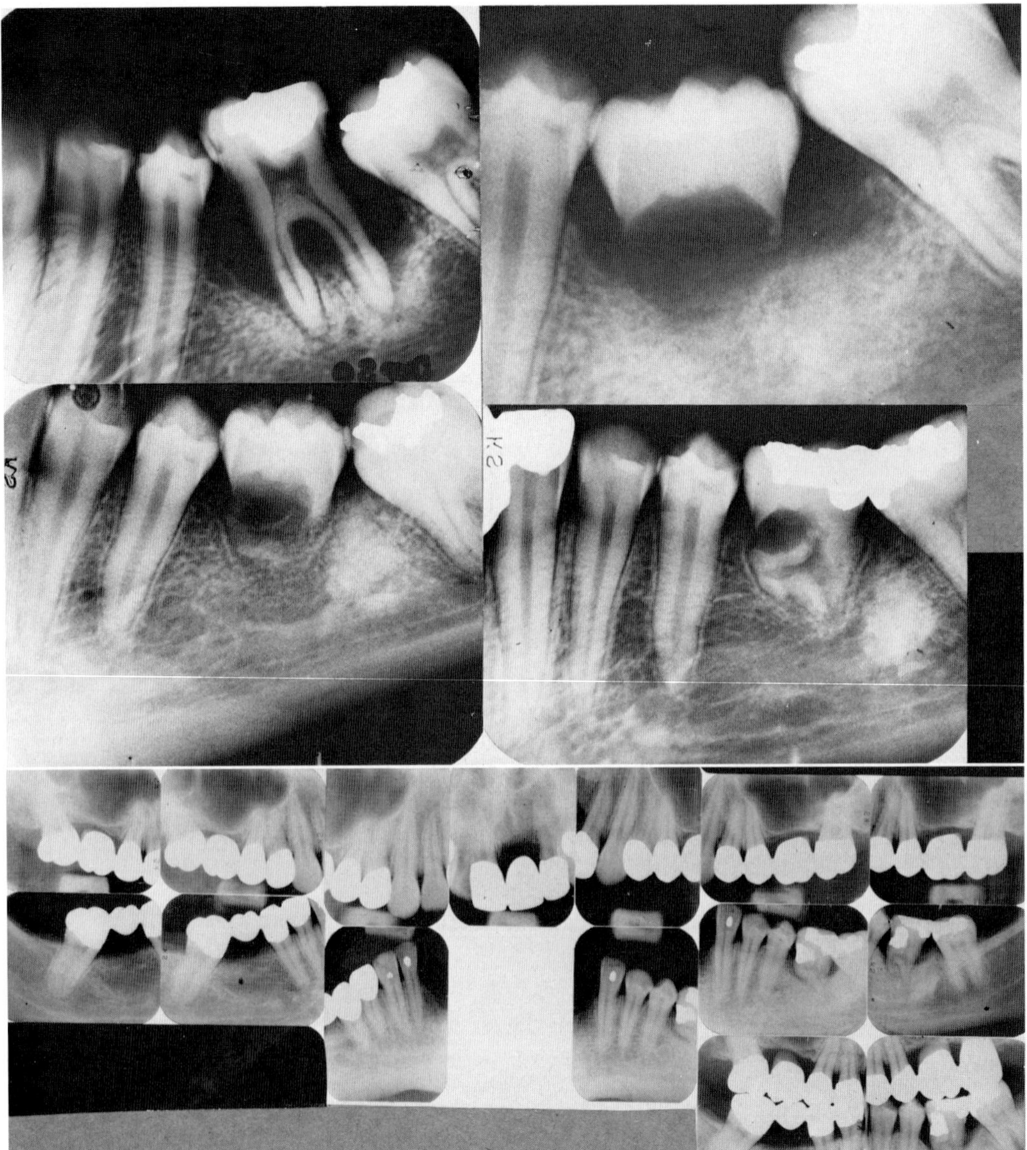

Fig. 10-35. *Top left.* The mandibular first molar of a 14-year-old girl.
Top right. A third molar transplant.
Center left. The same tooth approximately one year later.
Center right. Note the resorptive area on the mesial aspect of the transplant three years postoperatively.
Bottom. Nine-year postoperative results. The case is maintaining itself. Compare with the preoperative roentgenograms above. (Baer, and Gamble.)[3]

Clinical Characteristics. The chief complaint is pain and discomfort in the affected first molar area. Clinically the gingiva in the involved first molar area is within normal limits. However, upon probing, a deep infrabony type pocket can be found and a purulent exudate expressed. Roentgenographs will reveal a severe loss of bone if the lesion is on the proximal surface (Fig. 10-43) but will be negative if it is located on the buccal aspect. The infrabony lesion is unusual in that it is extremely wide and funnel-shaped (Fig. 10-43 and Fig. 10-44).

Treatment. Retraction of a buccal gingival flap and removal of all the granulomatous tissue within the bony defect usually results in a rapid healing of the lesion (see Fig. 10-43 *Bottom right* and *left*).

Prognosis. Excellent.

BRUXISM AND OCCLUSAL TRAUMA

Bruxism has been defined by some authorities as a nonfunctional, voluntary or involuntary mandibular movement which may occur during the day or night with manifestations of occasional or habitual grinding or clenching of the teeth.[31,32] Others feel that a differentiation should be

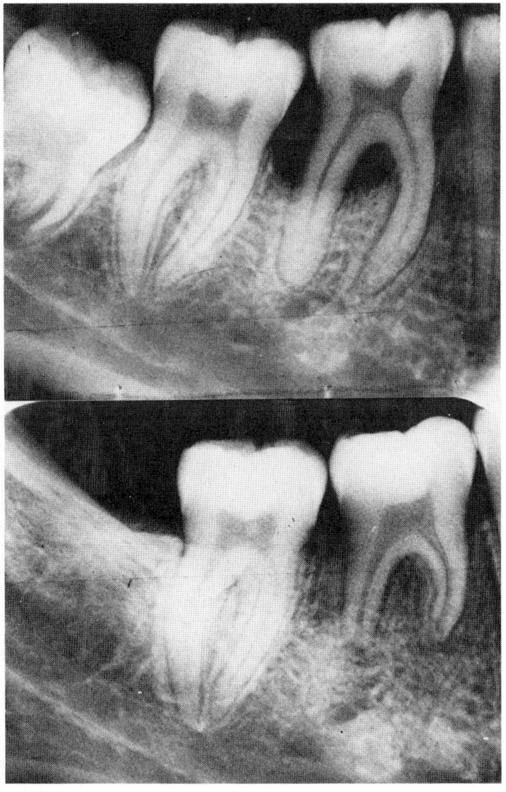

Fig. 10-36. *Top.* A preoperative view of the mandibular first molar.
Bottom. A postoperative view with the transplant in place showing healing of the bony defect. (Baer, and Gamble.)[3]

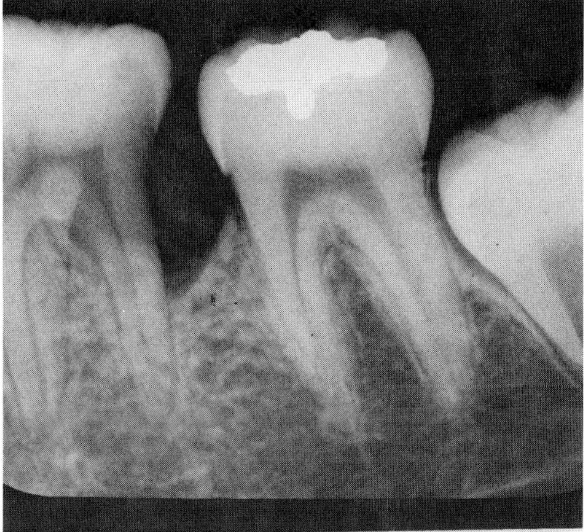

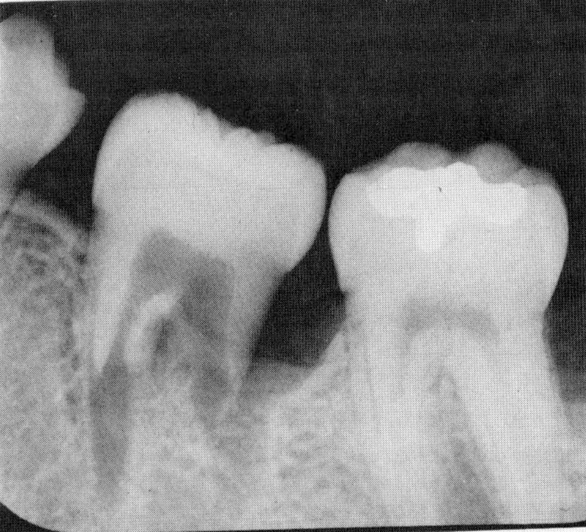

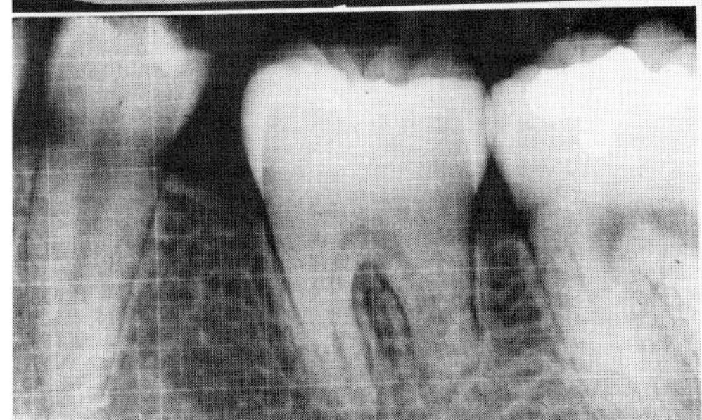

Fig. 10-37. *Top.* A preoperative roentgenograph.
Center. A third molar autotransplant in place.
Bottom. Healing eight years postoperatively.

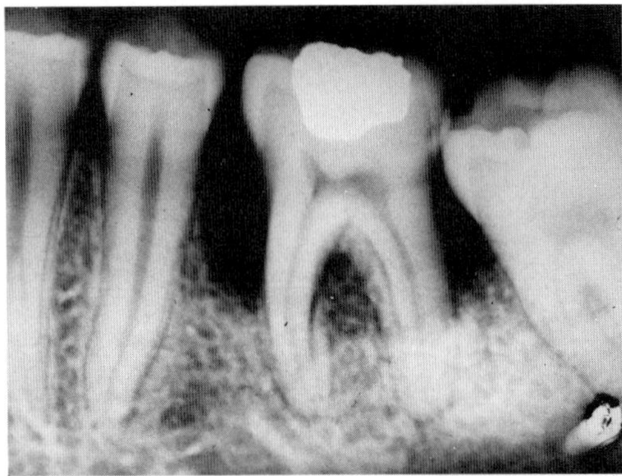

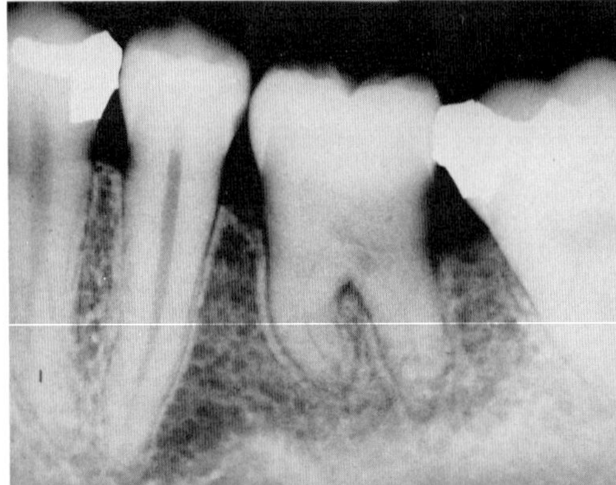

Fig. 10-38. *Top.* A preoperative roentgenograph of a mandibular first molar.
Bottom. A five-year postoperative view of a transplant.

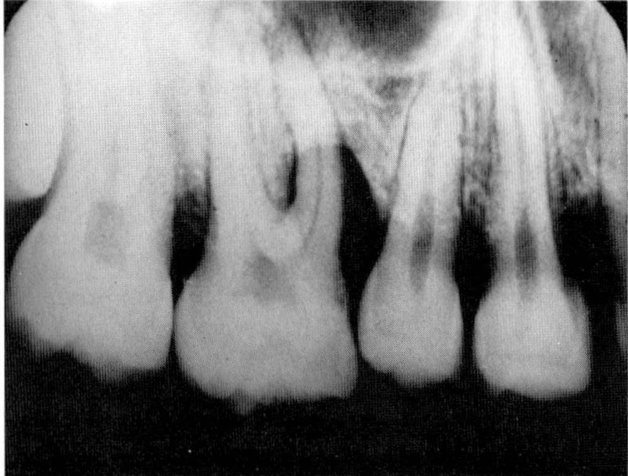

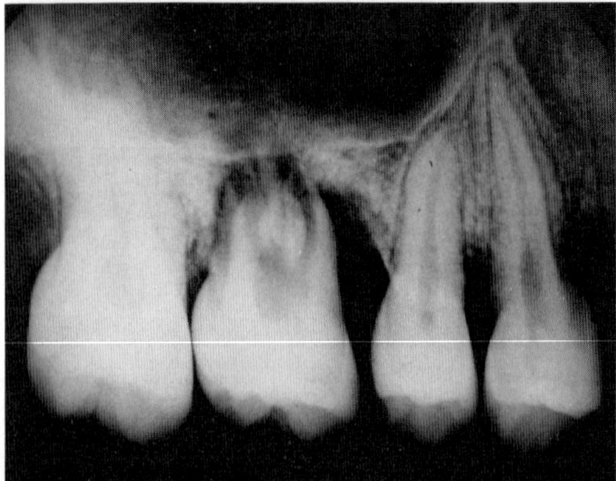

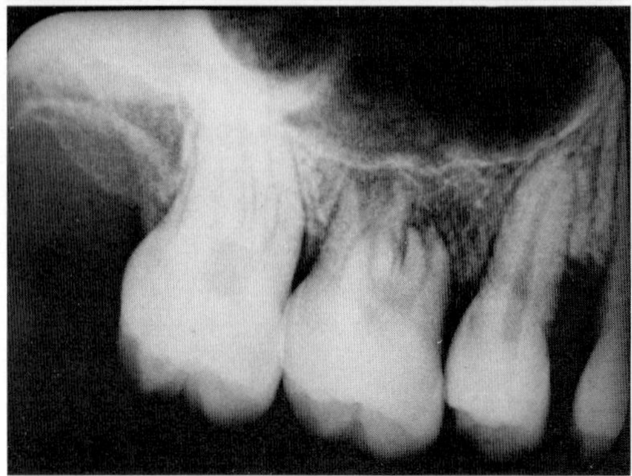

Fig. 10-39. *Top.* Note the lesion on the mesial of the maxillary first molar.
Center. The third molar autotransplant in position.
Bottom. A five-year postoperative result of an autotransplant.

made between tooth-grinding which occurs during sleep from that which occurs in the waking state, since on a priori grounds alone the two phenomena occur in different states of consciousness.[36,37] Furthermore, few individuals can produce tooth-grinding sounds while awake. Finally, there is no evidence that nocturnal bruxers practice diurnal bruxism or vice versa. The average duration of a grinding incident in a nocturnal bruxer has been found to be 9 seconds, with the average rate of grinding 40 seconds per hour of sleep. This invariably is accompanied by rhythmic contractions of the masseter muscle as diagnosed by EMG actively (Fig. 10-45) and by an increased heart rate.[36,37]

Prevalence. It is estimated that approximately 15 percent of elementary and high school students brux.[35] There is no apparent sex difference; age, however, does play an important role. From age 3 to 7 years,

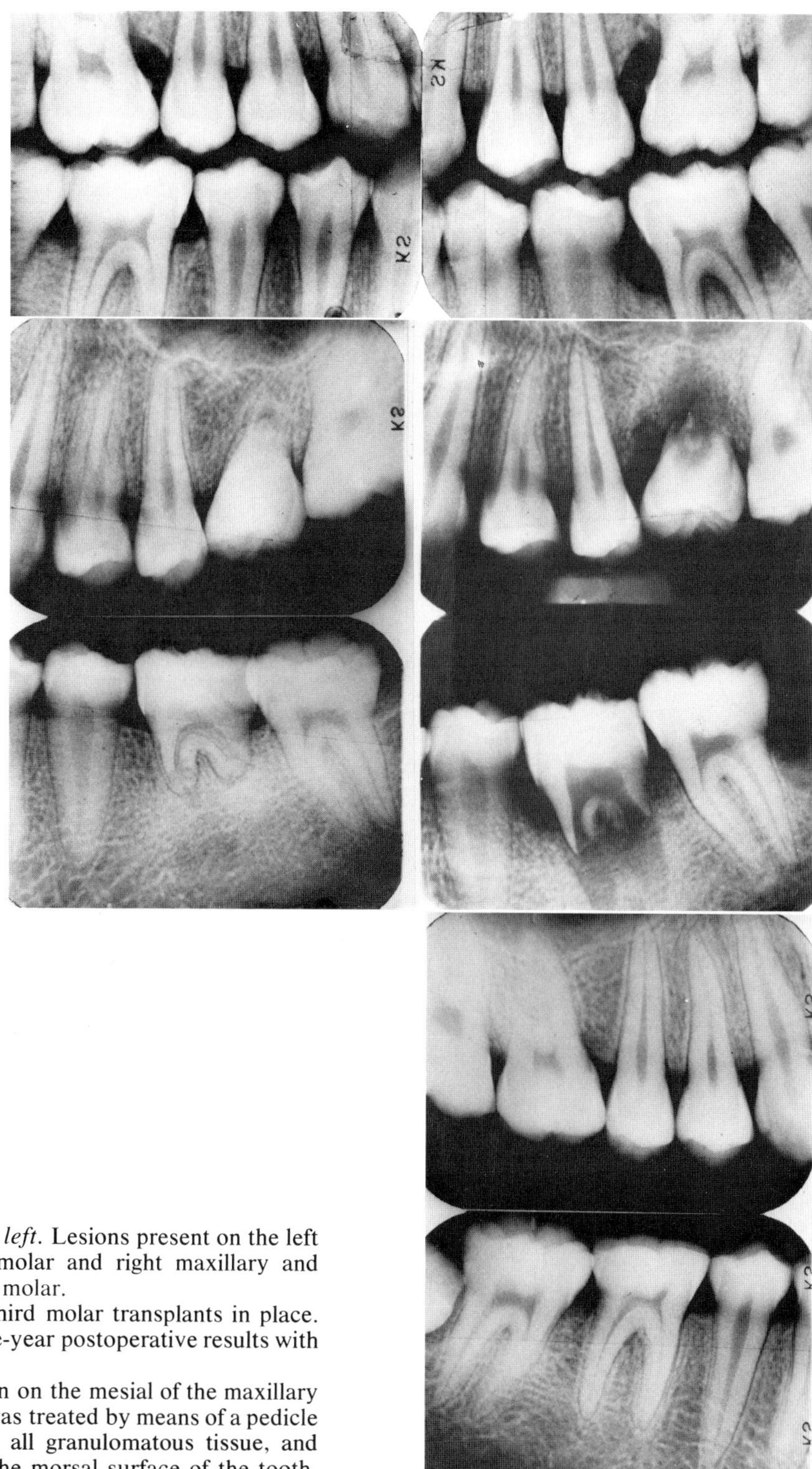

Fig. 10-40. *Top left.* Lesions present on the left maxillary first molar and right maxillary and mandibular first molar.
Center right. Third molar transplants in place.
Center left. Five-year postoperative results with transplants.
Bottom. A lesion on the mesial of the maxillary left first molar was treated by means of a pedicle graft to remove all granulomatous tissue, and by grinding of the morsal surface of the tooth. Compare with *Top left* roentgenograph.

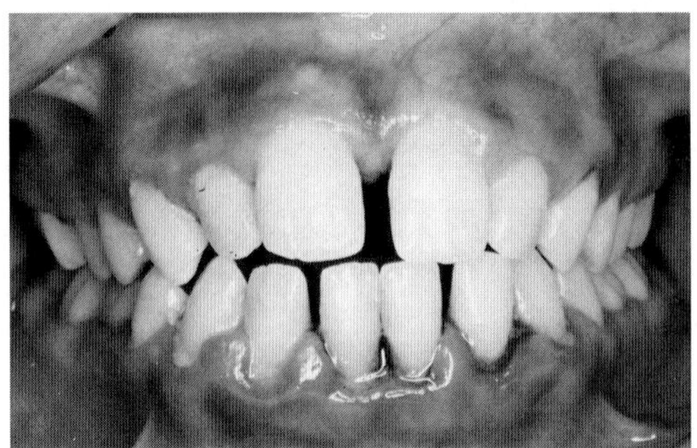

Fig. 10-41. Periodontitis, in a 15-year-old female, associated with obvious local etiologic factors.

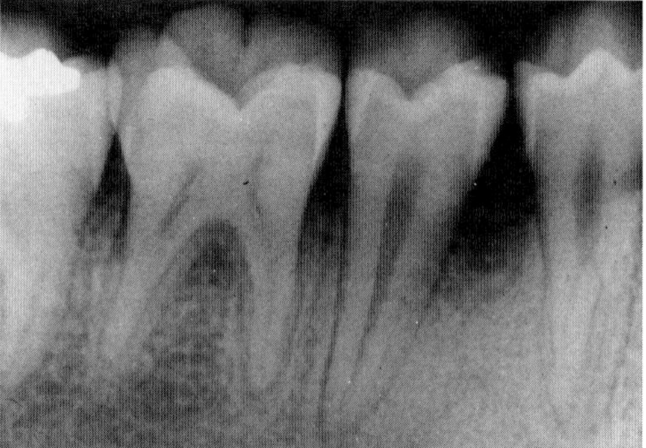

Fig. 10-42. Cupping as seen in the interdental region between the bicuspids is a diagnostic sign of periodontitis in this juvenile patient.

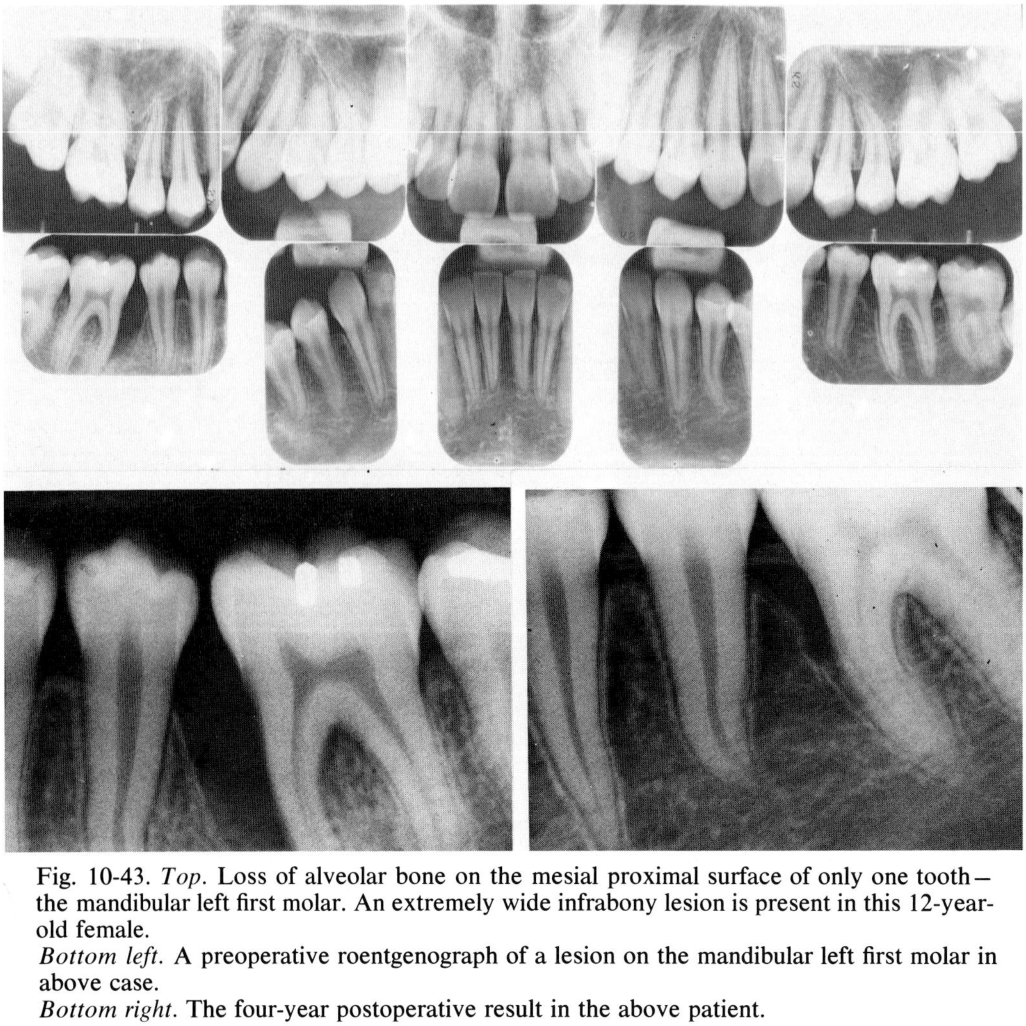

Fig. 10-43. *Top.* Loss of alveolar bone on the mesial proximal surface of only one tooth—the mandibular left first molar. An extremely wide infrabony lesion is present in this 12-year-old female.
Bottom left. A preoperative roentgenograph of a lesion on the mandibular left first molar in above case.
Bottom right. The four-year postoperative result in the above patient.

14.4 percent are estimated to be bruxers; from 8 to 12 years of age the percentage declines to 6.6 percent and this decline continues until only 1.2 percent brux by 13 to 17 years of age. A statistically significant association has been found of nocturnal bruxism among blood relatives of nocturnal bruxers.[35]

Etiology. In most instances bruxism has a dual etiology—psychic stress and occlusal interferences. In some cases the main etiologic factor is the psychological component, while in others it is the occlusal factor. In his night psychophysiologic studies on bruxism Reding[36,37] found a frequent association of nocturnal bruxing with body movement occurring during the transitional stages of sleep. If this be true, then bruxing may be symptomatic of a state of partial arousal from sleep and

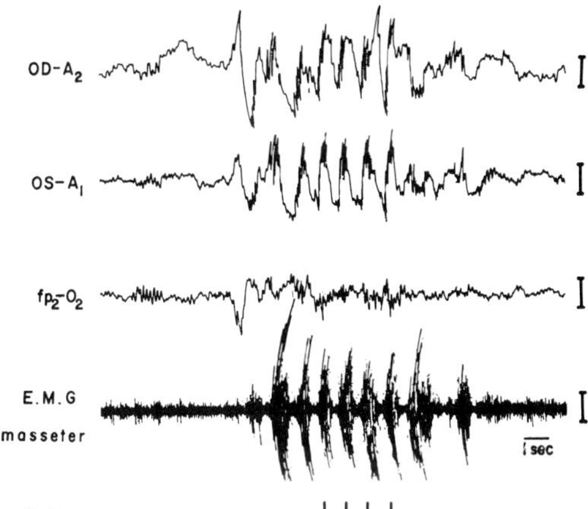

Fig. 10-45. Bruxism rhythmic contractions associated with sounds of grinding. $OD\text{-}A_2$ is the right referential alternating current electro-oculographic tracing. $OS\text{-}A_1$ is the left referential alternating current electro-oculographic tracing. $fp_2\text{-}O_2$ is the electroencephalographic reading (fronto-occipital), calibration. 50_uv. EMG (masseter) are the electromyographic tracings, direct (calibration 20_uv) and integrated. (Reeling, Zepelin, Robinson, Zimmerman, and Smith.)[36]

could conceivably be triggered by any external or internal physical or emotional stimuli.

Psychiatrically it has been found that bruxism occurs most often in hostile, dependent people who are involved in long-existing life problems, persons who have gradually built up to a more or less intolerable situation. As the rage and resentment increase, these people require additional need to control their anger in order to avoid conflict with people on whom they depend. The end result of all of this is exaggeration of their long-standing pattern of bruxing.[30] The following psychiatric consultation report will illustrate this point.

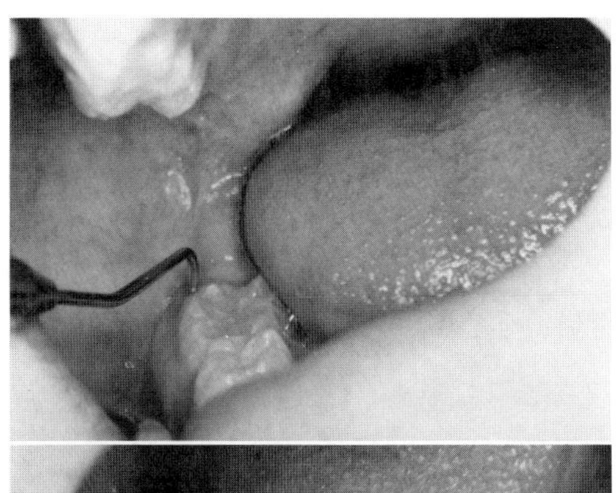

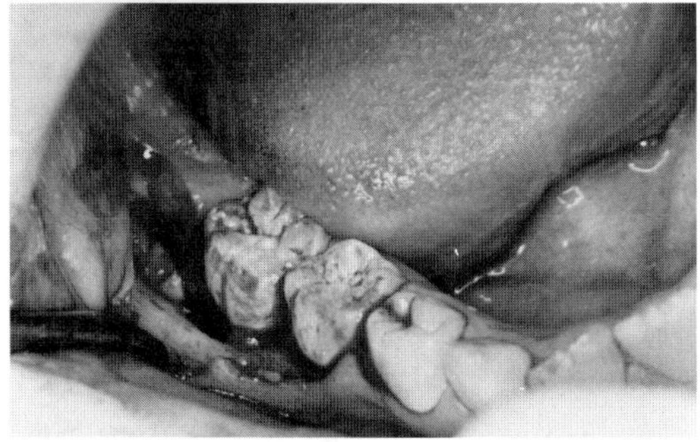

Fig. 10-44. *Top.* A deep infrabony pocket on the buccal and distal of the permanent mandibular right first molar in a 6-year-old boy.
Bottom. Note the unusually wide infrabony lesion in the above patient.

CASE HISTORY 5

Miss H., a 16-year-old female, was seen in psychiatric consultation with a request for suggestions regarding psychiatric aspects of

TABLE 10-1. BITING PRESSURE OF CHILDREN IN POUNDS

	Male			Female		
Age Years	No. Cases	Mean	Standard Error	No. Cases	Mean	Standard Error
6-7	18	53	4.3	6	52	4.2
7-8	23	55	4.0	16	53	4.6
8-9	29	56	3.1	29	63	4.4
9-10	46	61	3.2	31	59	4.2
10-11	45	78	3.8	34	67	3.3
11-12	46	80	2.9	41	73	3.5
12-13	66	80	2.9	41	84	3.5
13-14	54	90	3.4	20	90	6.0
14-15	70	105	3.8	14	99	11.4
15-16	92	109	3.5	4	103	10.9
16-17	57	111	4.3	1	90	

* After Brawley and Sedwick[28]

the management of her symptoms of bruxism. The patient understands that her teeth-grinding is the cause of progressive loosening of her lower front teeth. Miss H. states that her mother has said that she evidenced teeth-grinding even as an infant. She is unaware of any history of oral problems throughout her childhood and there is no evidence of feeding problems or current overconcern with food.

In discussing her symptoms, the patient quite directly relates her teeth grinding to her constant anger toward her 13-year-old sister who seems to continually antagonize the patient. This sister has an ulcer, and the family has apparently been instructed by her physician that the girl not be upset. The result is, the patient states, that her younger sister is allowed to "get away with" a great deal and her continual harassment of the patient and her parents

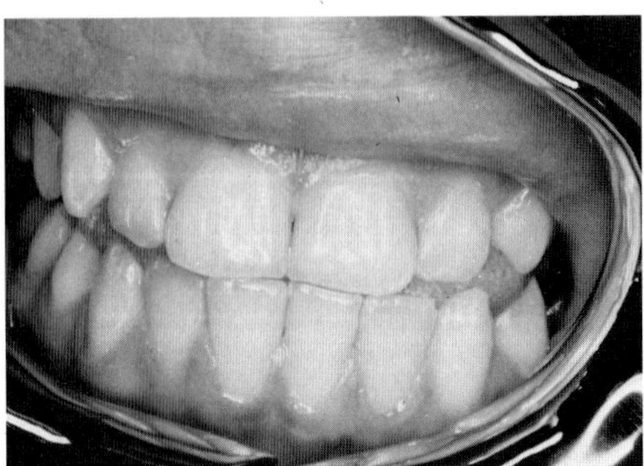

Fig. 10-46. Anterior bruxism in an 11-year-old female. Note that wear facets on mandibular anterior teeth match those on maxillary anterior teeth.

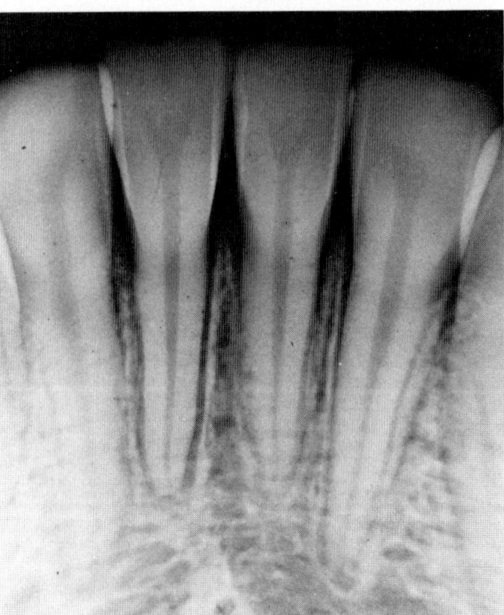

Fig. 10-47. Thickened periodontal ligament about the mandibular right central incisor is a result of the bruxism habit, in the 11-year-old female seen in Figure 10-46.

is attributed to the younger sister's problem with her ulcer.

The patient directly recalls frequent occurrences of being angry at her sister and, even after her anger is expressed, finding herself grinding her teeth. She is aware from her sore jaws on many mornings that she has been grinding her teeth during the night. She also notes that this occurs when she is taking examinations and concentrating on a lecture or a book. The patient denies that her younger sister is favored by her parents, yet she states that the family exerts less control over the younger sister, that the younger sister has her own horse (the patient claims she does not enjoy riding), and that the younger sister may be her father's favorite. The most outstanding observation was the patient's apparent emotional indifference to her symptoms in the face of her intellectual awareness of the cause and possible outcome of the situation. In other words, the patient did not reveal any emotional conflicts which might motivate her for further psychiatric treatment and in fact seemed emotionally indifferent to the implications of her symptom despite her apparently correct understanding of the cause and likely outcome.

There is some evidence to suggest that the patient's symptom may be related to feelings of rage of which she is entirely unaware and that possibly being unaware of certain feelings which are present on a deeper level may be one of her major defenses.

Diagnosis. While there is evidence to suggest that the patient's symptoms may be connected with unconscious anger and that she handles many of her feelings by "being unaware" of them, it appears that except for the symptom of bruxism she is satisfied with her life and is not motivated for further psychological exploration at this time. Therefore, I would not be in favor of any attempt to intervene in the patient's symptom at the level of her motivations.

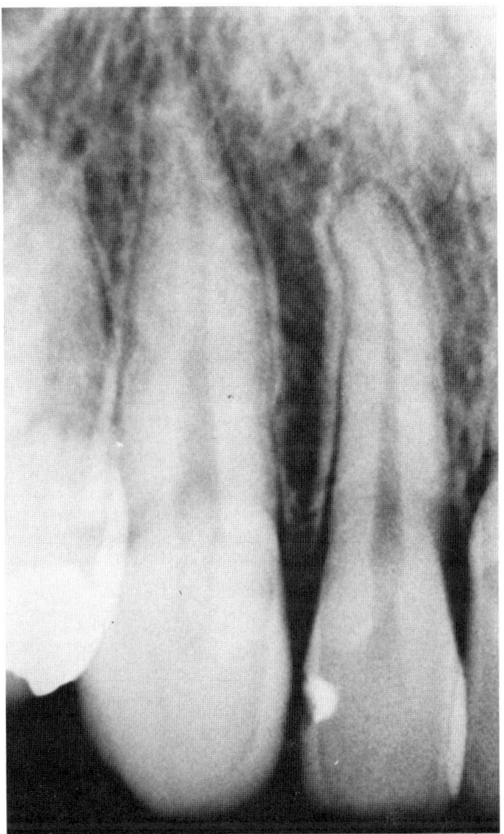

Fig. 10-48. Thickened periodontal ligament about the maxillary lateral incisor is a result of occlusal trauma in this 12-year-old female. (Courtesy of Dr. G. H. Ulrich, and J. W. Griffin.)

Biting Pressures. Biting pressures have been shown to increase gradually from 4 to 18 years of age at the rate of approximately 3 to 5 pounds per year. The pressures are greater in the molar area than in the incisor region[39] and range from 10 pounds to over 100 pounds. The highest values occur in the older age groups[28] (Table 10-1). Thus, it is possible for enough force to be generated on the teeth and periodontal structures by bruxing or clenching to cause damage. On the other hand, as Ramfjord[34] has so aptly pointed out, bruxism, particularly when started at a young age, does not necessarily lead to pathologic changes in the periodontal tissues. In fact when started early in life it most often results in a physiologic adaptation to the increased stresses. The end result in such instances is a thickening of the periodontal membrane with the development of heavy collagenous fibers, a thickening of the alveolar bone with an increased

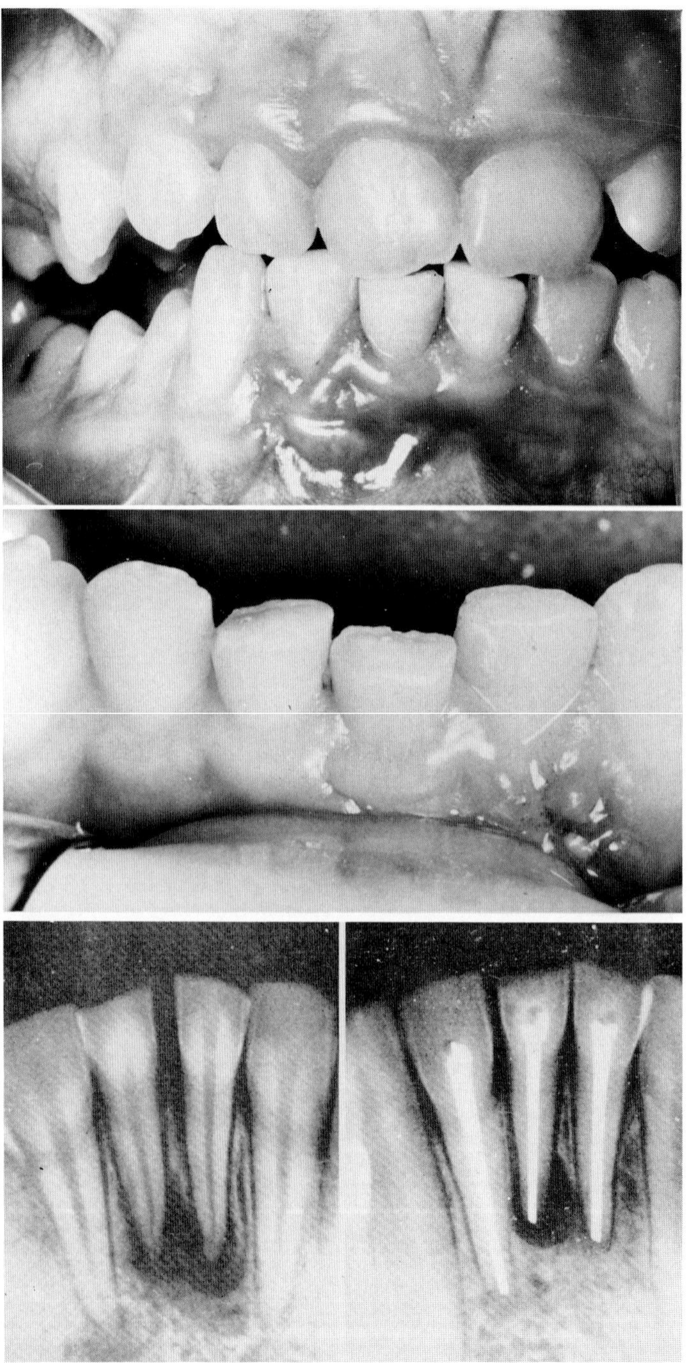

Fig. 10-49. *Top left.* Osteoporosis and pulpal death of the mandibular incisors in a 14-year-old female who compulsively grinds her teeth in protrusive excursion. *Center.* Extensive wear of the mandibular incisors is caused by the compulsive grinding. *Bottom left.* Pulps of three incisors have been devitalized by the force of the traumatic habit. An acute abscess has separated the central incisors. *Bottom right.* One year following root canal therapy, some repair has occurred. However, the persistent habit prevents complete healing. (Permission of Dr. Eugene Natkin, Dr. John Ingle, and the *Journal of the American Society of Periodontics.*)[33]

amount of trabeculation, and frequently localized thickenings of the cementum at the point of insertion of the principal fibers.

Clinical Characteristics. Where the forces of bruxism exceed the adaptive capacity of the individual, considerable injury to the teeth and supporting structures may occur. Some of these signs and symptoms are:

1. Abnormal wear or attrition of the teeth
2. Unexpected tooth mobility not accounted for by bone loss from chronic destructive periodontal disease
3. Obvious contractions of the muscles of mastication, particularly the masseters
4. Unexpected fractures of teeth or restorations
5. Audible sounds complained of by spouse, roommate or relative
6. Soreness of muscles of mastication
7. Temporomandibular joint symptoms.

CASE HISTORY 6

An 11-year-old girl was referred for a periodontal consultation because of marked mobility of one mandibular central incisor. Clinical examination revealed an absence of periodontal pockets, a crevicular depth and a gingival contour and color that were within normal limits. The incisal edges of the incisor teeth were abraded. When the patient was asked to protrude her mandible, it was found that the wear facets observed on the mandibular teeth matched those on the maxillary anterior teeth. (Fig. 10-46). A roentgenographic examination of the area revealed a thickened periodontal ligament (Fig. 10-47).

Diagnosis. Primary occlusal traumatism as a result of an anterior bruxing habit.

While this problem is observed most commonly on the mandibular incisor, it should be remembered that it can occur on any tooth[38] (Fig. 10-48).

ALVEOLAR OSTEOPOROSIS SYNDROME

A less common variation of ordinary bruxism is a syndrome characterized roentgenographically by one or more periapical radiolucencies, pulpal death of one or more of these teeth and compulsive bruxism.[29,33]

Etiology. While the real cause of this type of bruxism is presently unknown, Ingle contends that it is a manifestation of an underlying insecurity and anxiety in the environment.[29,33]

Clinical Characteristics. The signs and symptoms of this syndrome are:

1. Patients are all females between 13 and 16 years of age.
2. The chief complaint is usually discomfort in the mandibular incisor region. Occasionally a concomitant inflammatory swelling in the area is also present.
3. Roentgenographically there is a periapical radiolucency in the mandibular incisor region (Fig. 10-49).
4. The electric pulp tester may or may not show the dental pulps of the involved incisors to be vital.
5. In all cases there is definite evidence of marked bruxism. The mandibular incisors are severely abraded and highly polished facets are commonly found on the linguoincisal edges of the maxillary incisor and the labioincisal edge of the mandibular incisor.
6. One or more of the mandibular incisors invariably shows a high degree of mobility.
7. The gingival contour, color and crevicular depth are within normal limits.

Treatment. Occlusal adjustments should be tried first in all cases in which occlusal interferences are present. Sometimes it is a good idea to leave the teeth roughened after the occlusal adjustment to create an awareness that may make it possible for patients to control this habit. However, it is extremely difficult to treat a patient who has little occlusal interferences and a marked bruxing habit by means of an occlusal adjustment. In these instances a plastic night-guard may aid greatly in solving this problem. Unfortunately in those very patients where it might be most beneficial, a nightguard most often is rejected.

In the case of the compulsive bruxer who has caused a tooth to become nonvital, endodontic therapy of course will be required.

Finally, when nothing seems to work in relieving the problem, and when as a result of the bruxing severe pathologic changes are occurring to the teeth or periodontium, a psychiatric consultation might be worthwhile.

REFERENCES

Periodontosis

1. Atkins, J. P.: Conference on the implications of immune reactions in the pathogenesis of periodontal disease. J. Periodont., *41:*236, 1970.
2. Baer, P. N.: The case for periodontosis as a clinical entity. J. Periodont., *42:*516, 1971.
3. Baer, P. N., and Gamble, J. W.: Autogenous dental transplants as a method of treating the osseous defect in periodontosis. Oral Surg., *22:*405, 1966.
4. Baer, P. N., and Everett, F. G.: The maxillary sinus as a problem in the therapy of periodontosis. J. Periodont., *41:*476, 1970.
5. Basu. M. K., and Dutta, A. N.: Report on Prevalence of periodontal disease in the adult population of Calcutta, by Ramfjord's technique. J. All-India Dent. J., *35:*187, 1963.
6. Benjamin, S. D., and Baer, P. N.: Familial patterns of advanced alveolar bone loss in adolescence (periodontosis). Periodontics, *5:*82, 1967.
7. Butler, J. H.: A familial pattern of juvenile periodontitis (periodontosis). J. Periodont., *40:*51, 1969.
8. Cohen, D. W., and Goldman, H. M.: Clinical observations in the modification of human oral tissue metabolism by local intraoral factors. Ann. New York Acad. Sci., *85:*68, 1960.
9. Ennis, L. M., Berry, H. M. J., and Phillips, J. E.: Dental Roentgenology. 6 ed. Philadelphia, Lea & Febiger, 1967.
10. Everett, F. G., and Baer, P. N.: A preliminary report on the treatment of the osseous defect in periodontosis. J. Periodont., *35:*429, 1964.
11. Glauser, R. O., Humphreys, P. K., Stanley, H. R. and Baer, P. N.: Personal Communication.
12. Gottlieb, B.: Die Diffuse Alveolarknochens. Ztchr. Stomatol., *21:*195, 1923.
13. Gottlieb, B.: Paradentalpyorrhoe and Alveolaratrophie. Fortschr. Zhkde., *4:*398, 1928.
14. Jamison, H. C.: Prevalence of periodontal disease of the deciduous teeth. J.A.D.A., *66:*207, 1963.
15. Kaslick, R. S., and Chasens, A. I.: Periodontosis with periodontitis: a study involving young adult males. Part II. Clinical, medical and histopathologic studies. Oral Surg., *25:*327, 1968.
16. Miglani, D. C., and Sharma, O. P.: Incidence of acute necrotizing ulcerative gingivitis and periodontosis among cases seen at the government hospital, Madras. J. All-India Dent. J., *37:*183, 1965.
17. Miner, E. B., and Baer, P. N.: Studies in calcium metabolism in resorptive disease of alveolar bone (periodontosis). Report of three cases. Periodontics, *3:*301, 1965.

17A. Newman, M., Williams, R., Crawford, A., Manganiello, A. D., and Socransky, S. S.: Predominant cultivable microbiota periodontitis and periodontosis. III. Periodontosis. J. Dent. Res., *52*:131, 1973.

18. Nomenclature and Classification Committee Report. J. Periodont., *21:*40:1950.
19. Orban, B.: Classification of periodontal disease. Parodontologie, *4:*159, 1949.
20. Rao, S. S., and Tewani, S. V.: Prevalence of periodontosis among Indians. J. Periodont., *39:*27, 1968.
21. Russell, A. L.: Some epidemiological characteristics of periodontal disease in a series of urban populations. J. Periodont., *28:*286, 1957.
22. Russell, A. L.: The prevalence of periodontal disease in different populations during the circumpubertal period. J. Periodont., *42:*508, 1971.
23. Stallard, R. E.: The utilization of H^3 -proline by the connective tissue elements of the periodontium. Periodontics, *1:*185, 1963.
24. Stafne, W. C.: Oral Roentgenographic Diagnosis. ed 3. Philadelphia, W. B. Saunders, 1969.
25. Waerhaug, J.: Preliminary report on WHO periodontal survey in Ceylon, October-December 1960. World Health Organization MHO/PA175.62.

26. World Workshop in Periodontics. Ann Arbor, Michigan, 1966.
27. Worth, H. M.: Principles and Practice of Oral Radiologic Interpretation. Chicago, Year Book Medical Publishers, Inc. 1963.

Bruxism

28. Brawley, R. E., and Sedwick, H. J.: Studies concerning the oral cavity and saliva. II Biting pressure (2) measurements of biting pressure in children: Am. Jr. Orthodont Oral Surg., *26:*41, 1940.
29. Ingle, J. I.: Alveolar osteoporosis and pulpal death associated with compulsive bruxism. Oral Surg., *13:*1371, 1960.
30. Moulton, R.: Oral and dental manifestations in anxiety. Psychiatry, *18:*261, 1955.
31. Nadler, S. C.: Bruxism: A classification. Critical Review. J.A.D.A., *54:*615, 1957.
32. Nadler, S. C.: Detection and Recognition of Bruxism. J.A.D.A., *61:*472, 1960.
33. Natkin, E., and Ingle, J. I.: A further report on alveolar osteoporosis and pulpal death associated with compulsive bruxism. Periodontics, *1:*260, 1963.
34. Ramfjord, S. P., and Ash, Jr., M. M.: Occlusion. pp. 100, 111, 218. Philadelphia W. B. Saunders 1966.
35. Reding, G. R., Rubright, W. C., and Zimmerman, S. O.: Incidence of bruxism. J. Dent. Res., *45:*1198, 1966.
36. Reding, G. R., Zepelin, H., Robinson, J. E., Jr., Zimmerman, S. O., and Smith, V. H.: Nocturnal teeth-grinding: all night psychophysiologic studies J. Dent. Res., *47:* 786, 1968.
37. Robinson, J. E., Reding, G. R., Zepelin, H., Smith, V. H., and Zimmerman, S. O.: Nocturnal teeth-grinding: a reassessment for dentistry. J.A.D.A., *78:*1308, 1969.
38. Ulrich, G. H., and Griffin, J. W.: Atypical granuloma associated with compulsive bruxism in an adolescent female. J. Periodont., *38:*514, 1967.
39. Worner, H. R., and Anderson, M. N.: Biting force measurements in children. Aust. Dent. J., *48:*1, 1944.

11

Oral Manifestations of Systemic Diseases Associated with Resorptive Lesions of the Alveolar Bone

THE NEUTROPENIAS

Leukopenia refers to the condition where the total circulating white blood cell count falls below 4000 cells per cubic millimeter. When the leukopenia is due to a decrease in the number of circulating neutrophils, the condition is termed neutropenia. Neutropenia, however, may occur without leukopenia.

There are several types of neutropenia, of which 4 are of concern because of their oral manifestations.[22] Agranulocytosis or malignant neutropenia, cyclic neutropenia, chronic idiopathic neutropenia, and familial benign neutropenia.

Agranulocytosis (Malignant Neutropenia)

This condition is relatively rare in children, being found primarily in adults over 25 years of age. It is caused by a sudden decrease in circulating granulocytes. While drugs have been indicted in more than 50 percent of cases, there are instances where the cause remains unknown. The drugs most commonly associated with the onset of the disease are the coaltar derivatives, although many other drugs have also been implicated (Table 11-1). There is also a congenital form of agranulocytosis.

Etiology. Malignant neutropenia may be caused either by a decreased production of neutrophils by the bone marrow or an increased destruction of the neutrophils peripherally by the spleen or by leukocyte agglutinins. Various drugs utilize different pathways in causing the neutropenia. Amidopyrine, for example, produces a neutropenia by an immune mechanism which causes destruction of the peripheral leukocytes by leukocyte agglutinins. Chlorpromazine, however, acts directly on the marrow in a toxic dose related manner.

Clinical Characteristics. The oral lesions are an important diagnostic sign of the disease (Fig. 11-1). Ulcerative and/or necrotic lesions may appear anywhere on the gingiva. Unlike necrotizing ulcerative gingivitis, the lesions are not limited to the tips of the interdental papillae or even to the attached gingiva, but may appear on other parts of the oral cavity such as the tonsils and palate. There is a great deal of pain associated with the oral lesions, and the breath develops a foul odor from the presence of the necrotic tissue. A nonspecific systemic reaction—chills, high fever, malaise, sore throat and headache—is usually associated with the disease.

Laboratory findings. The total white blood count is generally less than 2000 cells per cubic millimeter with an almost complete absence of polymorphonuclear leukocytes. The total red blood cell and platelet count are within normal limits. The bone marrow shows an absence of granulocytes and plasma cells, but the lymphocytes and reticulum cells may be increased.

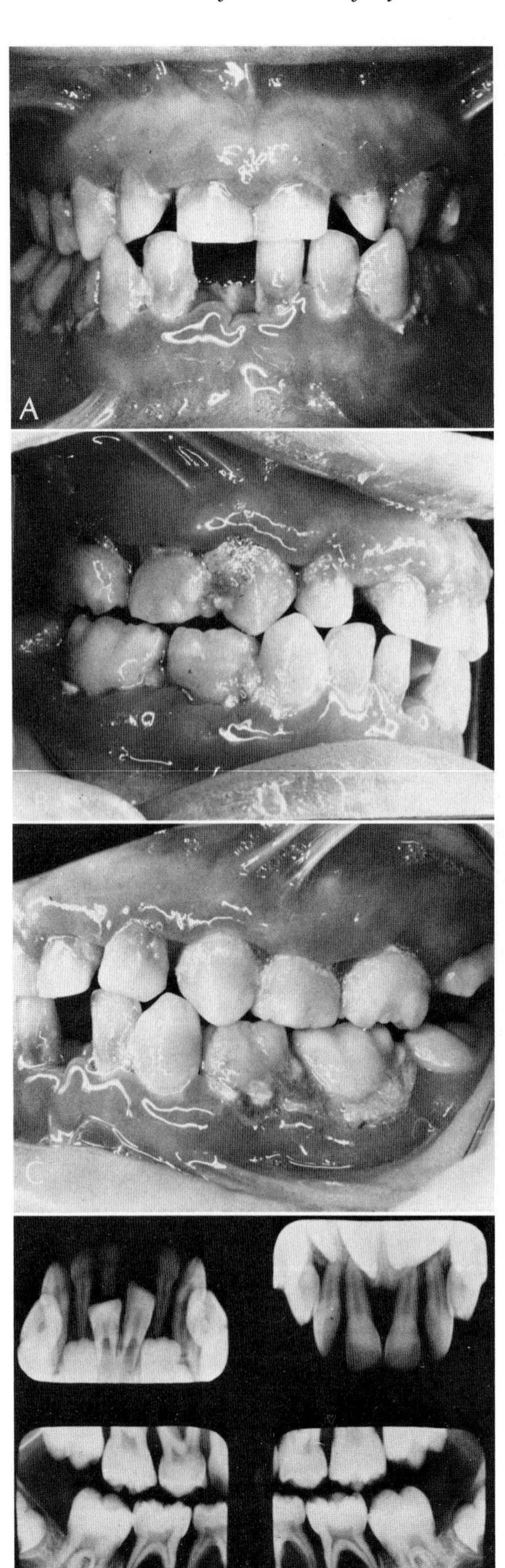

Fig. 11-1A. A 7-year-old girl with congenital agranulocytosis. Note the acute periodontitis and gingival ulcerations. Peripheral white blood cell counts since the age of 6 months have ranged between 5,000 and 7,000 cells per cubic millimeter. The differential counts ranged from 0 to 1 polymorphonuclear leukocytes with the remaining cells consisting primarily of lymphocytes and monocytes. Bone marrow studies revealed a maturation arrest of the neutrophil series.

Fig. 11-1B. In the left buccal area of the above patient, note the gingival ulcerations and areas of necrosis.

Fig. 11-1C. In the right buccal area, note the areas of gingival ulcerations and necrosis.

Fig. 11-1D. Radiographs of this patient showed extensive loss of bone about the primary teeth. Clinically all the teeth were very mobile.

(Fig. 11-1 through 11-4 courtesy of Dr. J. J. Awbrey, and E. D. Hibbard.)[1A]

TABLE 11-1 AGENTS ASSOCIATED WITH THE OCCURRENCE OF GRANULOCYTOPENIA

Analgesics	aminopyrine, dipyrone and drugs containing these compounds (Pyramidon, Cibalgine, Novaldin, Novalgin, antipyrine, Amidophen, Amytal, Causalin, neonal compound, Neurodyne, Peralga, Pyraminyl, Yeast-vite, Pyralgin, etc.)
	phenylbutazone (Butazolidin), oxyphenbutazone
Phenothiazines	chlorpromazine, promazine, mepazine, imipramine (Tofranil), prochlorperazine (Compazine), promethazine (Phenergan), thioridazine (Mellaril), etc.
Sulfonamides (antibacterial)	sulfanilamide, sulfisoxazole (Gantrisin) sulfamethoxypyridazine (Kynex), salicylazosulfapyridine, (Azulfidine) sulfapyridine, sulfathiazole, sulfadiazine, succinylsulfathiazole
Sulfonamide deriviatives (non-antibacterial)	chlorothiazides (Diuril), carbutamide, tolbutamide (Orinase), chlorpropamide, chlorthalidone, acetazolamide (Diamox)
Antithyroid drugs	thiouracil, propylthiouracil, methimazole (Tapazole), carbimazole
Tranquilizers	meprobamate (Miltown, Equanil)
Anticonvulsants	diphenylhydantoin sodium (Dilantin), trimethadione (Tridione) phethenylate, phenacemide, diethazine
Antihistaminics	Pyribenzamine, methaphenilene (Diatrin), thenalidine
Antimicrobial agents	chloramphenicol, thiosemicarbazone (Tibione), ristocetin, methicillin, organic arsenicals
Miscellaneous	dinitrophenol, phenindione penicillamine, metronidazole (Flagyl), thioglycolic acid ("cold wave"), novobiocin, mercurial diuretics, dichlorodiphenyltrichloroethane, antimony (Neostibosan), pyrithyldione (Presidon), quinine, cincophen, plasmochin, salol, procaine amide, barbiturates, New Allonal, acetophenetidin (phenacetin), acetanilid, ethacrynic acid.

From Wintrobe[22]

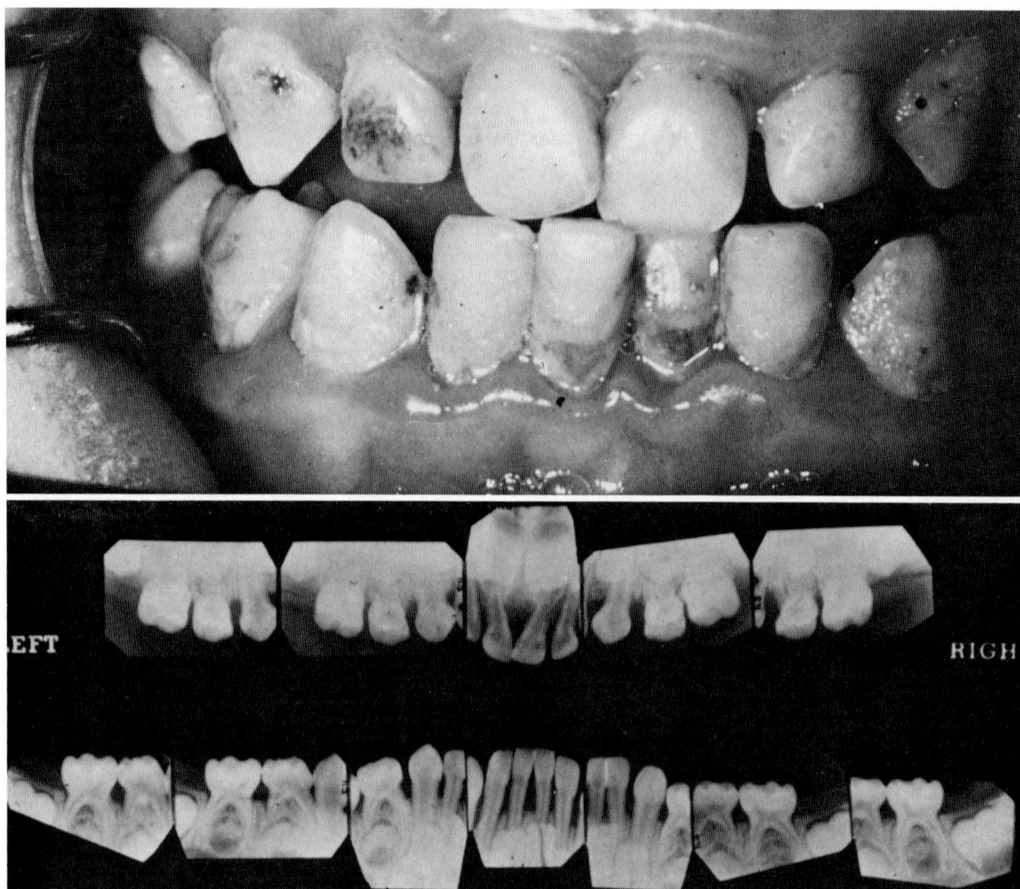

Fig. 11-2. *Top.* Cyclic neutropenia in a 4-year-old boy. Note gingival inflammation. *Bottom.* Roentgenograph of above patient demonstrating alveolar bone loss in the primary dentition.

Treatment. The oral symptoms are treated symptomatically

Prognosis. Generally favorable. In the past death was mainly due to overwhelming secondary infection, but it now can usually be prevented and/or controlled with antibiotics.

Cyclic Neutropenia

Cyclic neutropenia is an unusual disease characterized by neutropenia at approximately 21-day intervals and by a malaise, fever, arthralgia, oral ulcerations and in many instances, a severe loss of alveolar bone, gingival inflammation and the formation of deep periodontal pockets (Figs. 11-2 through 11-5).[5,6,11,19,20]

Etiology. Unknown. The hereditary aspects have not been well studied. The onset of the disease may occur at any age. There is no sex predilection.

Clinical Characteristics. The typical syndrome of cyclic neutropenia begins with a rapid diminution in the number of neutrophils in the blood, along with a disappearance of granulocytes and their precursors from the bone marrow. This is followed within the next few days by the appearance of ulcers on the lips, tongue, gingiva and buccal mucosa and is accompanied by chills, fever, malaise and

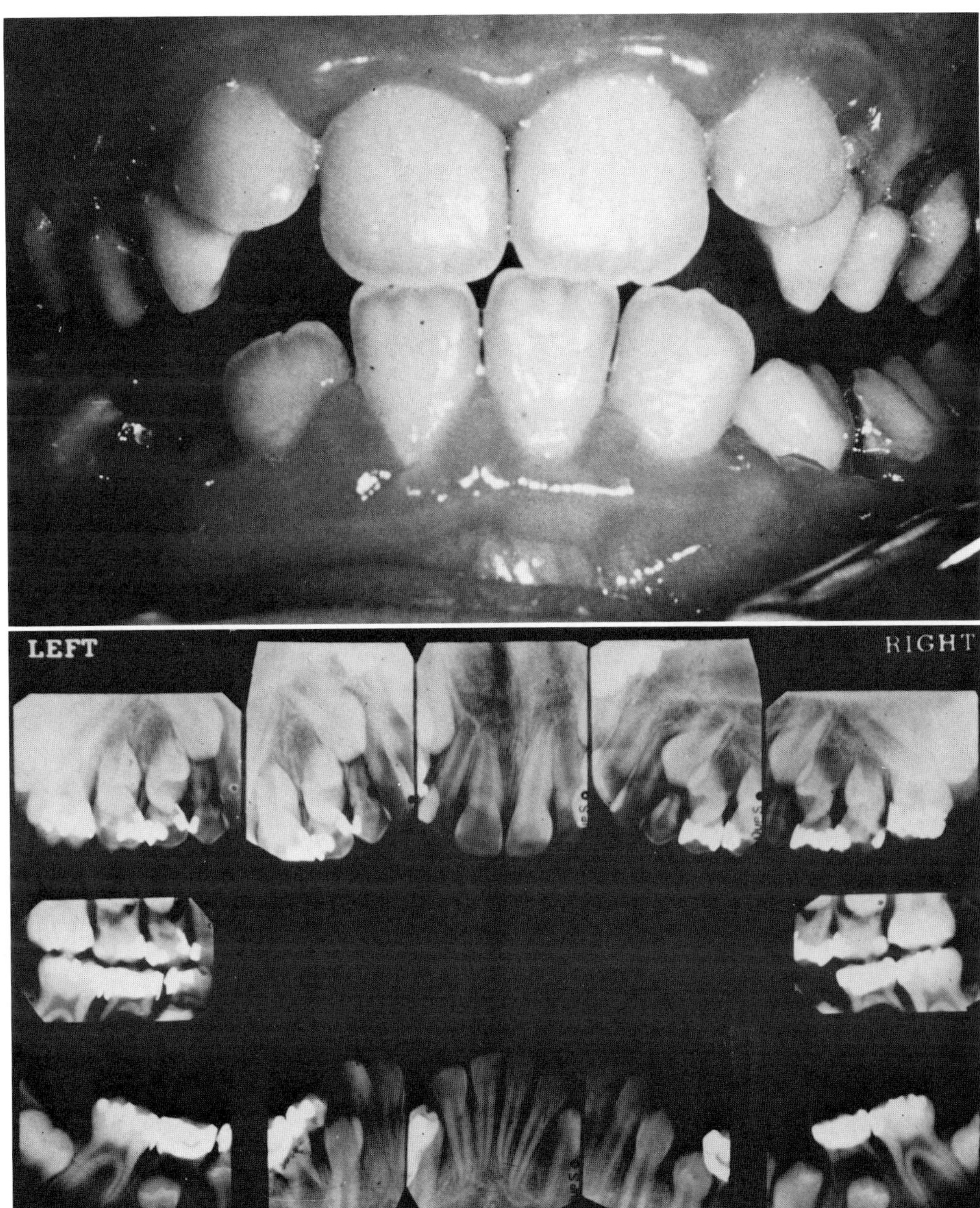

Fig. 11-3. *Top*. Cyclic neutropenia in a 7-year-old female. Gingival inflammation is an important diagnostic feature of this disease.
Bottom. Roentgenographs of the above patient.

anorexia. The majority of the patients also manifest skin lesions, such as furuncles, during the neutropenic phase of their disease. The patients also report a history of considerable upper respiratory infections. Whether this occurs during the neutropenic phase is often difficult to determine.

Periodontal manifestations. A review of the cases in the literature suggests that a relationship exists between the age of

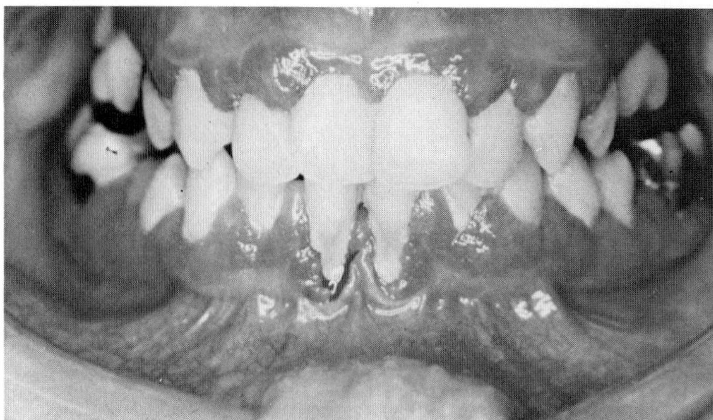

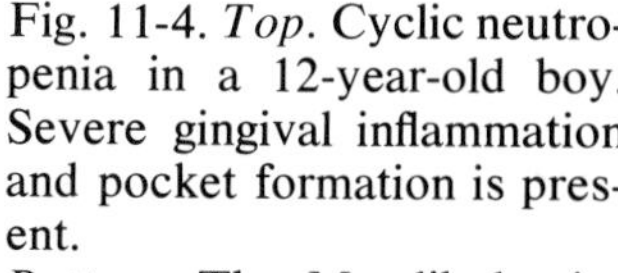

Fig. 11-4. *Top*. Cyclic neutropenia in a 12-year-old boy. Severe gingival inflammation and pocket formation is present.
Bottom. The Mandibular incisors in the patient shown above show marked loss of alveolar bone.

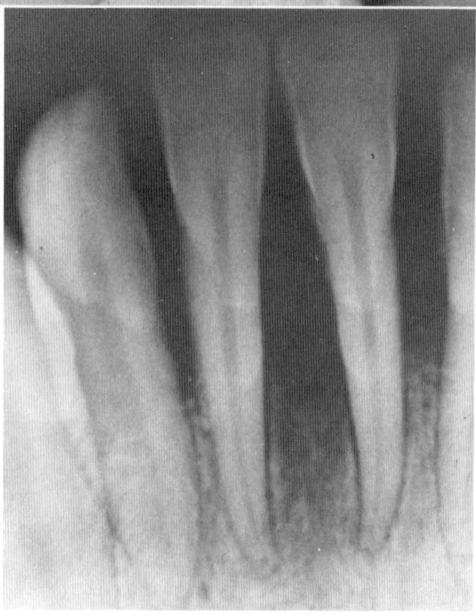

onset of the disease and the periodontal manifestations (Table 11-2). When the onset of symptoms has occurred in infancy, the children so affected generally seem to have a marked gingivitis about their primary teeth. Later, this is accompanied by loss of alveolar bone about the permanent teeth. Only two cases have been reported in which alveolar bone resorption was evident about the primary teeth. In the other published case reports the problem of the alveolar bone loss was either not mentioned or was actually not present.[8] However, since most of the reported cases have appeared in the medical literature, this omission is not surprising. When the clinical manifestations of the disease occur for the first time in adulthood, the oral ulcerations also usually occur, but the alveolar bone tends to be spared by the disease process.[2,3,14]

Laboratory findings. The principal laboratory finding is a fall in the neutrophil count that occurs periodically at intervals of approximately 21 days (Fig. 11-6). In the interval between the decreases, the blood picture may be normal. However, at all times the total white blood count tends to be a low normal. When the sudden marked decrease in neutrophils occurs, this is usually compensated for by an increase in the number of lymphocytes and/or monocytes. The neutrophils remain depressed for a period which ranges from

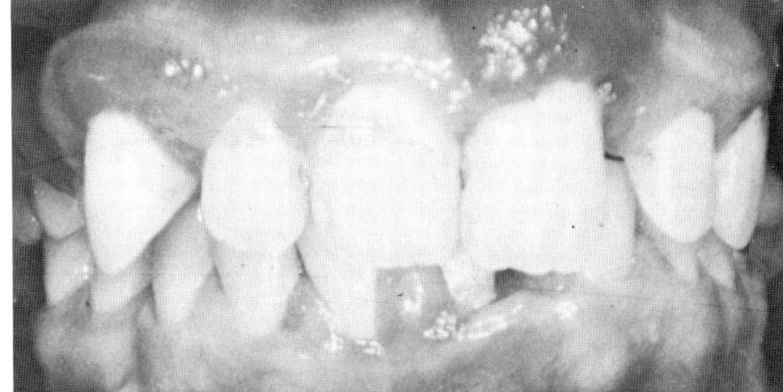

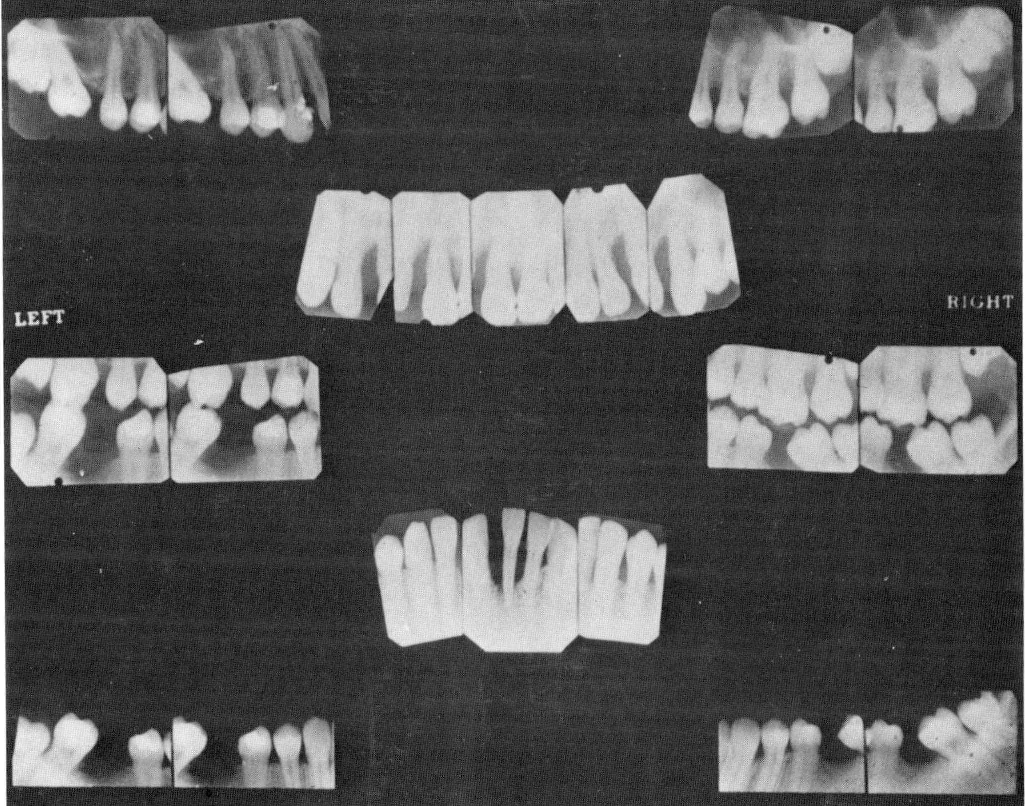

Fig. 11-5. *Top.* Cyclic neutropenia in a 15-year-old girl. Clinically there was a marked gingival inflammation and deep periodontal pockets. *Bottom.* Roentgenographs of the above patient.

2 to 6 days and reappear within a week or less, when the blood count also returns to within normal limits. During the peak of the depression period, the total white blood count usually ranges between 2500 to 3500 per cubic mm.

Because of the cyclic nature of the disease, a single blood count is inadequate for a diagnosis. Hematologic studies should be repeated at intervals of 2 or 3 times a week for 4 successive weeks to obtain an accurate diagnosis.

Treatment. Medical and dental therapeutic measures are usually disappointing. Therapy with corticotropin (ACTH) and corticosteroids does give symptomatic relief in some patients but has no effect on the neutropenic cycles. Splenectomy has been tried with some limited success, but is not recommended for patients under

TABLE 11-2 CYCLIC NEUTROPENIA WITH ALVEOLAR BONE RESORPTION

Case	Age of Patient	Age of Onset	Dentition Affected
Kaslick and Kutcher[11]	15	Infancy	Permanent
Cohen and Morris[6]	4	Infancy	Primary
	7	16 months	Primary
	16	13 years	Permanent
Levine[13]	14½	10 months	Permanent
Page and Good[17]	15	Infancy	Permanent
Cobet[5]	25	Infancy	Permanent
Owren[16]	23	5 years	Permanent
Coventry[7]	16	Infancy	Permanent
Smith[19]	20	6 years	Permanent
Telsey[20]	12	10 years	Permanent

25 years of age.[7] Supportive measures during the agranulocytic phase appear to be the best means of therapy at this time. For the periodontal problem, treatment should consist of occlusal adjustments, splinting of mobile teeth, curettage and plaque control. Periodontal surgery generally should be avoided and severely involved teeth extracted rather than an attempt being made to save them by surgery. However, minor surgical corrections may be done, such as a frenectomy, to relieve areas prone to inflammation. An antibiotic is usually administered postoperatively. The discomfort from the oral ulcerations can be relieved by topical application of triamcinolone acetamide with an oral adhesive (Kenalog in Orabase). The patient should apply this paste after each meal and before retiring. The use of tetracycline rinses also may be effective in reducing the discomfort. Tetracycline for oral suspension (Achromycin) containing uncoated tetracycline crystals, 250 mg. per 5 cc. (1 teaspoon) should be used. A teaspoonful of the suspension is held in the mouth over the area of the lesions and a flushing motion is maintained for a period of at least 2 minutes. The suspension is then expectorated.

Chronic Neutropenia and Familial Benign Neutropenia

Chronic idiopathic and familial benign chronic neutropenia have similar manifestations with the exception that the latter is inherited as a non-sex-linked dominant. Both are characterized by a consistent neutropenia associated with normal to decreased leukocyte counts, usually with a relative lymphocytosis and monocytosis and an absence of splenomegaly. In some patients clinical features are absent and the diagnosis results fortuitously from either a routine blood examination, a familial history of the disease, or from blood examination requested because of the unusual nature of the periodontal tissues.

Clinical Characteristics. The main clinical feature of this disease may be manifested as a severe periodontal problem.[1] In a child or adolescent so affected this can result in considerable discomfort. A tendency for repeated furuncles may also be present

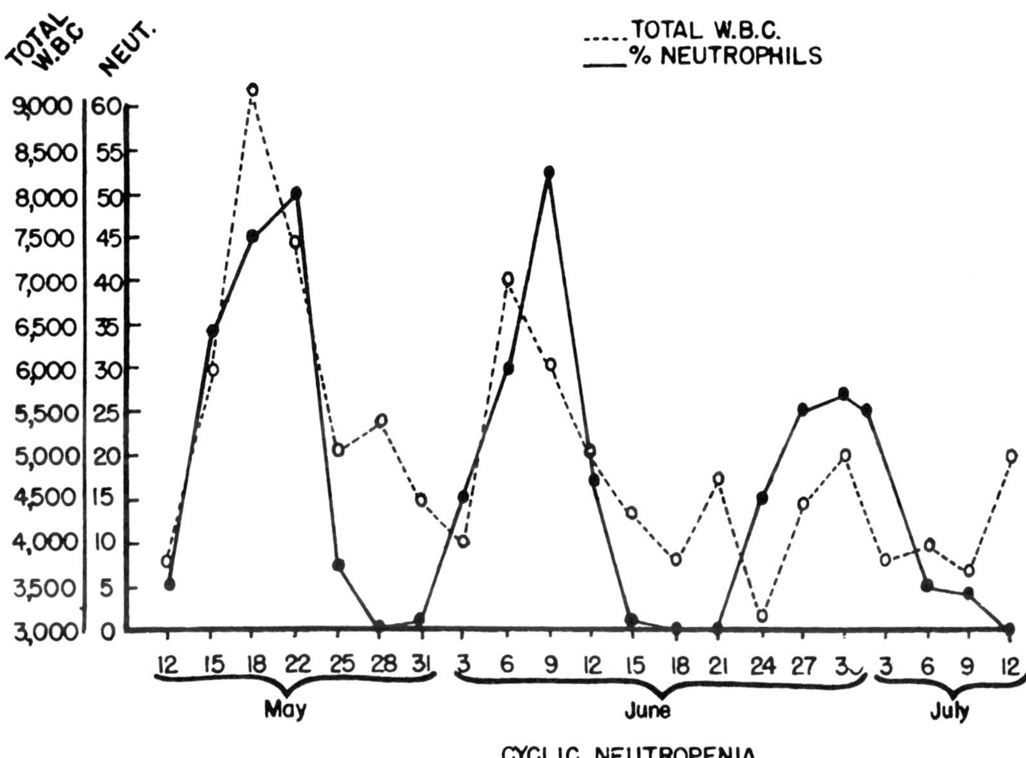

Fig. 11-6. The principal laboratory finding in cyclic neutropenia is a fall in the neutrophile count that occurs at intervals of approximately twenty-one days. (From Gorlin, and Chaudry.)[8]

along with a history of repeated upper respiratory infections.

Periodontal manifestations. The gingival has been described as being bright red in appearance,[22] or as being cherry-red, soft, swollen and edematous with areas of partial desquamation,[12] or as a bright red, jellylike hyperplastic gingivitis.[13] Cervically, a distinct granulomatous type of lesion, well demarcated from the rest of the attached gingiva, may be present (Fig. 11-7). These latter lesions disappear with exfoliation of the primary teeth and reappear with the eruption of the permanent dentition. Periodontal pockets are generally present and the alveolar bone loss can be quite marked (Fig. 11-8). Oral ulcerations are also usually present but all these manifestations are not present in all cases.

Laboratory findings. The total leukocyte count is rarely below 2000 cells per cubic millimeter. However, there is a marked neutropenia usually with a shift to the left and a relative or sometimes an absolute lymphocytosis.

Treatment. Generally, no systemic treatment is indicated despite the severe neutropenia, because overwhelming infections ordinarily do not occur. As in all disease there is some biologic variation. Corticosteroids do not influence the chronic neutropenia and therefore should not be given. Spontaneous remission has been reported to occur in several cases.[21] Periodontal therapy should be minimal with an effort made to remove local irritating factors where possible. Plaque control presents a problem to the patient in that the mouth is

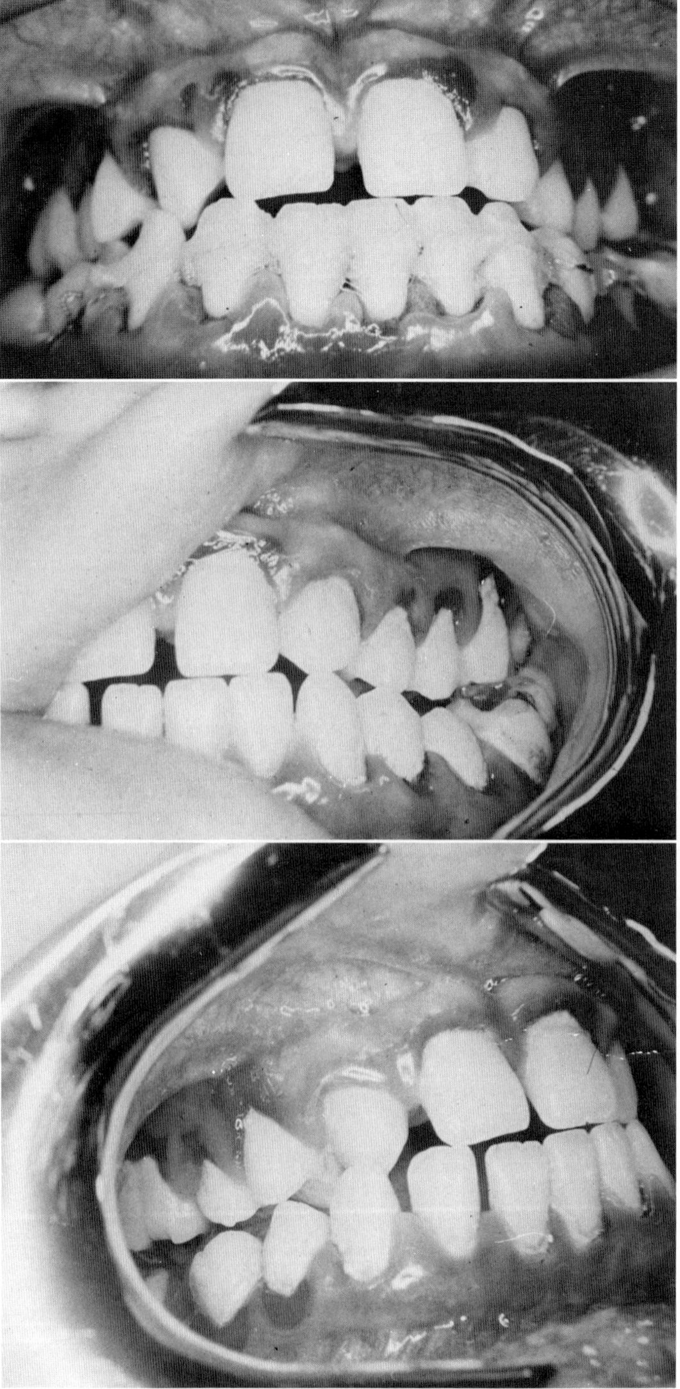

Fig. 11-7. Note the cervical granulomatous lesions present about the bicuspids and the maxillary central incisors in this patient with chronic neutropenia.

chronically sore and the patient has a tendency to avoid touching these areas. Reduction of the pain, therefore, is the first step in gaining patient cooperation. This can be accomplished by the use of topical anesthetic agents such as lidocaine hydrochloride (Xylocaine Viscous), diphenhydramine hydrochloride (Benadryl

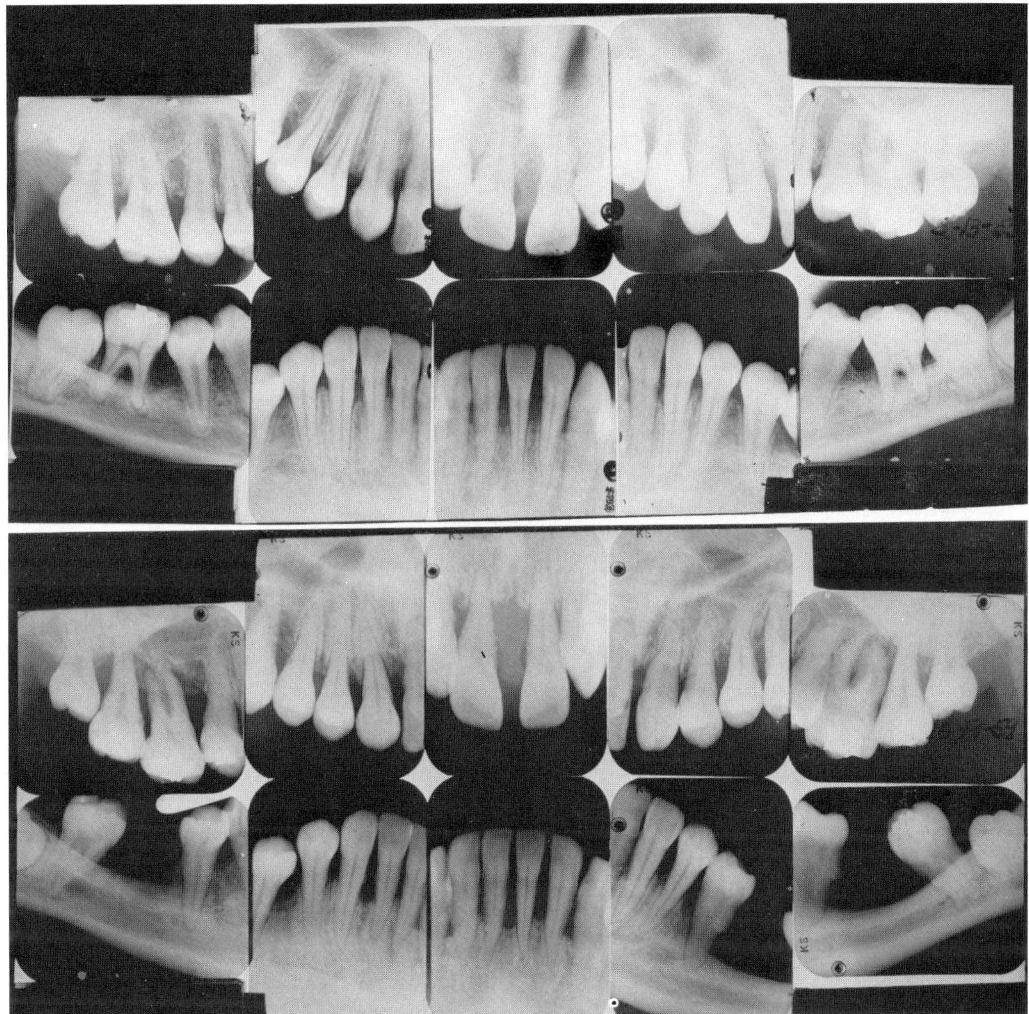

Fig. 11-8. *Top*. Roentgenographs of the patient shown in Figure 11-7 were taken when the patient was 13 years old. Total white blood cell count was 3300. Neutrophiles 1 to 10 percent, lymphocytes 65 to 90 percent. *Bottom*. The same patient four years later at 17 years of age. Rapid loss of alveolar bone has occurred.

elixir) or dyclonine hydrochloride (Dyclone hydrochloride). Once the areas have become anesthetized oral hygiene may be maintained by running a rubber stimulator tip along the gingival margin or by using a soft cotton swab in a like manner.

Pseudo Neutropenia

The accepted normal values for white blood cells in the peripheral blood are based almost entirely on values found in white populations. Recent studies, however, indicate that there are apparently true genetic differences between the races in regard to the granulocyte count.[4,10,15] It has been shown that more than 30 percent of American black men and 40 percent of American black women have leukocyte counts below 5000 per cubic millimeter, compared with less than 7 percent for white men and women.[10] This leukopenia is due to a granulocytopenia. Monocyte, eosinophil and basophil counts were the same in all groups studied. Means, ranges and standard deviations for age, hemoglobin and hematocrit values were nearly identical in both sexes for American blacks and whites. Similar findings have been reported for African Negroes.[9,18] A somewhat similar genetically determined neutropenia has been found among Jews of Yemenite origin.[18]

This entity has neither systemic, oral nor periodontal manifestations of clinical diagnostic significance.

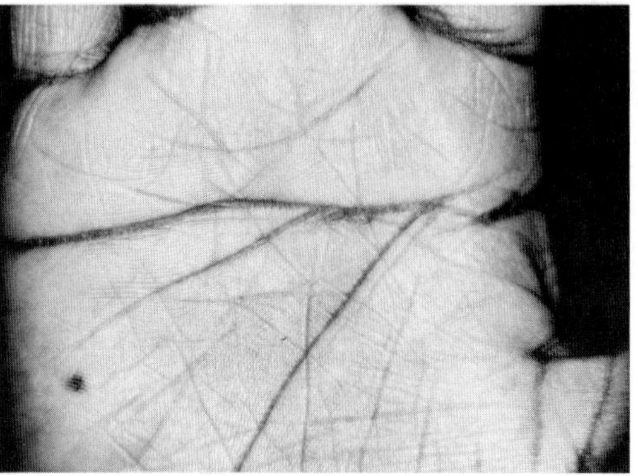

Fig. 11-9. The single transverse palmar flexion crease.

DOWN'S SYNDROME

Down's syndrome, which is frequently referred to as mongolism, was first described by Langdon Down in 1866.

Etiology. Unknown. It is associated with a chromosomal abnormality and has a direct relationship to the age of the mother.

Prevalence. It is safe to assume that in unselected material it occurs in 2 out of 1000 births.[24]

In maternal age group of 19 to 28 the incidence is estimated as 1 in 2300 births. At maternal age between 35 to 39 the incidence is somewhere between 3 and 8 per thousand births, after age 40 it increases to 10 to 20 children per thousand births and after maternal age 45 it doubles in number. A majority of the patients with Down's syndrome have a total number of 47 chromosomes as opposed to 46 for a normal individual, usually due to trisomy of the twenty first chromosome. However, in 2 to 3 percent of the patients, instead of trisomy of the twenty first chromosome there is a translocation, with a resulting normal number of 46 chromosomes. Translocation is more frequent in children born to young mothers. Clinically the translocation mongoloid shows very little difference from the standard trisomy patient.

There is some evidence from epidemiologic studies that the disease might be caused by an infective agent, possibly of viral origin.[28] Support for this idea is based on the following facts: There is a periodic variation in the incidence of mongolism, with a period of oscillation of from 5 to 6 years; a consistently higher incidence in urban areas as compared with rural areas; a "clustering" of cases in no fewer than 40 percent of mongoloid births (cluster indicating a group of such children born in a restricted area within a 12-month period). Kashgarian and Rendtorff in their study on the incidence of Down's syndrome in American blacks confirmed the presence of a clustering effect with the incidence varying periodically in 5- to 6-year cycles.[34] These authors also found no difference between the rate of Down's syndrome in white and black populations. While the mechanics of trisomy can be traced to nondisjunction, the etiology of nondisjunction has not been established and can be suspected only in general terms. The present evidence suggests that Down's syndrome is not due to so-called hereditary factors but is due to an error in cell metabolism which must be traced back to such environmental conditions as radiation, nutrition or a virus, that interferes with normal cell division.[24] The most likely way virus-induced damage might be related to the etiology of Down's syndrome is in the induction of nondisjunction by persistent nucleoli or as the result of gene mutation. It is also possible that virus-induced mitotic delay could result

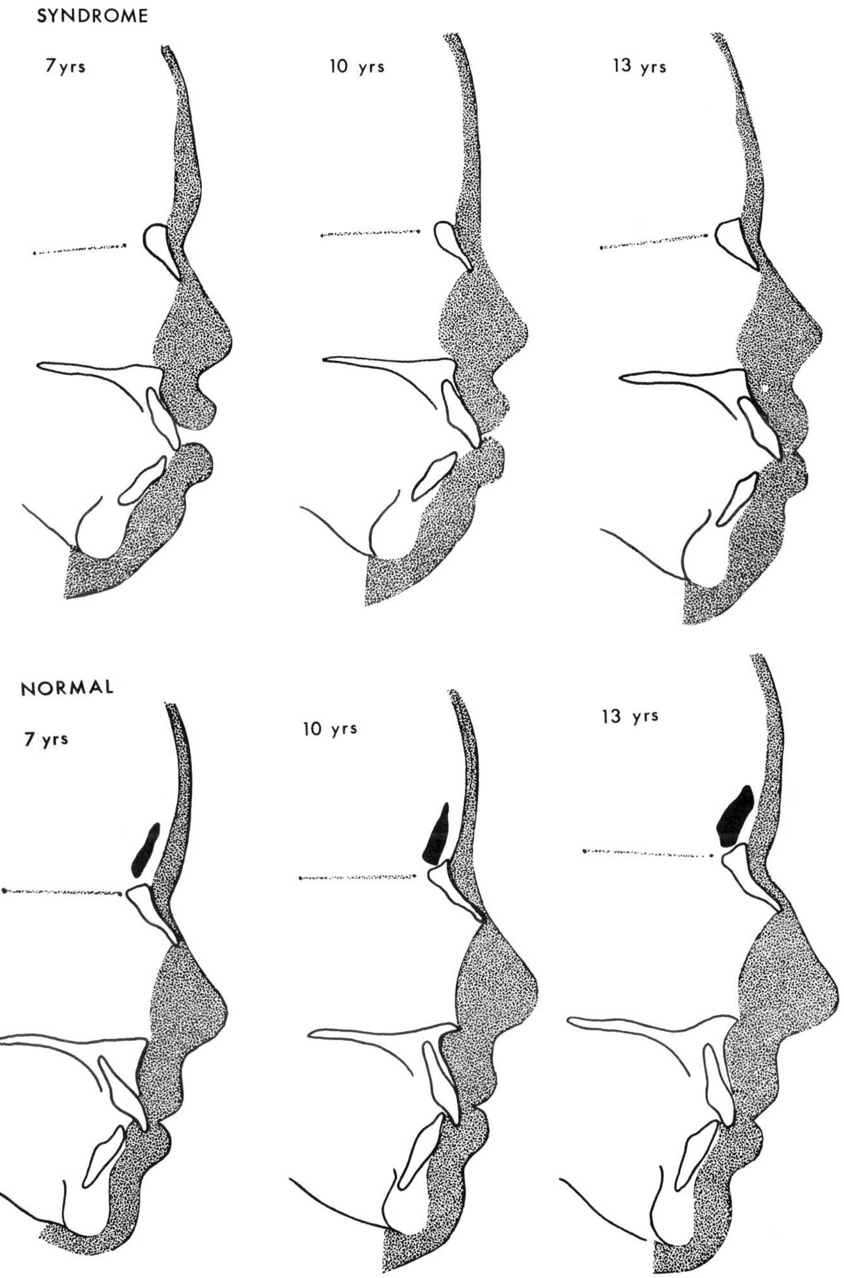

Fig. 11-10. *Top.* The soft-tissue and skeletal profile of a subject with Down's syndrome at three different ages. Included is the linear dimension of the anteroposterior limits of the cribriform plate of ethmoid bone. Note the absence of a frontal sinus.
Bottom. The soft-tissue and skeletal profile of a normal subject at three different ages. Included is the linear dimension of the anteroposterior limits of the cribiform plate of ethmoid bone. Note the progressive morphologic changes of the frontal sinuses at different age levels. (Baer.)[23]

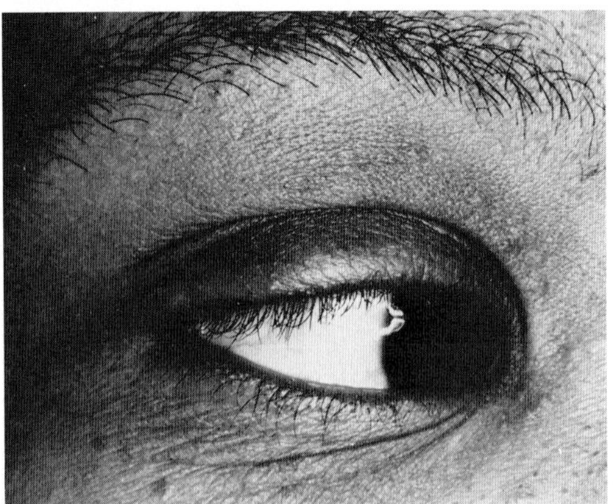

Fig. 11-11. The best-known sign of Down's syndrome is the anomaly of the direction of slant and the size and shape of the palpebral fissure.

in the production of an over-ripe egg with its consequent abnormalities.[40]

Clinical Characteristics. In addition to some degree of mental subnormality, and the oral manifestations which will be discussed later, there are 3 physical characteristics that may help the dentist to establish a diagnosis:

1. A single transverse palmar flexion crease (Fig. 11-9).

2. Anomalies in the area of craniofacial development[45,47] such as small head, smaller linear dimensions of cranium, short cranial base, flattened occiput, smaller orbital cavities, underdeveloped bones within region of nasal cavity, depressed bridge of the nose, short and arched palate and partial or complete absence of frontal sinuses. The characteristic brachycephalic skull is due to a marked lack of growth in length. The width of the skull is only slightly below normal. In a recent study[23] it was shown that the area of the skull most affected in Down's syndrome is the region of the cribriform plate, ethmoid and nasal bones (i.e., the area most affected was the face), resulting in an infantile skull with abnormal proportions (Fig. 11-10).

3. The anomaly of the direction of slant, the size and shape of the palpebral fissure, perhaps the best known of the Down's syndrome signs[46] (Fig. 11-11). The slant of the eyes in Down's syndrome is the result of slanting openings in the skull. The Mongolian race, on the other hand, does not exhibit such an upward curvature of the orbital margin of the skull.[24] The up-and-out slanting palpebral fissure occurrence, however, is not ubiquitous but occurs in about 75 to 88 percent of the affected individuals. Actually the most characteristic configuration is the even arch of the upper eyelid margin, with its highest point occurring in the center of the lid. This is contrary to the configuration of the normal eyelid in that the high point of the arch is at the junction of the inner and middle third.[32] The epicanthus is reported to occur in only about 28 percent of cases of Down's syndrome. Many other various signs and symptoms constituting the diagnosis of Down's syndrome are shown in Table 11–3.

Oral signs and symptoms. The tongue is frequently fissured but not usually enlarged and the lips may frequently be fissured and dry. These patients also exhibit a tendency for xerostomia. The widely held view that a high narrow palate is a common characteristic of people with Down's syndrome has not been substantiated by a recent study.[42]

Eruption of the primary teeth is invariably retarded. Normally, the incisors erupt at about 6 months of age, while in Down's syndrome this rarely occurs before the ninth month and the primary dentition is generally not completely erupted before the fourth or fifth year.[41, 43]

Microdontia is the most common morphologic defect. McMillan and Kashgarian noted that the defects of abnormal morphology and congenitally missing teeth were present in both the primary and permanent dentitions and tended to be confined to the maxillary and mandibular incisors.[39]

The prevalence of missing teeth in Down's syndrome is at least 4 to 5 times greater than in the general population or

TABLE 11-3. SYMPTOMS CONSTITUTING THE DIAGNOSIS OF MONGOLISM

	Percent		Percent
Skull		Nose	
Open fontanel (beyond 1½ yrs.)	16	Flat nose	44
Open sutures	4	Small nose	54
Flat occiput	82	Flat nasal bridge	62
		Mouth	
Face		Constantly open mouth	62
Wrinkled	14	Small mouth	32
Red cheeks	66	Broad lips	36
Rough and scaly cheeks	74	Irregular lips	28
		Dry lips	32
Eyes		Fissured lip	56
Slanting eyes	88	Small teeth	56
Epicanthus	50	Conical lateral incisors	46
Blepharitis	38	Irregular alignment	68
Strabismus	14	Widely spaced teeth	28
Nystagmus	14	Crowded teeth	38
Speckling of iris	30	Large tongue	30
Double zone in iris	22	Furrowed tongue	44
		Protruding tongue	32
Ears		High-arched palate	74
Prominent	50	Narrow palate	52
Malformed	48	Cleft uvula	4
Small or absent lobule	80	Raucous voice	54
		Low-pitched voice	20

After Levinson, Friedman, and Stamps[37]

TABLE 11-4. PREVALENCE OF PERIODONTAL DISEASE

			Periodontal Disease %	
	No.	Age	Slight	Severe
	10	1 - 7	6–60	1–10
Male	12	8–12	10–83	2–16
	25	13–18	16–65	9–36
	28	19–Up	2 - 7.1	26–92.2
	8	1–77	5–62.5	2–25
Female	15	8–12	12–80	1 - 6.6
	25	13–18	15–60	10–40
	28	19–Up	5–17.6	23–82.1

After Dow[31]

in nonmongoloid mental retardates.[43] One or more permanent teeth were found to be congenitally absent in about 25 to 35 percent of the Down's syndrome patients sampled.[41] Anodontia, however, is extremely rare.[38]

A relatively low prevalence of caries was originally reported in these patients.[26] McMillan and Kashgarian found that 34 percent of the 95 patients they examined with the aid of a mirror and explorer were estimated to be caries free.[39] More recently Cutress in New Zealand did a survey and found that trisomy-21 persons resident in institutions had significantly fewer DMF teeth than congenitally mentally defective (CMD) persons, in institutions, but this difference was not apparent at a significant level between trisomy-21 persons and congenitally mentally defective subjects living at home.[30] In all instances, institutionalized people had fewer DMF teeth than their counterparts living at home. This is probably due to the lower sucrose intake of institutionalized people. Kroll, *et al.* also found no significant difference in the occurrence of dental caries between mongoloid and nonmongoloid patients.[36] He found that the average DMF teeth of patients through 18 years of age was 6.2 for the mongoloid group and 6.5 for the nonmongoloid group.

Periodontal Disease

Individuals with Down's syndrome have a high prevalence of periodontal disease. Nash reported a prevalence of 90 percent in his patients.[24] Dow examined 151 Down's patients and reported the prevalence according to age groups and severity[31] (Table 11–4).

McMillan and Kashgarian found that 62 percent of their 95 patients had periodontal disturbances characterized by inflammation of the gingivae in the region surrounding the mandibular incisors and early loss of their teeth.[39]

Kisling and Krebs found the prevalence of gingivitis to be 100 percent in a group of 71 male patients 19 to 25 years of age.[35] Cohen, in a group of 100 mongoloid patients, 57 males and 43 females, found severe periodontal disease in 96 percent.[26] In a roentgenographic study he found that the most frequent sites of bone loss were the maxillary and mandibular anterior regions.[27] The alveolar bone loss, however, was more severe in the anterior segments than in the posterior segments, even though the incidence was about the same in both regions (Fig. 11-12). Others have also noted that the mandibular anterior segment has the most severe periodontal destruction.[33] Johnson and Young also found periodontal disease in 96 percent of their mongoloid patients.[38] In comparing the periodontal

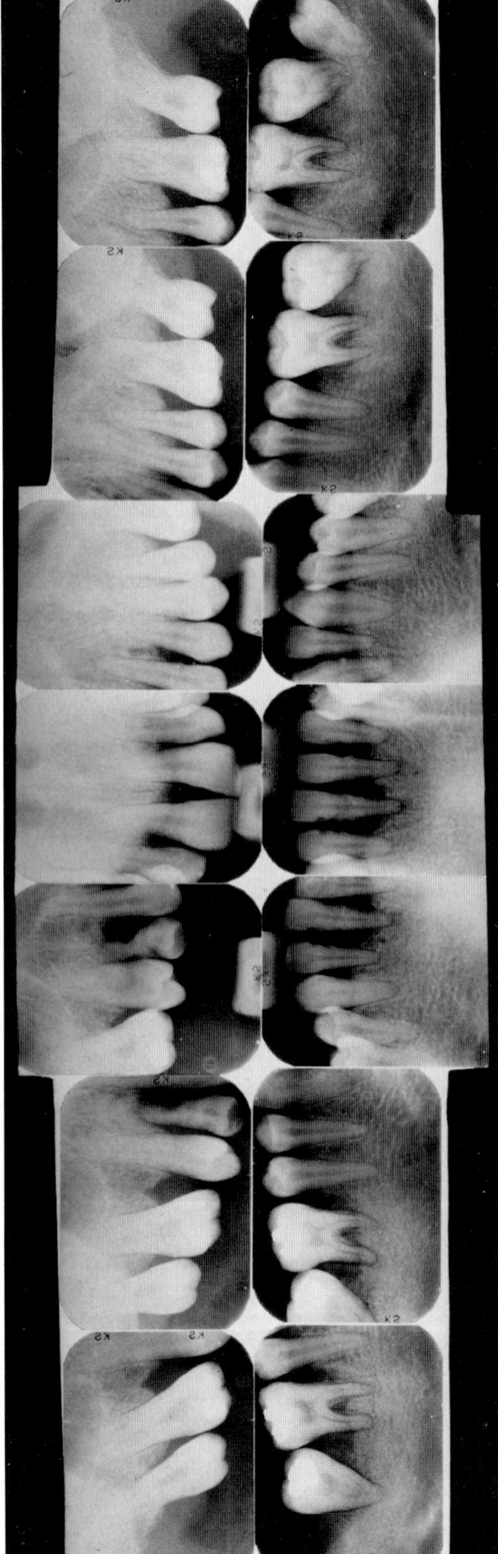

Fig. 11-12. Alveolar bone loss tends to be more severe in anterior segments.

TABLE 11-5. ALVEOLAR BONE LOSS IN MONGOLS AND IN CONGENITAL MENTAL DEFECTIVES

Group	Total Number Examined	Alveolar Bone Loss			
		None	Slight	Moderate	Severe
Mongoloids	25	1	6	8	10
Mental Defectives (Non-mongoloids)	25	7	9	9	0

After Johnson and Young.[33]

conditions in a group of trisomy-21 patients with other congenital mental defectives, they found that the severity of the disease in the trisomy-21 group was approximately twice that seen in the other congenital defectives. In fact, among the nonmongoloid congenital mental defective children there were no cases with excessive loss of alveolar bone (Table 11-5). These results have been confirmed by Sznajder, *et al.* in Argentina and Cutress in New Zealand.[49,30] For example, in comparing mongoloid with cerebral palsy children, Sznajder found that both groups had poor oral hygiene and similar plaque indices—(2.27 ± 0.75) for the trisomy-21 and (2.56 ± 0.75) for the cerebral palsy children—yet the cerebral palsy children had a low periodontal index (1.74 ± 1.32) without periodontal pocket formation, while the mongoloids had a high periodontal index (2.27 ± 0.75) with deep pocket formation and alveolar bone loss. Alveolar bone loss has been reported to occur about the teeth in both dentitions, although it is a more common occurrence in the permanent dentition. From some of the reports there is some indication that males may have more severe alveolar bone loss than females. This is based on the fact that male patients exhibit a higher rate of premature loss of their permanent teeth than do females.[35, 39]

There is also some evidence to indicate that the disease is more severe in institutionalized patients than in those attending training centers and living at home.[48] No significant correlation between bone loss and blood citrate levels was found in Down's syndrome patients with periodontal disease.[29, 44]

Another interesting feature is the high prevalence of acute necrotizing ulcerative gingivitis. Cohen reported its presence in 29 out of the 100 cases in his study, while Johnson and Young noted that some of the children in their series had grayish overlying ulcerated interdental papillae suggestive of a necrotizing ulcerative gingivitis, but in no instance could a definitive diagnosis be made.[26,33] Brown compared the clinical records of 68 patients with Down's syndrome with 99 other congenital mental defectives, all under 21 years of age, and found that 32.4 percent of the Down's patients had experienced necrotizing ulcerative gingivitis compared with 7.1 percent of the control group.[25]

Calculus. Kisling and Kreb and Sznajder, *et al.* found that the amount of calculus was fairly small, while Johnson and Young reported that the gross calculus was much more evident among mongoloids, in which it occurred in 85 percent of the patients as against 67 percent of the nonmongol mental defectives.[33,35,49] This latter group, they felt, showed more calculus than would be expected in normal noninstitutionalized children. Cutress reported on a comparison of the calculus among institutionalized versus noninstitutionalized mongols and found that groups resident in institutions had higher calculus scores than those resident at home.[30]

Treatment and Prognosis. Institutionalized patients with extremely low IQ's are unmanageable without premedication, and no cooperation can be expected from them. On the other hand some limited therapeutic procedures can be done on the noninstitutionalized patient who is willing to cooperate and who has a higher IQ. The prognosis, however, is poor for the severely involved teeth with deep periodontal pockets and bone loss. The alveolar bone loss in such instances should probably be regarded as another manifestation of the systemic problem. Extensive and heroic periodontal procedures, therefore, are not indicated.

HYPOPHOSPHATASIA

In 1948 Rathbun described a patient with low alkaline phosphatase activity in serum and with skeletal abnormalities. He established this as a syndrome, hypophosphatasia.[59,60] By 1957, when Fraser reviewed 35 cases reported in the literature, increased urinary excretion of phosphorylethanolamine was recognized as a third important feature.[62,63] Also, at this time the disorder was characterized as a genetically determined metabolic disease. In several families recently studied genetically, it was revealed that all the affected persons were heterozygous carriers of the gene.[58] The pattern of distribution and number of heterozygotes were compatible with transmission of the trait by an autosomal recessive gene. There have also been reported 3 cases of this disease with exfoliation of the primary teeth occurring in twins.[51,56,58]

Fraser[55] divided the phenotypic expressions of hypophosphatasia into 3 types: Type 1 starts in utero or within the first 6 months of life and is associated with severe skeletal abnormalities, craniostenosis, hypercalcemia and, occasionally, renal insufficiency. It usually results in death during the first year of life. The immediate cause of death is usually attributable to either renal damage resulting from hypercalcemia or from pulmonary or cardiac failure secondary to maldevelopment of the thorax. The few who survive the neonatal period usually develop premature synostosis of the skull, which can lead to oxycephaly unless artificial sagittal sutures are created surgically.

Type 2 is a less severe expression of the disease in which the lesions gradually become apparent after the age of 6 months. It may include rachitic skeletal changes and premature loss of the primary teeth. However, there may be an absence of clinical and roentgenographic evidence of bone disease in some patients. In these cases the only manifestations of the disease are the dental findings. This does not necessarily indicate that the bones in these latter patients are completely normal. It is possible that a slight abnormality of bone does exist or that bone lesions that were present earlier in life and not now detectable have healed.[58]

Type 3 hypophosphatasia patients are usually healthy asymptomatic adults in whom the diagnosis is frequently made fortuitously. Some of these patients may have undue fragility of the long bones. None appears to have periodontal problems related to the disease. In a few rare instances, some of these patients have had an enamel hypoplasia of their permanent teeth and some abnormality in crown morphology.[56] Since only in Type 2 are there persons who have periodontal problems, this will be the type discussed here.

While most reports have suggested that an enzyme deficiency exists not only in the skeletal tissues but also in all tissues in which alkaline phosphatasia is normally found, recent investigations indicate that this may not be so. The low activity of alkaline phosphatase in the serum probably reflects the low activity mainly in bone. There is no decrease in alkaline phosphatase activity, for instance, in the mucosa of the small intestine or liver.[54,61]

Clinical Characteristics. The dental findings that are diagnostic of this disease are premature exfoliation of one or more anterior primary teeth, either spontaneously or as a result of very slight trauma, roentgenographic evidence of "shell" teeth, loss of alveolar bone, usually limited to the anterior primary teeth, and absence of severe gingival inflammation (Fig. 11-13).[50,52] There have been a few cases reported in which the posterior primary teeth were also affected by loss of alveolar bone.[53,56,57] A low serum alkaline phosphatase and/or phospho-ethanolaminuria, and histologic evidence of hypocementogenesis of the affected teeth should be present before a definitive diagnosis is made.

Laboratory findings. Confusion in the alkaline phosphatase must be guarded against, since misinterpretations may occur because of the different normal values for children and adults. The range for a normal adult is from 4 to 13 King-Armstrong units; for a child, from 13 to 20 King-Armstrong units. Since this disease is believed to have a genetic basis and to be inherited through the action of an autosomal recessive gene, the serum alkaline phosphatase values should be ascertained wherever possible for the parents and siblings. In addition, when possible, the urines should be tested for the presence of ethanolamine phosphate, since present evidence suggests that there is usually a reciprocal relation between the serum alkaline phosphatase level and the excretion of phosphoethanolamine.

Differential Diagnosis. Although there are several systemic diseases which result in premature loss of primary teeth, the only disease which, from a strictly dental standpoint, resembles hypophosphatasia is Papillon-Lefèvre syndrome. The differential clinical diagnosis of these two diseases, therefore, is given in Table 11-6.

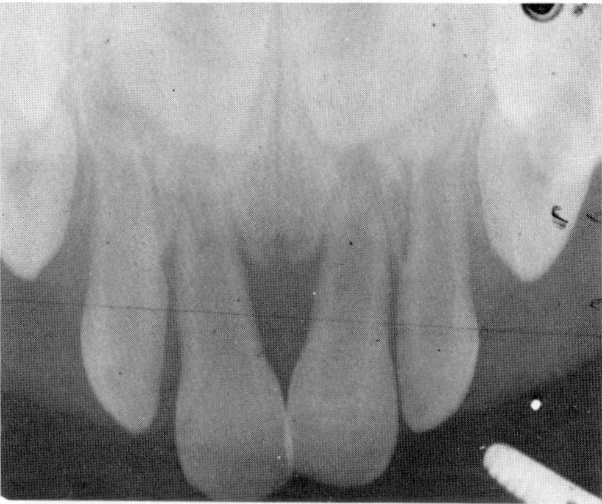

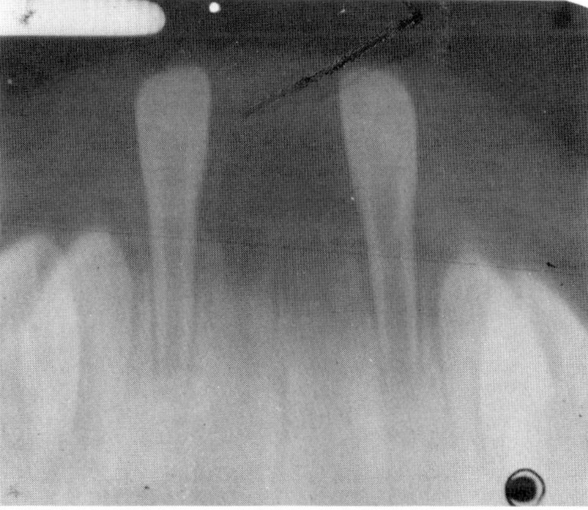

Fig. 11-13. Loss of alveolar bone and exfoliation of primary teeth tends to be limited to the anterior region.

The other systemic diseases which may result in loss of primary teeth are Down's syndrome, acrodynia, cyclic and noncyclic neutropenia. The physical findings are so distinctive in these 4 diseases, however, that a differential diagnosis should not be difficult to make. Children with neutropenia generally have very sore mouths owing to the presence of extensive ulcerations of the lips, tongue, palate, gingiva and buccal mucosa. In addition, they tend to have low-grade fever with malaise and arthralgia. Acrodynia is believed to be due to mercury poisoning; thus loss of hair, abdominal cramps and gastrointestinal upsets are prominent diagnostic features. The Down's syndrome patient is of course physically distinct.

TABLE 11-6. DIFFERENTIAL CLINICAL DIAGNOSIS OF PAPILLON-LEFÈVRE SYNDROME AND HYPOPHOSPHATASIA

Clinical Sign or Symptom	Papillon-Lefèvre	Hypophosphatasia
Gingival inflammation	Prominent feature	Usually absent
Roentgenograms of teeth	Normal	"Shell" teeth
Roentgenograms of alveolar bone	Extensive loss affecting entire primary dentition	Alveolar bone loss generally limited to anterior primary teeth
Prognosis	Poor, since both primary and permanent dentitions affected. Patients usually edentulous before years of age.	Good, since only primary dentition is affected

CASE HISTORY 1

In February 1964 a 2-year-old girl was referred for evaluation of loss of her 2 primary mandibular central incisors.

Late in September of 1963, at 19 months of age, the patient ate some pokeberries and was taken to the local hospital to have her stomach lavaged. After this procedure, the mother noted that there was "blood on the patient's gums." Thereupon she was taken to her dentist who noted that the 2 mandibular central incisors were quite mobile and that there was a loss of alveolar bone about them (Fig. 11-14).

In October 1963 her dentist extracted these 2 incisors and placed a space maintainer in this region. In an attempt to treat an excessive finger-sucking habit the patient was placed on 15 mg. of phenobarital, twice a day. From mid-November to mid-December, however, she had received not more than a single 15 mg. dose per week. There was no exposure to other drugs or toxic agents.

Laboratory tests of her fasting sugar, BUN, calcium, phosphorus and alkaline phosphatase were reported as normal.

The child's first cousin, through her mother, lost her lower central incisors, secondary to trauma, at the age of 2 years. She was reputed to have lost some of her other primary teeth, all secondary to trauma. Apparently her permanent teeth had erupted normally.

The patient's father had a full-mouth extraction at the age of 21 because of advanced dental caries. The mother's teeth are normal. There was no other family history of early loss of either primary or secondary teeth.

The patient was 84 cm. tall and weighed 10.5 kg. She was thin, well-nourished, intelligent and did not appear ill.

She was noted to have prominent metopic and coronal sutures on her skull. The remainder of the general physical and neurological examinations revealed no abnormalities.

Roentgenograms obtained from her referring dentist, plus the ones taken at our clinic, re-

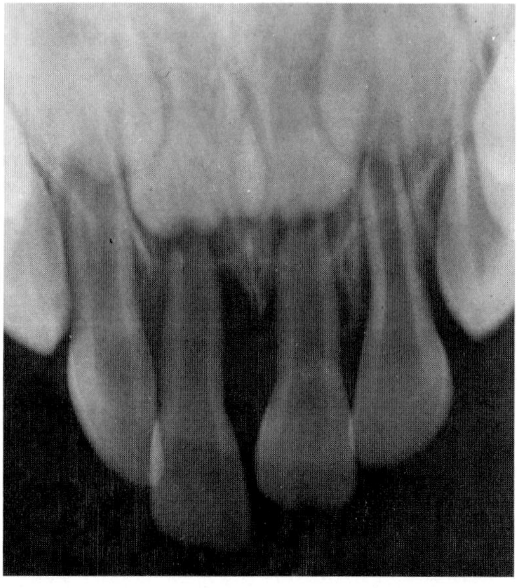

Fig. 11-14. There is severe loss of alveolar bone in this 19-month-old girl with hypophosphatasia.

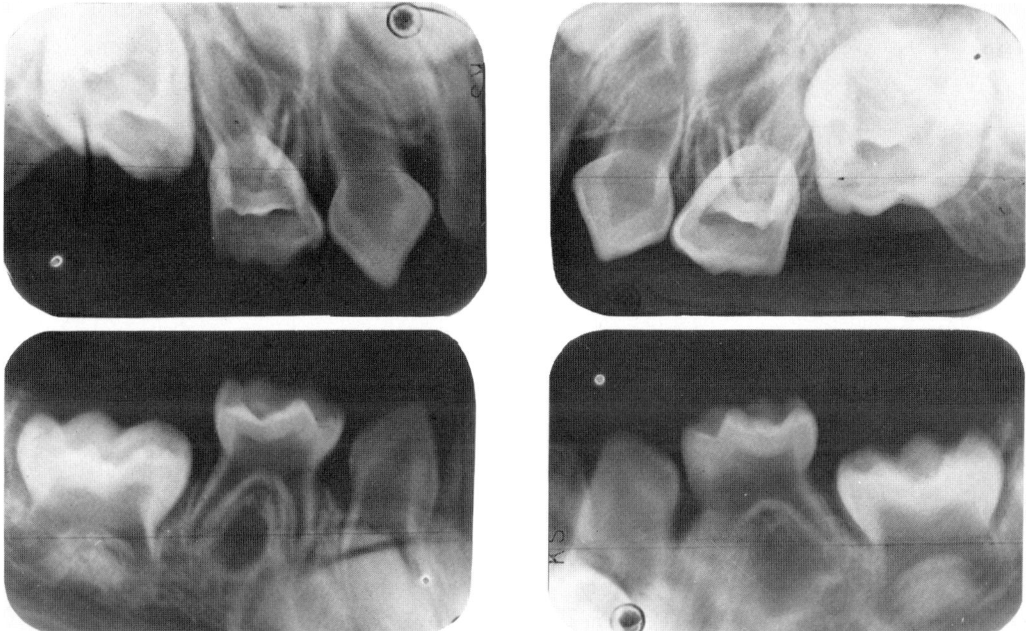

Fig. 11-15. "Shell" teeth are another diagnostic signs of hypophosphatasia.

vealed that all the primary teeth had large pulp chambers (i.e., "shell" teeth) (Fig. 11-15). A loss of alveolar bone had occurred about the primary mandibular central incisors. In all other areas the alveolar bone appeared to be within normal limits.

A clinical examination of the patient showed the gingiva and mucous membranes to be normal.

Urinalysis revealed specific gravity 1.022, pH 7, protein 0, sugar 0, sediment-rate white blood cell. On 2-18-64 the hemoglobin was 12.0 Gm., and hematocrit 37, white count 13,900, differential count–76 polymorphonuclears, 19 lymphocytes, 5 monocytes. Morphologically there was a question of anisocytosis. A repeat hemogram gave values of hemoglobin 10.9, red blood count 3.84 million, hematocrit 35, white count 12,000, differential count–70 polymorphonuclears, 16 lymphocytes, 11 monocytes, 3 eosinophils and mean corpuscular volume 92, mean corpuscular hemoglobin concentration 31, mean corpuscular hemoglobin 29. Fasting blood sugar was 92 mg.%, BUN 17 mg.% calcium 5.5 mg./eq. phosphorus 5.7 mg.% alkaline phosphatase 7 King-Armstrong units, total protein 6.4 Gm.%, albumin 3.6, globulin 2.8, creatinine 0.6 mg.%. Repeat calcium phosphorus and alkaline phosphatase was calcium 5.35 mg./Eq. phosphorus 4.3 mg.%, alkaline phosphatase 7 King-Armstrong units. Other serum electrolyte values were sodium 138 MEq/liter, potassium 4.4 MEq./liter, chloride 104 MEq./liter, CO_2 25 MEq./liter.

A roentgenographic survey of the skeleton, including the spine, hands, wrists, chest, knees and skull was made. No significant abnormalities were noted in any of these areas.

The patient was evaluated as to the etiology of her premature loss of 2 primary mandibular incisor teeth. Alkaline phosphatase on 2 repeat determinations was 7 King-Armstrong units. Normal for a child of 2 years of age is 13 to 20 King-Armstrong units, in our laboratory. When this was considered, along with the presence of premature loss of her primary teeth, the presence of "shell" teeth and the presence of prominent metopic and coronal sutures, a diagnosis of hypophosphatasia was made.

In addition, a 24-hour urine collection from the patient was positive for phosphoethanolamine. This is another feature which is characteristic of this disease.

The patient's mother's serum alkaline phosphatase was 3 King-Armstrong units, which is below the lower limit of normal, and her urine was positive for phosphoethanolamine.

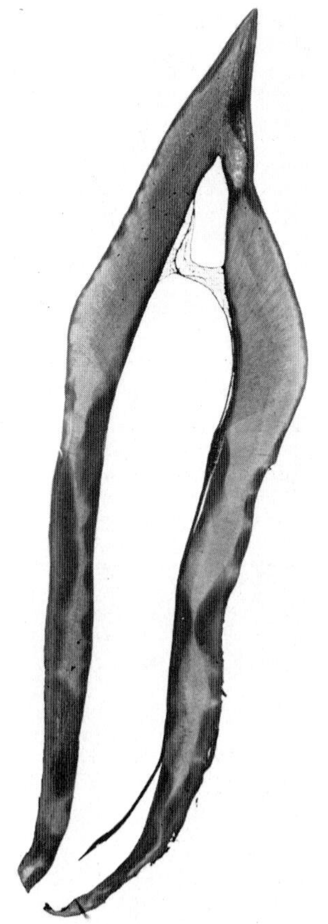

Fig. 11-16. The pulp chamber is enlarged.

The 2 primary mandibular incisor teeth, which had been extracted from the patient, were received in a dried state. The crowns of the teeth appeared to be normal but gross areas of resorption were present on the roots.

The specimen consisted of the primary maxillary left central incisor tooth that demonstrated an enlarged pulp chamber (see Fig. 11-16). The width of the dentin was reduced but it maintained a normal tubular form. The root surface was etched by external resorption and the amount of cementum was reduced (Fig. 11-17). Few periodontal fibers demonstrated cemental attachment.

Diagnosis. Hypocementogenesis, compatible with hypophosphatasia.

HYPERKERATOSIS PALMOPLANTARIS

This is primarily a dermatologic disorder which may exist in one of 3 forms—Meleda's disease, keratosis palmaris et plantaris (KPP or tylosis) or Papillon-Lefèvre. Only the Papillon-Lefèvre syndrome is associated with a marked gingival inflammation and the premature exfoliation of both the primary and permanent teeth.

The 3 forms of hyperkeratosis palmoplantaris may be differentiated as follows:

Meleda's Disease[66,76,79]

This disease has the following characteristics:

1. There is a marked degree of hyperkeratosis of the palms of the hands and the soles of the feet with deep fissures and a marked hyperhidrosis of these affected parts.
2. The hyperkeratosis usually extends excentrically in a glovelike manner. In

Fig. 11-17. Hypocementogenesis and external root resorption. (Baer, Brown, and Hamner.)[50]

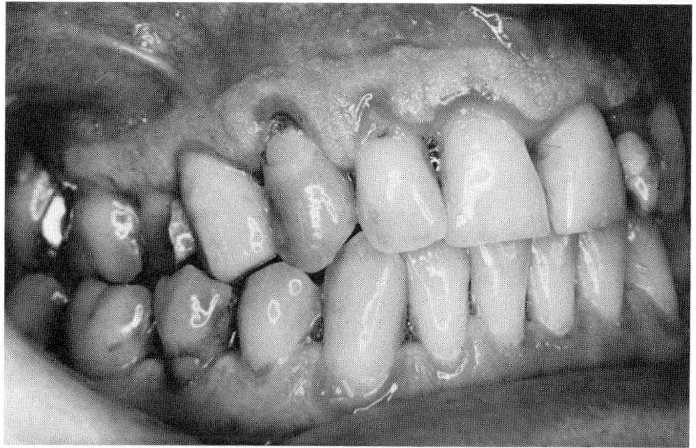

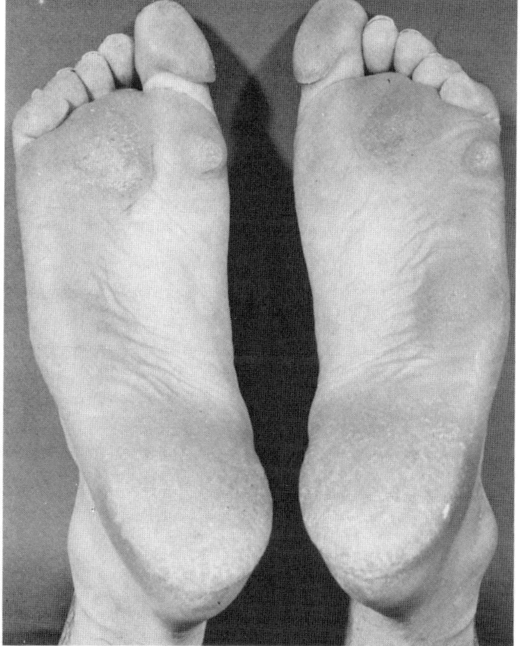

Fig. 11-18. (*Top*) Hyperkeratinization of attached gingiva. (*Bottom*) Hyperkeratinization of plantar surfaces. There was no palmar involvement in this patient. (Courtesy of Raphael, Baer, and Lee.)[81]

a great number of cases the hyperkeratosis may even involve the distal parts of the extremities and or elbows and knees. Occasionally it may even affect the axilla and trunk.

3. The degree of hyperkeratosis usually progresses with advancing age.

4. The disease is transmitted as a recessive genetic disorder.

5. Oral findings are not an integral part of this disorder.

6. It is found primarily in the inhabitants of the island of Meleda off the Dalmatian coast.

Keratosis Palmaris et Plantaris (KPP or tylosis)[66,70,74,76,81,86]

This disease differs from the above form in 2 ways:

1. It is believed to be inherited as an autosomal dominant trait rather than as an autosomal recessive trait.

2. Occasionally the gingiva and other

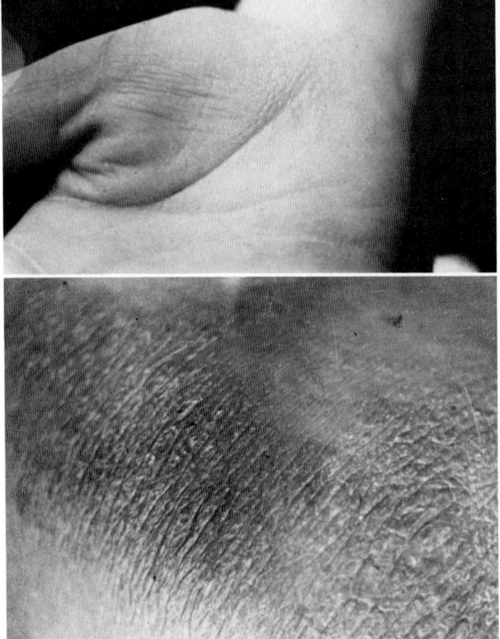

Fig. 11-19. *Top.* A hyperkeratotic lesion on the palm.
Bottom. A hyperkeratotic lesion on the knee. (Courtesy of Dr. F. A. Carranza, Jr.)

parts of the oral cavity may be involved with hyperkeratosis and even the esophagus may become involved. In some instances carcinoma of the esophagus has been reported to develop.[74]

Many other anomalies may also be present with this syndrome.

3. Unlike the Papillon-Lefèvre syndrome, the gingiva does not become inflamed and neither the primary nor the permanent teeth are prematurely exfoliated.[66,69,70,81,86]

4. The onset is usually at the third or fourth month of life, but initial detection may vary from birth to the second decade.

Recently we have seen 2 patients with what we believe is a variant of this disease in that hyperkeratinization of the gingiva and the soles of the feet were present without the palmar involvement (Fig. 11-18).[81]

Papillon-Lefèvre Syndrome

The following characteristics are typical of this disease:

1. It is inherited as an autosomal recessive trait. In many cases there is evidence of parental consanguinity.

2. It is associated with gingival inflammation and exfoliation of both the primary and permanent dentition.

3. The hyperkeratotic skin lesions tend to be well demarcated and limited to the palms of the hands and the soles of the feet, although at times they may be diffuse or punctate (Fig. 11-19).

4. The degree of hyperkeratosis tends to be light. The soles of the feet usually

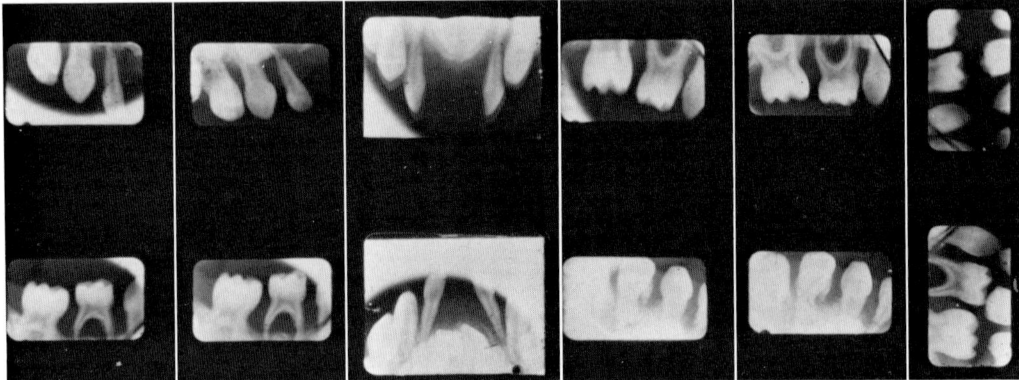

Fig. 11-20. Severe loss of alveolar bone in a 3-year-old boy with Papillon-Lefèvre syndrome.

are more severely affected than the hands, but rarely do they become excessively fissured and troublesome to the patient. The onset of the dermatologic involvement occurs at about the same time that the periodontal involvement first occurs, that is, some time between the second to fourth year of life, although it may start earlier.

5. The degree of hyperkeratosis present does not usually increase in severity with increase in the patient's age. The degree of involvement tends to fluctuate. It is usually worse in the winter, but some degree of hyperkeratosis palmoplantaris remains throughout life.

Etiology. Unknown. Recently collagen obtained from gingiva of clinically healthy and clinically inflamed areas of otherwise healthy young people was compared by disc electrophoresis with that from a 14-year-old boy with Papillon-Lefèvre syndrome. A comparison of the results indicated that it differed from that obtained from otherwise healthy individuals in that it was reminiscent of, but not identical with, that of published electrophoretic patterns of collagens digested by animal collagenases. On the basis of these results it was postulated that the periodontal involvement may be the result of a functional imbalance of the collagenolytic activity in that area. With regard to the dermatologic aspects of this syndrome, it was hypothesized that this might be due to an interenzymatic imbalance between proteolytic and mucoproteolytic enzyme systems in the skin without any change in the molecular integrity of the dermal collagens.[84]

Onset of Dental Changes.[67,68,72,73,75,77,82,85,87] The gingival inflammation, pocket formation and loss of alveolar bone are believed to start between the second and third years of age and to progress rapidly thereafter so that by the fourth to fifth year of age all the primary teeth are lost (Fig. 11-20). The severity of the inflammation is an important diagnostic feature of this disease

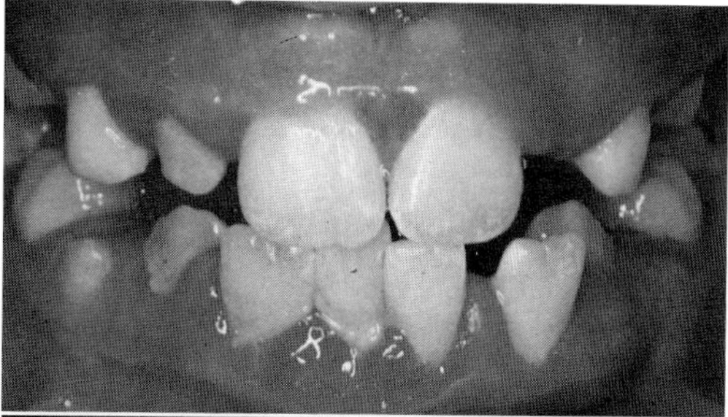

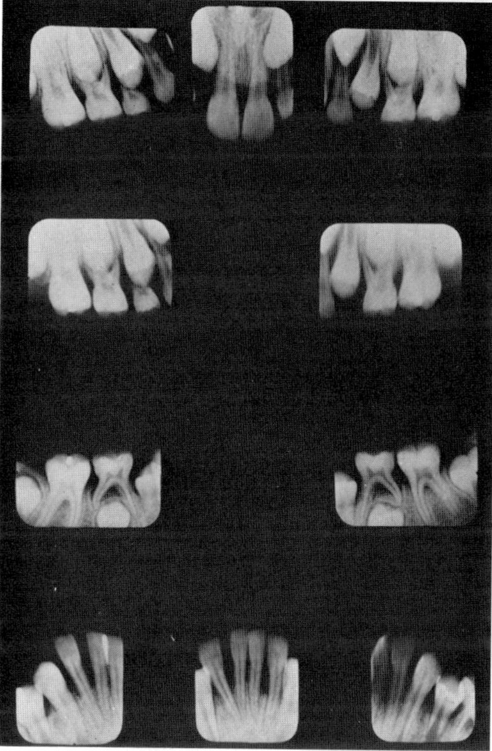

Fig. 11-21. *Top.* Severe gingival inflammation in an 8-year-old girl.
Bottom. Alveolar bone loss of patient shown above.

(Fig. 11-21). The gingival inflammation subsides after the teeth are exfoliated or extracted and remains so until the eruption of the permanent dentition. Tooth eruption itself is not interfered with, and the teeth in both dentitions erupt in a normal manner. With eruption of the permanent teeth, however, the process is initiated all over again. The gingiva becomes very red and inflamed, followed by severe alveolar bone loss that leads to a premature exfoliation

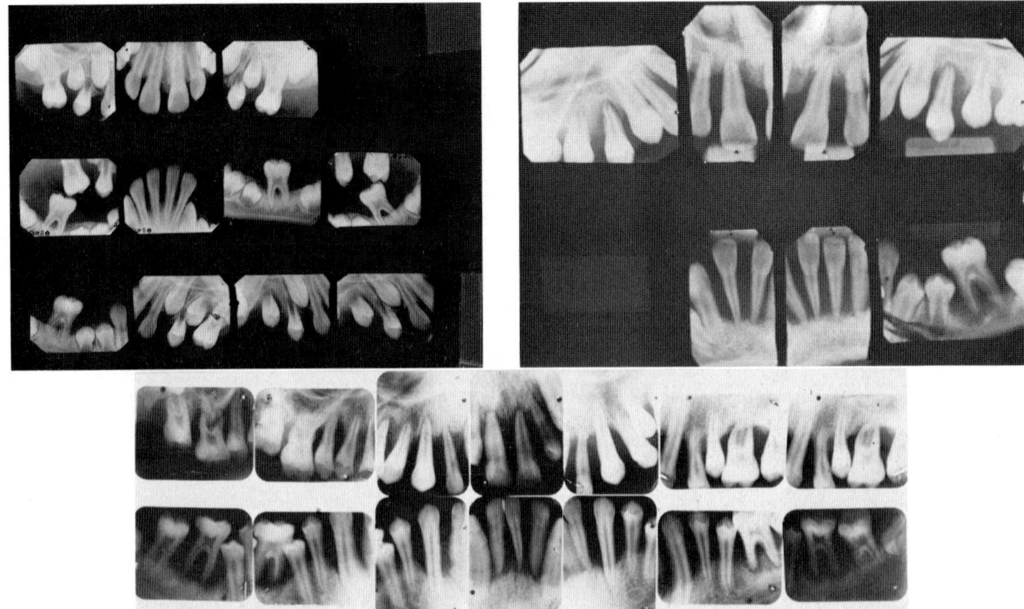

Fig. 11-22. *Top Left.* Roentgenographs of a 7-year-old boy with Papillon-Lefèvre syndrome. (Courtesy of Dr. Dennis R. Galanter.)
Top Right. Roentgenographs of a 9-year-old boy with Papillon-Lefèvre syndrome. (Courtesy of Dr. Dennis R. Galanter.)
Bottom. Roentgenographs of a 12-year-old boy with Papillon-Lefèvre syndrome. (Courtesy of Dr. F. A. Carranza, Jr.)

of the entire permanent dentition except for the third molars, which are usually not involved (Fig. 11-22). However, there has recently been reported a case where the third molars followed the same fate as the other teeth. Shortly after eruption they became loose and were exfoliated in periods ranging from 2 to 4 years.[64] The teeth in both dentitions are usually exfoliated in the same sequence as their time of eruption. The gingival and periodontal tissues only are affected by the disease. The oral mucous membranes of the lips, cheek, palate and floor of the mouth remain normal in size, shape and appearance. The patient usually becomes edentulous before the age of 20 years. Once the patient has become edentulous the gingival tissues return to normal and he generally does not have any unusual difficulty in wearing dentures. Healing, following exfoliation or extraction of the teeth, occurs at a normal rate and in a normal manner. The rapid destruction of alveolar bone which accompanies the disease leads to an edentulous mandible with very little vertical height. This leads to an interesting speculation. One wonders if, when the diagnosis of the disease is established, the permanent teeth were extracted as soon as they erupted, and before the onset of the destructive inflammatory changes, some of the vertical height of the mandible might not be preserved.

Histopathologic Findings.[77] A biopsy was taken of a block of tissue in a 12-year-old boy, containing the lower left premolar. Because of severe periodontal disease this tooth had to be extracted. Microscopic study of these tissues revealed complete destruction of the entire periodontal membrane along the labial wall and its

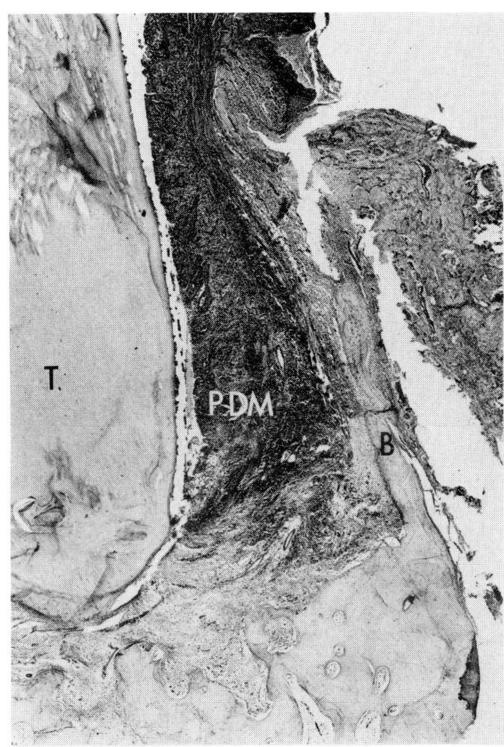

Fig. 11-23. Note the chronic granulation tissue filling entire periodontal ligament space. *T* is the tooth; *B* is the bone; and PDM is the periodontal ligament space.

replacement with chronic granulation tissue (Fig. 11-23). Acute osteoclastic activity and an apparent lack of osteoblastic activity was noted. The cementum along most of the root surface was very thin or almost absent except in the apical area where an area of cellular cementum was seen.

Other findings. Several authors have reported the finding of calcification in the attachment of the tentorium and choroid of the skulls of these patients.[72,76,88] Gorlin feels that this is a common finding and should be included as an additional component of this syndrome.[72] However, a review of the literature indicates that it is present in only 50 percent of the reported cases.[64,65,71,78,80,83] Predispositions to infectious diseases have also been noted in these patients. A regional adenopathy is also common, particularly during the acute periodontal episodes.

Genetic Analysis. A genetic analysis[64] reveals that the syndrome results from homozygosity for autosomal recessive genes (Fig. 11-24). The frequency of the disorder in the general population is believed to be 1 to 4 per million persons, and the carrier frequency is estimated to be 2 to 4 per 1,000 of the population.[72]

HISTIOCYTOSIS X

Reticuloendotheliosis

Letterer-Siwe, Hand-Schüller-Christian disease and eosinophilic granuloma at one time were considered to be distinct disease entities which could easily be clinically and histologically differentiated. However, it is now generally agreed that these are all variants of a single entity that belong to the broad group of diseases known as reticuloendotheliosis. The reason for this turnabout in point of view is based on

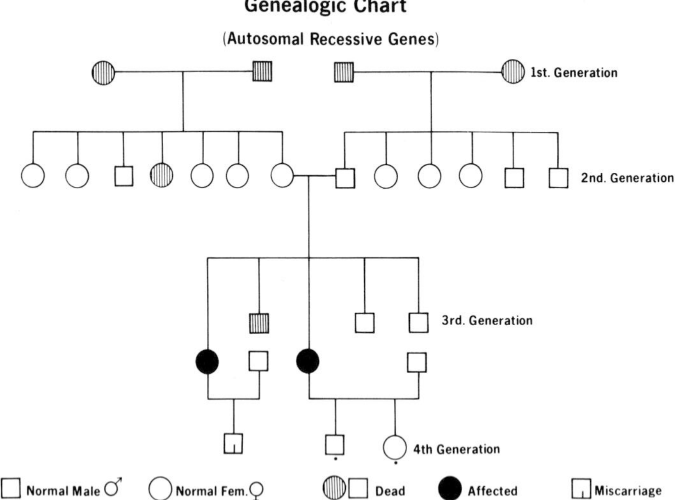

Fig. 11-24. Genealogic chart. (Courtesy of Dr. R. I. Carvel.)

several facts. First, the pathologist, looking at a single biopsy, cannot state categorically in which classification a given patient belongs. In one area the cells may resemble an eosinophilic granuloma, while in the same patient another area may consist almost entirely of foam cells. It used to be thought that the presence of these latter cells was diagnostic of Hand-Schüller-Christian disease. It is now known that this is not so. From a pathologist's point of view all that can safely be said of such lesions is that they belong to the broad group of reticuloendotheliosis with one or another cell predominating in the particular section being examined.

Second, the clinician is no longer certain of the subsequent course of the disease in a patient seen with a single lesion. After some months, however, it usually becomes apparent whether the lesion will remain limited to the skeleton or become disseminated to other organs. In those cases where the lesions remain confined to the skeleton, the prognosis is generally excellent. When the disease becomes systemic but the course is not rapidly progressive, the prognosis remains good. However, in those instances where the disease disseminates rapidly to multiple organs, the outlook is guarded to poor.

For these reasons, Lichenstein has suggested the following terminology for these three clinical states:

Eosinophilic granuloma—histiocytosis localized in bone; Hand-Schüller-Christian disease—chronic disseminated histiocytosis X; and Letterer-Siwe disease—acute disseminated histiocytosis X.[94,95]

Age of Onset. This is primarily a disease of children, adolescents and young adults, although the onset may occur at any age, with males being more frequently affected than females.

Clinical Characteristics. There may be no physical signs or symptoms in the mild form of this disease. In these instances the disease is diagnosed fortuitously through roentgenographic findings. The most common initial complaint is unilateral otitis media that does not respond to therapy.[89,96] Radiographs of the skulls of these patients generally reveals lytic lesions of the mastoid process. Oral lesions also occur frequently in the disease. In 30 to 40 percent of the patients they are actually the first manifestation of the disease process, and well over 60 percent of all patients have oral symptoms at some time during the course of the disease.[97,98]

Hand-Schüller-Christian variant. Actually fewer than 10 percent of the patients exhibit what used to be thought of as the classic triad of symptoms—skull lesions, exophthalmos and diabetes insipidus. The diabetes insipidus results from an infiltration of the pituitary by histiocytes, while the exophthalmos results from an infiltration of histiocytes into the orbit. Other common soft tissue locations which may become infiltrated by histiocytes are the liver, viscera, skin, lymph nodes, pulmonary tract and mucous membranes.[92]

Oral signs and symptoms. Pain, soreness and loosening of the teeth may be one of the early signs. Examination of the oral cavity may reveal an ulcerative necrotizing lesion of the gingiva with root exposure of the tooth in the affected area (Fig. 11-25). In some instances the gingiva and roentgenographic appearance of the lesion may resemble those seen in periodontal disease.[91,92,93] The most common roentgenographic finding is destruction of the alveolar bone, which gives the appearance that the involved tooth is "floating" in soft tissue. The margin of the radiolucency is sharp without evidence of a reactive sclerosis. The mandible is affected more frequently than the maxilla.[90] Generally two or more quadrants are affected by the destructive process. Almost invariably the molar or premolar regions are the sites of the initial involvement. In young children, the first evidence of the alveolar destruction is usually evidenced in the furca areas of the primary molars. The destructive process may then extend around the roots of the molar teeth and progress to involve the body, angle and ascending portion of the ramus of the mandible. In other patients, the failure of an extraction site to heal may be the first indication of an abnormality. Many times the skeletal involvement is limited to the jaws. If the skull becomes involved, then roentgenographically the lesions have a punched-out appearance without a reactive sclerosis. The skull lesions frequently tend to perforate the cortex and inner and outer tables, respectively. If the lesions involve the long bones, then radiographically they have an irregular, lobulated appearance and may be expansile. Laboratory tests are of little value in establishing a diagnosis of histiocytosis X.

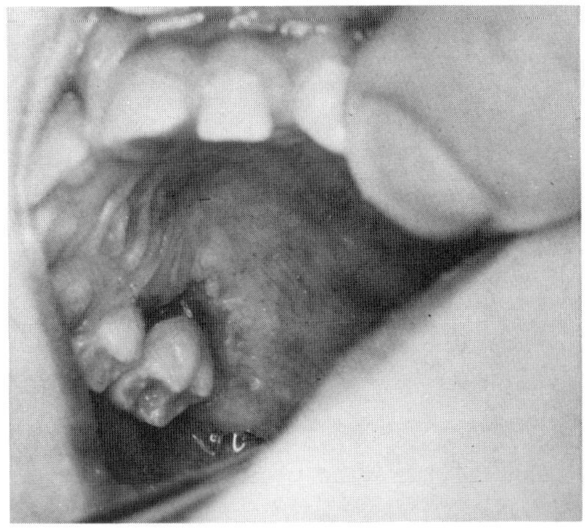

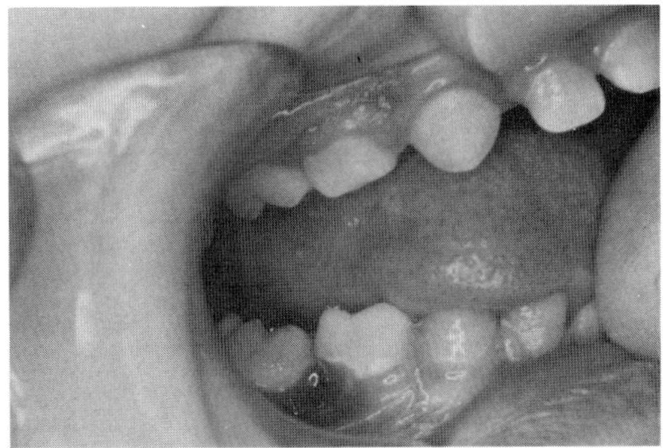

Fig. 11-25. *Top.* A lesion about the marginal gingiva of the palatal surface of the maxillary primary second molar in a 3-year-old girl. Biopsy of the gingival lesion was consistent with the diagnosis of histiocytosis X. *Bottom.* The root exposure on the buccal aspect of the primary first molar is the result of a gingival lesion in a 3-year-old girl with histiocytosis X.

Treatment. Treatment has been much more successful in recent years, even for the rapidly disseminating form of Letter-Siwe disease seen in young children. Steroids used in conjunction with antibiotics to combat secondary infections have proven to be of great value in tiding over the patient in critical situations. Roentgen therapy has been extremely beneficial in suppressing

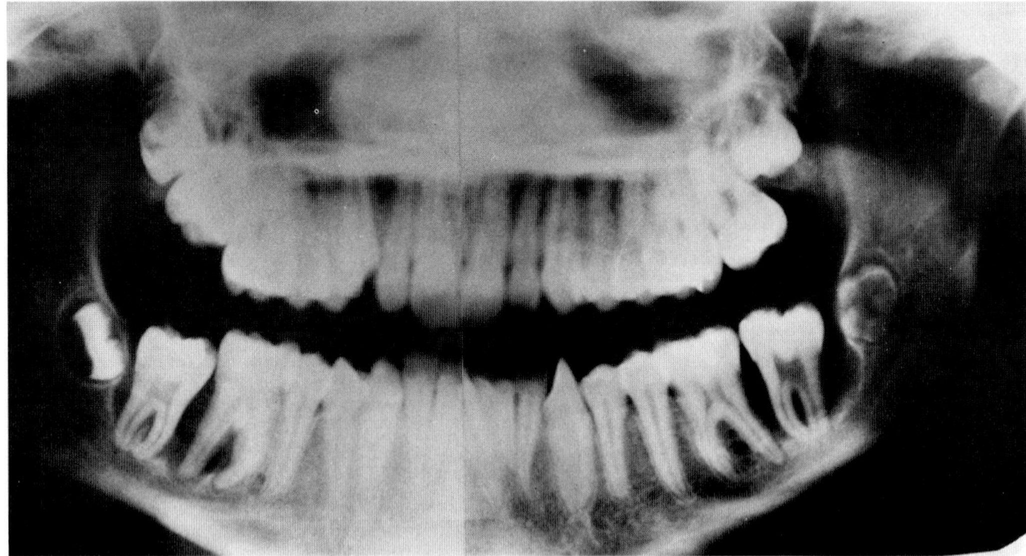

Fig. 11-26. Note the osteolytic lesions about the mandibular left and right first and second molars in 16-year-old boy. (See Case History 2.)

the mucocutaneous and skeletal lesions. The isolated skeletal lesions usually respond well to curettage and radiation. However, lone-term studies have shown that the disseminated form must still be considered to be a serious disease.[89,96] The mortality rate is still 13 percent for even the chronic disseminated, Hand-Schüller-Christian variant of this disease.

CASE HISTORY 2

The patient was the product of a normal full-term delivery and weighed 7 pounds, 3 ounces at birth. He apparently had a normal early growth and development with good weight gain and normal stature. At age 3½ years he was noted to have a painful area in the right parietotemporal region which was found to be a lytic bone lesion on x-ray examination. He was admitted to Children's Hospital in Pittsburgh for a biopsy of this area with a diagnosis of Hand-Schüller-Christian disease. He was treated with local excision of the lesion as well as radiation therapy and had a good clinical response. At about this same time the patient was noted to have the onset of severe polyuria and polydipsia and a diagnosis of vasopressin sensitive diabetes insipidus was made. The patient was treated with posterior pituitary extract with apparently good control of the diabetes insipidus.

Over the next several years the patient was admitted on at least 5 occasions to Children's Hospital in Washington, D.C. for radiotherapy of new bone lesions located in the skull, right posterior ribs and scapular areas. All of these responded well to radiotherapy. The patient's last such treatment was approximately 4 years ago for lytic lesions in the right posterior rib area. At age 13, the patient was noted to be below the fifth percentile in height and was noted to have no sign of puberty. Therefore, following an evaluation, he was started on methyltestosterone 10 mg. b.i.d. which was maintained over the next 4 years and finally discontinued about one year ago. During that period the patient was noted to grow approximately 3 inches in height.

At age 16, the patient's dentist noted abnormal development of his mandibular molars bilaterally and the boy was subsequently found to have lytic bone lesions in this area (Fig. 11-26). The patient was treated with extraction of the mandibular first and second molars on the right and the second molar on the left side. No radiotherapy was required. The final pathologic diagnosis confirmed the diagnosis of histiocytosis of the mandible.

REFERENCES

The Neutropenias

1. Andrews, R. G., Benjamin, S., Shore, N., and Canter S.: Chronic benign neutropenia of childhood with associated oral manifestations. Oral Surg., *20:*719, 1965.

1A. Awbrey, J. J., and Hibbard, E. D.: Abbreviated case report. Congenital agranulocytosis. Oral Surg., *35:*526, 1973.

2. Barling, B.: Chronic cyclical granulopenia. Proc. Roy. Soc. Med., *41:*653, 1948.
3. Barton, G. M. G.: Recurrent agranulocytosis: report of a case. Lancet, *254:*103, 1948.
4. Brown, G. O., Herbig, F. K., and Hamilton, J. R.: Leukopenia in Negroes. N. Eng. J. Med., *257:*1410, 1966.
5. Cobet, R., and Schilling, V.: Periodischezidivierende Neutropenie mit Monocytose. Folia Haematol., *70:*286, 1951.
6. Cohen, D. W., and Morris, A. L.: Periodontal manifestations of cyclic neutropenia. J. Periodont., *32:*159, 1961.
7. Coventry, W. D.: Cyclic neutropenia: report of a case treated by splenectomy. JAMA, *153:*28, 1953.
8. Gorlin, R. J., and Chaudhry, A. P.: The oral manifestations of cyclic (periodic) neutropenia. AMA Arch. Derm., *82:*344, 1960.
9. Howell, D. P. N.: Neutropenia in people of African origin. Lancet, *1:*1318, 1971.
10. Karayalcin, G., Rosner, F., and Sawitsky, A.: Pseudo-neutropenia in American Negroes. Lancet, *1:*387, 1972.
11. Kaslick, R., and Kutscher, A. H.: Cyclic neutropenia. Clinical Stomat. Conf. Columbia University, *4:*56, 1963.
12. Kyle, R. A., and Linman, J. W.: Gingivitis and chronic idiopathic neutropenia: report of two cases. Mayo Clin. Proc., *45:*494, 1970.
13. Levine, S.: Chronic familial neutropenia with marked periodontal lesions. Oral Surg., *12:*310, 1959.
14. Levy, E. J., and Schetman, D.: Cyclic neutropenia. Arch. Derm., *84:*429, 1961.
15. Orfanskis, N. G., Ostlund, R. E., Bishop, C. R., and Athens, J. W.: Normal blood leukocyte concentration values. Am. J. Clin. Pathol., *53:*647, 1970.
16. Owren, P. A.: Cyclic agranulocytoses. Acta. Med. Scand., *134:*87, 1949.
17. Page, A. R., and Good, R. A.: A clinical and experimental study of the function of neutrophils in the inflammatory response. Am. J. Pathol., *34:*645, 1958.
18. Shaper, A. G., and Lewis, P.: Genetic neutropenia in people of African origin. Lancet, *2:*1021, 1971.
19. Smith, J. F.: Cyclic neutropenia. Oral Surg., *18:*310, 1964.
20. Telsey, B.: Oral manifestations of cyclical neutropenia associated with hypergammaglobulinemia: report of a case. Oral Surg., *15:*540, 1962.
21. Vahlquist, B. C., and Anjou, N.: Granulocytopénie chronique bénigne. Acta Haematol., *8:*199, 1952.
22. Wintrobe, M. M.: Clinical Hematology. ed. 6. Philadelphia, Lea & Febiger, 1967.

Down's Syndrome

23. Baer, P. N., Coccaro, P. J., Baer, M. J., and Kilham, L.: Craniofacial manifestations of virus-induced mongolism in the hamster and Down's syndrome in man. Am. J. Orthodont., *60:*221, 1971.
24. Benda, C. E.: Down's Syndrone. Mongolism and Its Management. ed 2. New York, Grune & Stratton, 1969.
25. Brown, R. H.: Prevalence of ulcerative gingivitis in institutionalized mongoloid and non-mongoloid retarded individuals. J. Dent. Res., *49:*663, 1970.
26. Cohen, M. M.: Periodontal Disturbances in the mentally subnormal child. Dent. Clin. North Am., July, 1960.
27. Cohen, M. M. Winer, R. A., Schwartz, S., and Shklar, G: Aspects of mongolism. 1. Periodontal disease in mongolism, Oral Surg., *14:*92, 1961.

28 Collman, R., and Stoller, A.: A survey of mongoloid births in Victoria, Australia. Am. J. Public Health, *52:*813, 1962.

29. Cutress, T. W.: The prevalence of dental disease in trisomy-21 (mongolism). J. Dent. Res., *648:*(Suppl.) 1150, 1969.
30. Cutress, T. W., and Suckling, G. W.: Periodontal disease and serum citric acid levels in trisomy-21 (mongolism). Arch. Oral Biol., *14:*1129, 1969.
31. Dow, R. S.: Preliminary study of periodontoclasia in mongolian children at Polk State School. Am. J. Ment. Defic., *55:*535, 1951.

32. Falls, H. F.: Ocular changes in mongolism. N.Y. Acad. Sci., *171*:627, 1970.
33. Johnson, N. P., and Young, M. A.: Periodontal disease in mongols. J. Periodont., *34*:41, 1963.
34. Kashgarian, M., and Rendtorff, R. C.: Incidence of Down's syndrome in American Negroes. J. Pediatr., *74*:468, 1969.
35. Kisling, E., and Krebs, G.: Paradontale Forheld Hos Vokone Patients Med Down's Syndrom. (Periodontal disease in men with mongolism) Tandlaegebladet., *67*:101, 1963.
36. Kroll, R. G., Budnick, J., and Kobren, A.: Incidence of dental caries and periodontal disease in Down's syndrome. New York State Dent. J., *36*:151, 1970.
37. Levinson, A., Friedman, A., and Stamps, F.: Variability of mongolism. Pediatrics, *16*:43, 1955.
38. MacGillivary, R. C.: Anodontia in mongolism. Br. Med. J., *2*:282, 1966.
39. McMillan, R. S., and Kashgarian, M.: Relation of human abnormalities of structure and function to abnormalities of the dentition. II. Mongolism. J.A.D.A., *63*:368, 1961.
40. Nicholas, W. W.: Viruses and chromosomal abnormalities. N.Y. Acad. Sci., *171*:478, 1970.
41. Roche, A. F., and Barkla, D. H.: Development of the dentition in mongoloids. Australian D. J., *12*:12, 1967.
42. Shapiro, B. L.: Prenatal anomalies in mongolism. Ann. N.Y. Acad. Sci., *171*:562, 1970.
43. Shapiro, B. L., Gorlin, R. J., Redman, R. S., and Bruhl, H. H.: The palate and Down's syndrome. N. Engl. J. Med., *276*:1460, 1967.
44. Shapiro, S., Gedalia, I., Hofman, A., and Miller, M.: Periodontal disease and blood citrate levels in patients with trisomy-21. J. Dent. Res., *48*:1231, 1969.
45. Spitzer, R.: Observations on congenital dentofacial disorders in mongolism and microcephaly. Oral Surg., *24*:325, 1967.
46. Spitzer, R., and Mann, I.: Congenital malformations in the teeth and eyes of mental defectives. J. Ment. Sci., *96*:681, 1950.
47. Spitzer, R., and Quilliam, R. L.: Observations on congenital abnormalities in teeth and skull in two groups of mental defectives: a comparative study. Br. J. Radiol., *32*:596, 1958.
48. Swallow, J. N.: Periodontal disease in children with Down's disease. J. Dent. Res., *42*:1096, 1963.
49. Sznajder, N., Carrare J. J., Otere, E., and Carranza, F. A., Jr.: Clinical periodontal findings in trisomy 21 (mongolism). J. Periodont. Res. *3*:1, 1968.

Hypophosphatasia

50. Baer, P. N., Brown, N. C., and Hamner, J. E.: Hypophosphatasia: report of two cases with dental findings. Periodontics, *2*:209, 1964.
51. Baysal, M. C.: Premature loss of deciduous teeth in identical twins with congenital hypophosphatasia—case report. Dent. Dig., *71*:536, 1965.
52. Brucker, R. J., Rickles, N. H., and Porter, D. R.: Hypophosphatasia with premature shedding of teeth and aplasia of cementum. Oral Surg., *15*:1351, 1962.
53. Casson, M.: Oral manifestations of primary hypophosphatasia. Br. Dent. J., *127*:561, 1969.
54. Danovitch, S. H., Baer, P. N., and Laster, L.: Intestinal alkaline phosphatase activity in familial hypophosphatasia. N. Eng. J. Med., *278*:1253, 1968.
55. Fraser, D.: Hypophosphatasia. Am. J. Med., *22*:730, 1957.
56. Houpt, M. I., Kenny F. M., and Listgarten, M.: Hypophosphatasia: case reports. J. Dent. Child., *37*:126, 1970.
57. McCormick, J., and Ripa, L. W.: Hypophosphatasia. N. Eng. J. Med., *281*:604, 1969.
58. Primstone, B., Eisenberg, E., and Silverman, S.: Hypophosphatasia: Dental studies. Ann. Int. Med., *65*:722, 1966.
59. Rathbun, J. C.: Hypophosphatasia. Am. J. Dis. Child., *75*:882, 1948.
60. Rathbun, J. C.: Hypophosphatasia. Helv. Paediatr. Acta, *14*:548, 1959.
61. Scaglione, P. R., and Lucey, J. F.: Further observations on hypophosphatasia. Am. J. Dis. Child., *92*:493, 1956.
62. Sobel, E. H., Clark, L. C., and Robinson, M.: Report on a disorder of the skeleton resembling rickets, associated with loss of teeth and deficient alkaline phosphatase activity in a 2-year-old child. Am. J. Dis. Child., *83*:410, 1952.
63. Sobel, E. H., Clark, L. C., Fox, R. P., and Robinson, M.: Rickets, deficiency of alka-

line phosphatase activity and premature loss of teeth in childhood. Pediatrics, *11:* 309, 1953.

Hyperkeratosis Palmoplantaris

64. Carvel, R. I.: Palmo-plantar hyperkeratosis and premature periodontal destruction. J. Oral Med., *24:*73, 1969.
65. Coccia, C. T., McDonald, R. E., and Mitchell, D. F.: Papillon-Lefèvre syndrome: precocious periodontosis with palmar-plantar hyperkeratosis. J. Periodont., *37:* 408, 1966.
66. Cockayne, E. A.: Inherited Abnormalities of the Skin and Its Appendages. pp. 186–206. London, Oxford University Press, 1933.
67. Corson, E. F.: Keratosis palmaris et plantaris with dental alteration. Arch. Derm., *40:*639, 1939.
68. Dekker, G., and Jansen, L. H.: Periodontosis in a child with hyperkeratosis palmoplantaris, J. Periodont., *29:*266, 1958.
69. Dowling, G. B.: Congenital ectodermal defect: hyperkeratosis of palms; atrophy of nails and adjoining skin over dorsum of terminal phalanges; microdontismicatrical alopecia. Proc. Soc. Med., *29:*1633, 1936.
70. Fred, H. L., Gieser, R. G., Berry, W. R., and Eibard, J. M.: Kertosis palmaris et plantaris. Arch. Int. Med., *113:*866, 1964.
71. Galanter, D. R., and Bradford, S.: Hyperkeratosis palmoplantaris and periodontosis. The Papillon-Lefèvre syndrome. J. Periodont, *40:*40, 1969.
72. Gorlin, R. J., Sedano, H., and Anderson, V. E.: The syndrome of palmar-plantar hyperkeratosis and premature periodontal destruction of the teeth. J. Pediot., *65:*895, 1964.
73. Haim, S., and Munk, J.: Keratosis palmoplantaris congenital with periodontosis, arachnodactyly, and a peculiar deformity of the terminal phalanges. Br. J. Dermatol., *77:*42, 1965.
74. Howel-Evans, W., McConnell, R. B., Clarke, C. A., and Sheppard, P. M.: Carcinoma of the oesophagus with keratosis palmaris et plantoris (tylosis). A study of two families. Q. J. Med., *27:*13, 1958.
75. Ingle, J. I.: Papillon-Lefèvre syndrome: precocious periodontosis with associated epidermal lesions. J. Periodont., *30:*230, 1959.
76. Jansen, L. H., and Dekker, G: Hyperkeratosis palmo-plantaris with periodontosis (Papillon-Lefèvre). Dermatologica, *113:*207, 1956.
77. Martinez, L. R. R., López, O. R., and Carranza, F. A., Jr.: A case of Papillon-Lefèvre syndrome. Periodontics, *3:*292, 1965.
78. Naik, D. N., Velou, A., Alavandar, G., *et al.:* Papillon-Lefèvre syndrome. Oral Surg., *25:*19, 1968.
79. Niles, H. D., and Klumpp, M. M.: Mal de Meleda: review of the literature and report of four cases. Arch. Derm. Syph., *39:*409, 1939.
80. Perriman, A. O. M.: Papillon-Lefèvre syndrome. Br. Dent. J. *123:*484, 1967.
81. Raphael, A. L., Baer, P. N., and Lee, W. B.: Hyperkeratosis of gingival and plantar surfaces. Periodontics, *6:*118, 1968.
82. Rosenthal, S. L.: Periodontosis in a child resulting in exfoliation of the teeth. J. Periodont., *22:*101, 1951.
83. Schaffer, A. L., and Pearlstein, H. H.: Hyperkeratosis palmoplantaris with periodontosis (Papillon-Lefèvre syndrome). Oral Surg., *25:*180, 1967.
84. Shosen, S., Finkelstein, S., and Rosenzweig, K. A.: Disc electrophoretic pattern of gingival collagen isolated from a patient with palmoplantar hyperkeratosis. J. Periodont. Res., *5:*255, 1970.
85. Smith, P., and Rosenzweig, K. A.: Seven cases of Papillon-Lefèvre syndrome, Periodontics, *5:*42, 1967.
86. Touraine, A.: Congenital polykeratosis. Br. J. Dermat., *66:*294, 1954.
87. Wilson, F. M.: Papillon-Lefèvre syndrome. Report of a case. Oral Surg., *28:*488, 1969.
88. Ziprkowski, L., Ramon, Y., and Brish, M.: Hyperkeratosis palmoplantaris with periodontosis (Papillon-Lefèvre). Arch. Dermatol., *88:*207, 1963.

Histiocytosis X

89. Avery, M. E., McAfee, J. G., and Guild, H. G.: The course and prognosis of reticuloendotheliosis eosinophiles granuloma, Schüller-Christian disease and Letter-Siwe disease: study of forty cases. Am. J. Med., *22:*636, 1957.
90. Blevins, C., Dahlin, D. C., Lovestedt, S. A., and Kennedy, L. J.: Oral and dental manifestations of histiocytosis X. Oral Surg., *12:*473, 1959.

91. Carraro, J. J., DeSereday, M., De Sznajder, N.: Oral manifestation of histiocytosis X. J. Periodont., *38:*77, 1967.

92. Johnson, R. P., and Mahrac, A. M.: Histiocytosis X: report of 7 cases. J. Oral Surg., *25:*7, 1967.

93. Jones, J. C., Lilly, G. E., Marlette, R. H.: Histiocytosis X. J. Oral Surg., *28:*461, 1970.

94. Lichtenstein L.: Histiocytosis X: integration of eosinophilic granuloma of bone, "Letterer-Siwe disease," and "Schüller-Christian disease" as related manifestations of a single nosologic entity. A.M.A. Arch. Path. *56:*84, 1953.

95. Lichtenstein, L.: Histiocytosis X: (eosinophilic granuloma of bone, Letterer-Siwe disease, and Schüller-Christian disease). Further observation of pathological and clinical importance. J. Bone Joint Surg., *46A:*76, 1964.

96. Oberman, H. A.: Idiopathic histocytosis. A clinicopathologic study of 40 cases and review of the literature on eosinophilic granuloma of bone. Hand-Schüller-Christian disease and Letter-Siwe disease. Pediatrics, *28:*307, 1961.

97. Sedano, H. O., Cernea, P., Hosxe, G., and Gorlin, R. J.: Histiocytosis X. Oral Surg., *27:*760, 1969.

98. Sleeper, E. L.: Eosinophilic granuloma of bone. Oral Surg., *21:*896, 1951.

12

Systemic Diseases Associated with Miscellaneous Changes of the Alveolar Bone

FIBROUS DYSPLASIA

Fibrous dysplasia of bone is primarily a disease of childhood but, because of its insidious onset and slow progress, is usually not diagnosed until adolescence or young adulthood.[11] The disease can occur in 3 forms: The *monostotic,* involving a single bone; the *polystotic,* involving several bones; and *Albright's syndrome,* occurring rather uncommonly and consisting of polystotic bone lesions in combination with cutaneous melanotic pigmentation in the form of café-au-lait spots and an endocrine abnormality that results in precocious sexual development in the female. The monostotic type, the commonest form, occurs about equally in both sexes.[3,4,5,7,8] The polystotic form, on the other hand, has a predilection for females. In the polystotic form, although any bone can become affected, the most frequently involved are

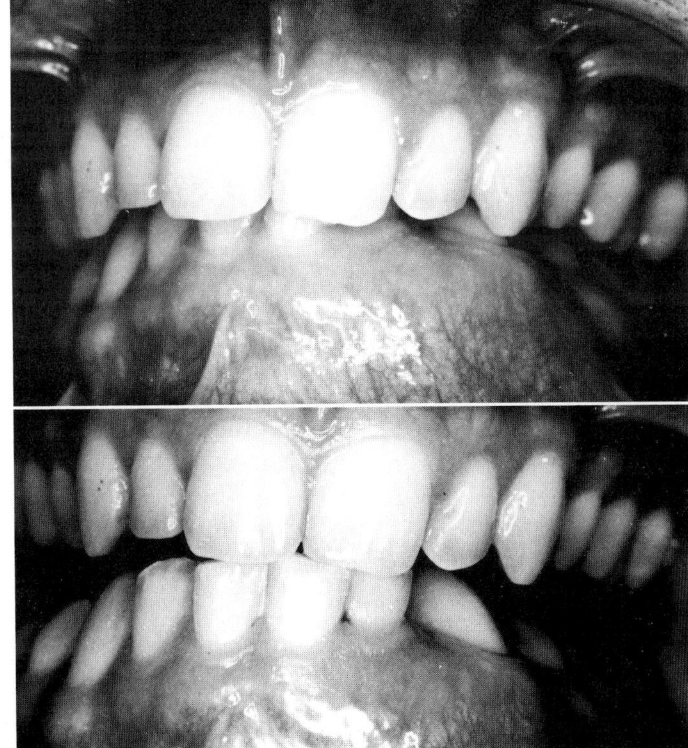

Fig. 12-1. *Top.* A painless, hard enlargement covered with a normal oral mucosa conceals the mandibular left anterior teeth.
Bottom. Enlargement is limited to the mandibular left central-cuspid area.

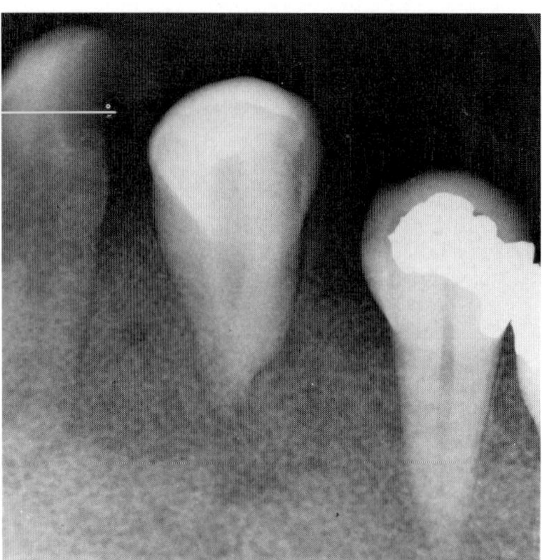

Fig. 12-2. Arrested root development and resorption in the area of the fibrous dysplasia. Roentgenographs of patient shown in Fig. 12-1. Also note the ground-glass appearance of the alveolar bone.

the femur, tibia, fibula, pelvis, humerus, radius and ulna in that order.[2] In those patients with severe polystotic lesions, the skull is almost invariably affected.[11] About 15 percent of all patients with the polystotic disease also have jaw lesions.[12]

Etiology. Unknown. There is no evidence that the disease is familial or has a genetic basis.[4] Many investigators feel that it is the result of a developmental defect.

Clinical Characteristics. In the jaws the first sign of the lesion is usually a painless, bone-hard enlargement covered with a normal appearing oral mucosa (Fig. 12-1). The swelling invariably affects the labial and buccal plate and results in a facial asymmetry. Only rarely is the lingual plate affected. On the other hand, in the polystotic form the complaints depend on the particular bones involved and the severity of their involvement. The earlier in life the skeletal lesions become pronounced, the more likely it is that they will give rise to clinical complaints. When the lower limbs are affected the result may be a limp, a bowing deformity, a pathologic fracture and pain in the hip.[4,5] In the maxilla, the antrum frequently becomes affected and may lead to exophthalmos.

Radiographic findings. In young patients where the lesion has been present for only a short period of time, the roentgenogaphic appearance may be cystic in nature. Later on the lesion becomes more calcified and has a mottled appearance. As the lesion matures, calcification increases and the alveolar bone assumes a ground-glass appearance. The roots of the teeth in the area of the fibrous dysplasia frequently become arrested in their development or show resorption (Fig. 12-2). The region where the lesion appears tends to be poorly demarcated from the surrounding areas of normal bony trabeculation (Fig. 12-3). In the skull, as elsewhere, the early lesions are frequently cystic, assume a ground-glass appearance as they mature and are poorly circumscribed.[6] There also may be some evidence of swelling and expansion of some part of the calvarium.[5] In the advanced case there is a tendency toward the formation of sclerotic dense bony deposits which is most marked when the disease extends to the base of the skull, paranasal sinuses or nasal cavity.[11]

Treatment. Because the main problem is usually an esthetic one resulting from a facial asymmetry, removal of that portion of the bony lesion causing the obvious deformity is the treatment of choice. Radiation is contraindicated, since it may lead to malignant change in the bone.[9]

Prognosis. The lesions tend to become quiescent or progress at an extremely slow rate after adolescence.

OSTEOPETROSIS

(Albers-Schonberg Disease, Marble Bone Disease)

This rare hereditary bone disease can occur in 2 forms with equal frequency: A malignant childhood form, transmitted as an autosomal recessive trait; and a benign form, transmitted as an autosomal dominant trait.[14] The disease is characterized by failure of bone resorption while bone formation continues, resulting in generalized increase in bone density. The bone formed, however, has an abnormal composition and an abnormal architecture.[13,14] All the clinical features of the disease can be explained on this increase in bone formation.

Malignant Form. This form has its onset before or shortly after birth and leads frequently to an early death. In fact no known case of this type has ever been reported to survive past the age of 20 years.[14] A replacement of the marrow spaces by the overgrowth of bone results in a reduction of the hematopoietic tissue and a severe anemia; this in turn leads to an increased susceptibility to infection and resultant death. The increased bone formation also causes a narrowing of the foramina which may cause deafness, impairment of vision or blindness and facial paralysis. The anemia usually results in a compensatory hyperplasia of the lymphoid tissue, especially of the lymph nodes and spleen. The commonly occurring clinical features in the malignant form are[14]

	Percent
Optic atrophy	78
Splenomegaly	62
Hepatomegaly	48
Poor growth	36
Frontal bossing	34
Fractures	28
Loss of hearing	22
Mental retardation	22
Large head	22
Osteomyelitis	18
Lymphadenopathy	18
Facial palsy	10
Genu valgum	16
Pectus deformities	8

Benign Form. These cases have their onset later in childhood and are most often discovered after the age of 15 but before 30 years of age. The abnormality is frequently discovered fortuitously, since the radiographic picture may be the only detectable sign in a large percentage of the affected patients. However, there may be

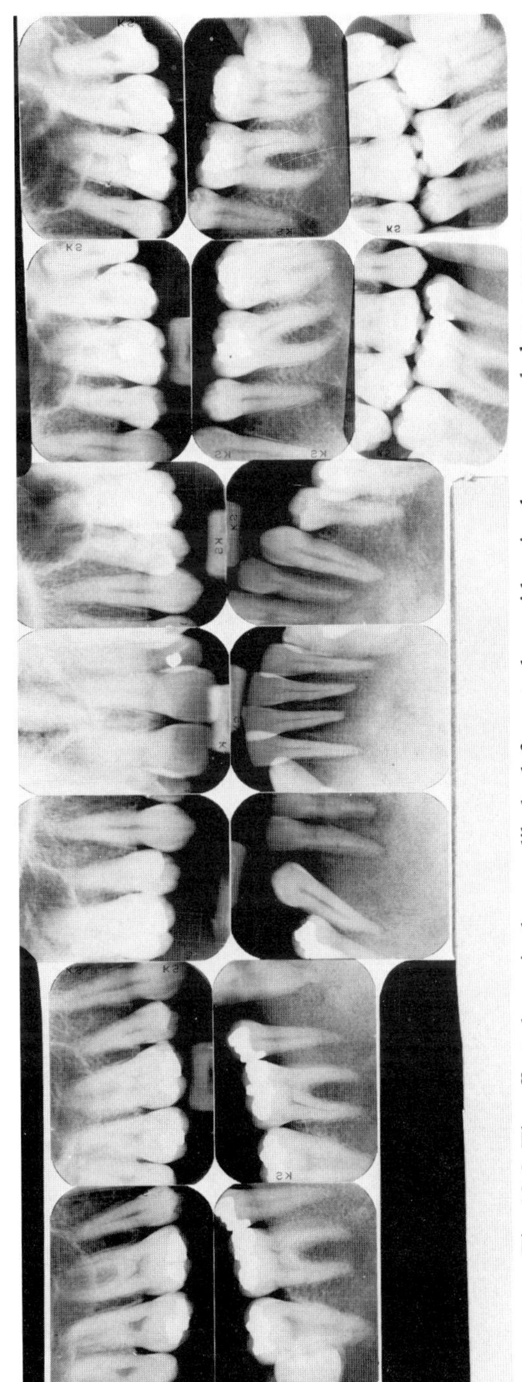

Fig. 12-3. The affected area in the mandibular left central-cuspid region has a ground-glass appearance.

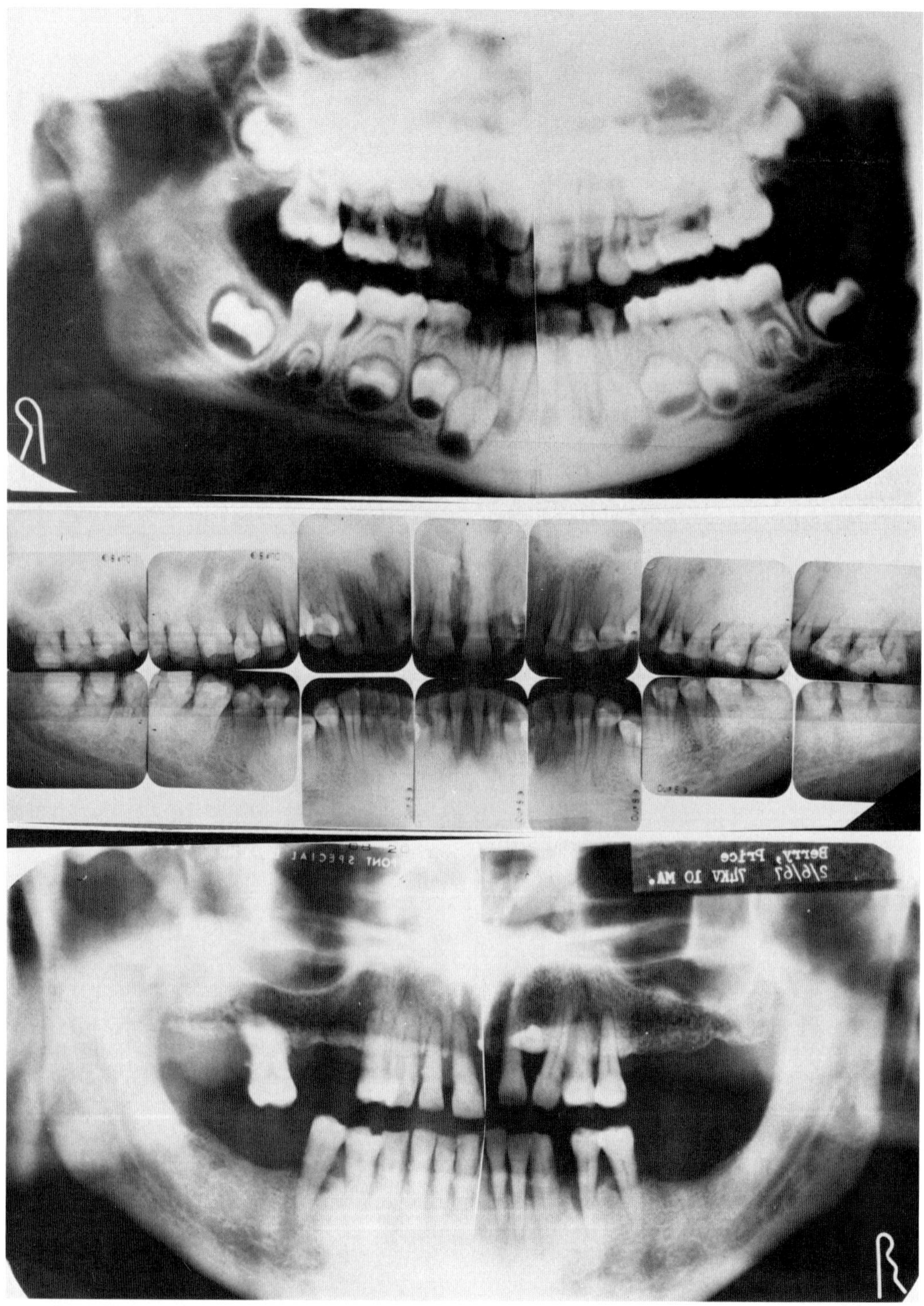

Fig. 12-4. *Top*. Dense sclerotic bone in the mandibular anterior segment of a 6-year-old boy.
Center. The father of the 6-year-old boy.
Bottom. The grandfather of the 6-year-old boy.

a tremendous variability in the clinical characteristics in this form of the disease, even within a pedigree. The formation of an excessive amount of an abnormal type of bone leads to easy fracture of the long bones. Osteomyelitis is a frequent complication following fracture, because the overgrowth of bone causes poor nutrition to the few viable remaining bone cells. The poor nutrition may also explain, in part at least, the lack of normal resistance to infection. The vast majority of the cases of osteomyelitis occur in the jaws following tooth extraction or an infectious process in the oral cavity, such as a pericoronal infection. The mandible has been found to be more susceptible to osteomyelitis than the maxilla, probably because there is a more abundant nutrient supply in the maxilla than in the mandible. Normally there is also a much greater percentage of cortical bone in the mandible than in the maxilla.

Comment on Periodontal Therapy. Periodontal treatment, if needed, should be limited. Extensive surgical procedures should be avoided because these patients are very susceptible to osteomyelitis of the jaws. The prophylactic use of antibiotics, therefore, is indicated in all dental procedures of a surgical nature.

Clinical Characteristics. The most common clinical features in the dominantly inherited benign form are[14]

	Percent
Asymptomatic	50
History of fracture	40
Osteomyelitis	10
Cranial palsy	15
Bone pain	20

Radiographic findings. Tooth eruption may be retarded because of the presence of sclerotic bone and a uniform dense sclerotic bone may result in a radiopacity that may completely obliterate not only the trabecular pattern in the alveolar bone but also the roots of the teeth (Fig. 12-4).[15,16] Fractures of the long bones are common and their marrow cavities become obliterated, giving a homogenous radiopacity to the bones; hence the name marble bone. In the skull there is an increased density of the calvaria with disappearance of the diploë. A thickening of the base of the skull occurs with clubbing of the anterior and posterior clinoid processes. The maxillary sinuses also gradually become obliterated.

Treatment. None.

Prognosis. This is variable and largely depends on whether it is the malignant or benign form of the disease which has been inherited. The age at onset also is important. In general, when the onset is discovered at an early age, the prognosis is poor, the cause of death being anemia, frequently complicated by secondary infection. On the other hand, when the onset develops in later life, the prognosis is much more favorable.

REFERENCES

Fibrous Dysplasia

1. Fairbank, H. A. T.: Fibrocystic disease of bone. J. Bone Joint Surg., *32B:*403, 1950.
2. Gorlin, R. J., and Goldman, H. M.: Thoma's Oral Pathology. St. Louis, C. V. Mosby, 1970.
3. Houston, J. W. O.: Fibrous dysplasia of maxilla and mandible clinicopathologic study and comparison of facial bone lesions with lesions affecting general skeleton. J. Oral Surg., *23:*17, 1965.
4. Jaffe, H. L.: Fibrous dysplasia of bone. J. Mt. Sinai Hosp., *12:*364, 1945.
5. Lichtenstein, L., and Jaffe, H. L.: Fibrous dysplasia of bone: a condition affecting one, several or many bones, the graver cases of which may present abnormal pigmentation of skin, premature sexual development, hyperthyroidism with other extra-skeletal abnormalities. Arch. Path., *33:*777, 1942.
6. Reed, R. J., and Hagy, D. M.: Benign nonodontogenic fibro-osseous lesions of the skull. Oral Surg., *19:*214, 1965.
7. Schlumberger, H. G.: Fibrous dysplasia (ossifying fibroma) of the maxilla and

mandible. Am. J. Orthodont. Oral Surg., *32*:579, 1946.

8. Shafer, W. G., Hine, M. K., and Levey, B. M.: A Textbook of Oral Pathology. pp. 576-578. Philadelphia, W. B. Saunders, 1963.
9. Tanner, H. C., Dahlin, D. C., and Childs, D. S., Jr.: Sarcoma complicating fibrous dysplasia; probable role of radiation therapy. Oral Surg., *14*:837, 1961.
10. Waldron, C. A.: Fibro-osseous lesions of the jaws. J. Oral Surg., *28*:58, 1970.
11. Windholz, F.: Cranial manifestations of fibrous dysplasia of bone. Their relation to leontiosis ossea and to simple bone cysts of the vault. Am. J. Roentgen., *58*:51, 1947.
12. Zimmerman, D. C., Dahlin, D. C., and Stafne, E. C.: Fibrous dysplasia of the maxilla and mandible. Oral Surg., *11*:55, 1958.

Osteopetrosis

13. Gomez, L. S. A., Taylor, R., Cohen, M. M., and Shklar, G: The jaws in osteopetrosis (Albers-Schonberg disease). J. Oral Surg., *24*:67, 1966.
14. Johnston, C. C. Jr., Lavy, N., Lord T., Vellios, F., Merritt, A. D., and Press, W. P.: Osteopetrosis. Medicine, *47*:149, 1968.
15. Kaslick, R. S., and Brustein, H. C.: Clinical evaluation of osteopetrosis. Oral Surg., *15*:71, 1962.
16. Wittich, H. C., Chaudry, A. P., Gorlin, R. J., and Stoesz, A. R.: Osteopetrosis. J. Dent. Child., *24*:41, 1957.

13
The Juvenile Diabetic

Diabetes Mellitus

Diabetes mellitus can be defined as a genetically determined metabolic disease characterized by polyuria, polydipsia, polyphagia, weight loss, ease of fatigue, changes in the retinal blood vessels and a fasting hyperglycemia and glycosuria. The term diabetes mellitus, therefore, means more than the mere finding of glucose in the urine and a hyperglycemia in the fasting state 2 or 3 hours after a carbohydrate-rich meal of 100 Gms. or more of carbohydrate. The diabetic neuropathy and the cause of the vascular disease which accompanies diabetes mellitus is not understood. The hyperlipemia, the reduced lipogenesis, the atherosclerosis and the intimal and medial alterations of the large and small vessels may occur in these patients at rates and in ways which are often independent of the state of control of the carbohydrate metabolism. While the administration of insulin may correct most of the apparent biochemical disturbances that occur in insulin deficiency, it does not appear to prevent the tissue changes which affect the ground substances, mucopolysaccharides, lipids and proteins. The most misleading of all is a classification of diabetic patients based on insulin requirement, where patients are referred to as "severe," "moderate," or "mild" because they require large, moderate or small doses of insulin. Such a classification is not warranted, since prognosis, complications or tendency to ketoacidosis are not related to insulin requirement in insulin-dependent diabetic individuals.

The Prediabetic

Another problem is the prediabetic, that is a person who, before real diabetic signs or symptoms appear, has a somewhat abnormal metabolic response to glucose loading. There are no definitive studies to show how many such subjects ever become true diabetics, or are any routine diagnostic tests available to detect such an individual. However, there are 3 groups of patients who might be considered as prediabetics: Offspring of a diabetic father and a diabetic mother, an identical twin of a diabetic, and a mother who gives birth to a large baby.[5] In no instance has any conclusive evidence shown that "prediabetics" are more susceptible to periodontal disease than normal controls. In fact, some experts in the field believe that the term "prediabetes" should not be used as a clinical diagnosis at all, since such a diagnosis can be made only in retrospect (i.e., after diabetes is established in an individual by the presently accepted criteria).

Juvenile Diabetic

Juvenile diabetes as a rule differ from maturity-onset diabetes in that the patients are insulin-deficient, while most post-maturity diabetics tend to be insulin-resistant.[42] Of course, there are always exceptions to this rule because some juvenile patients exhibit the same characteristics adult diabetic patients do and vice versa. There are a number of clinical features of diabetes in children which distinguish it from maturity-onset diabetes. The

TABLE 13-1. COMPARISON OF JUVENILE AND ADULT DIABETES

Juvenile	*Adult* (Maturity-onset)
1. Approximately 15 years of age or less at onset	More than 16 years of age at onset
2. Sudden onset of symptoms	Gradual onset of symptoms
3. Patient thin or normal in weight	Patient usually obese
4. Ketosis prone	Not prone to ketosis
5. Control by insulin	Control by oral hypoglycemic drugs and/or diet
6. Unstable – many insulin reactions	Fairly stable – few insulin reactions
7. Decreased insulin in plasma	Increased insulin in plasma
8. No sex difference or slight preponderence of males	Females in majority with 2-1 ratio to men in older age groups

diabetic child is more sensitive to hyperglycemic and hypoglycemic influences and therefore more labile and more difficult to control.

Oral hypoglycemic drugs have limited value in the management of juvenile diabetes. All diabetic children require insulin, whereas a substantial percentage of maturity-onset diabetic patients can be controlled by diet alone or by hypoglycemic oral drugs and diet. The differences between juvenile and adult diabetes are shown above, Table 13-1.

Juvenile diabetics comprise between 3.5 to 5.0 percent of the diabetic population. While the mean age at onset is 8 years, the commonest age is 11 years. True congenital diabetes, if it occurs, is extremely rare. The height and weight of children with reasonably controlled diabetes is usually within normal limits. There is nothing to suggest that the intelligence or school records of such children is significantly different from the average normal child.

Chinical Characteristics and Course. The onset is usually acute with emphasis on polyuria and polydipsia as the initial symptoms of the disease; thus, enuresis may be the presenting complaint.[19] After the initial severe symptoms have been controlled by insulin, remission is common. The nature of the remission is obscure, since it was also seen in the days before insulin was available and dietary restriction was the only mode of treatment available. However, after a variable period, and frequently following an infection, the diabetes relapses and insulin dependency is established. Vascular lesions in the first 5 years of diabetes in children are usually absent and few are observed during the first 10 years. White found, however, that after 15 years, 10 of those examined had retinopathies, and by 35 years of age nearly all showed such lesions.[45] Life expectancy is short and usually does not extend much beyond 25 years of age. While there are few satisfactory records for long-term follow-ups of juvenile diabetics, White also found that for those who lived longer than 25 years the median age at subsequent death was 32 years.

The Glucose Tolerance Test

The oral glucose tolerance test is performed after a fast of from 12 to 14 hours. In adults, the test dose may be either 100 Gm. of glucose or 1.75 Gm. of glucose per kilogram of body weight dissolved in 250 cc. of water. The dose of glucose for the oral test for children is as follows:

Age	*Amount of Glucose*
0-18 months	2.5 gm./Kg. body weight
1½-3 years	0.2 gm./Kg. body weight
3-12 years	1.75 gm./Kg. body weight
12 years +	1.25 gm./Kg. body weight

The glucose content in the blood and urine is then determined in the fasting state, and at intervals of 30 minutes, 1 hour, 2 hours and 3 hours.

Prolonged starvation or restriction of carbohydrates may cause a temporary impairment of glucose tolerance which is reflected in hyperglycemia and glycosuria on refeeding or the administration of glucose. To avoid an erroneous diagnosis of diabetes in nondiabetic persons, therefore, a diet containing at least 150 Gm. of carbohydrate daily is given for from 3 to 5 days preceding the test. Also, before and during the test the subject should be made comfortable, and tension and excitement avoided, since they may cause a rise in the blood glucose. Physical activity may lower the blood glucose and therefore should be reduced to a minimum shortly before and during the test.

Glucose Tolerance Curves

The results of an oral glucose tolerance curve in a normal adult are shown in Figure 13-1.

Mosenthal and Barry stress two key readings—the fasting level, and the level 2 hours after administration of glucose. The characteristic of the deranged carbohydrate metabolism in diabetes is the high and prolonged tolerance curve after the test dose of glucose.[23] Thus, a fasting true blood glucose of 120 mg./100 ml., a 2-hours' value of 120 mg./100 ml. or more and 110 mg. per 100 ml. or more at the 3-hour period is diagnostic of diabetes mellitus. A peaking of the curve during the first 30 minutes, or one hour only, is not an adequate criterion of diabetes, because such a value may occur from a rapid absorption of sugar from the intestinal tract.

Instead of using a standard 3-hour oral glucose tolerance test, many investigators have tried using a standard 2-hour oral glucose tolerance test. It has been stated by proponents of this modified test that it can detect early derangements of carbohydrate metabolism in individuals with a normal fasting blood sugar. In adequately prepared subjects, failure of the blood sugar to return to 100 mg.% true glucose within 2 hours after an oral glucose load has been commonly interpreted as evidence of diabetes mellitus or prediabetes. In the dental field, the failure of the blood sugar to return to 100 mg.% within the 2-hour period has been related to various periodontal and oral disturbances.[34,35] The objections to the use of a standard 2-hour glucose tolerance test, however, are that gastrointestinal factors, unrelated to peripheral utilization of glucose, play too great a role in determining the configuration of the curve. Variations in gastric emptying time, particularly when nausea occurs following glucose ingestion, may influence the blood sugar level at 2 hours. Variations in the time of intestinal absorption may also alter the results of the test.[24] Soskin has expressed strong doubts as to the validity of the test as a measure of carbohydrate utilization and considered it a poor diagnostic tool in the borderline group, the very group for which it was designed.[36] Mirsky has stated that anyone can be labeled "diabetic" if a sufficient number of oral glucose tolerance tests are performed.[22]

In addition, there is evidence that repeated oral glucose tolerance tests done in the same individuals under similar conditions in respect to diet, exercise and other controllable factors may yield dissimilar results. Finally, Unger showed that in 152 normal subjects, the 2-hour oral glucose tolerance resulted in 54.6 percent of them having blood sugar levels at 2 hours which exceeded the widely accepted Mosenthal standard normal, 100 mg.% and 39.4 percent exceeded this standard by more than 10 percent.[44] Duplicate 2-hour tests in these same individuals under similar circumstances demonstrated that variations in 2-hour blood sugar levels were not unusual. He concluded, "that the test, as commonly performed and interpreted, is variable, and that in persons

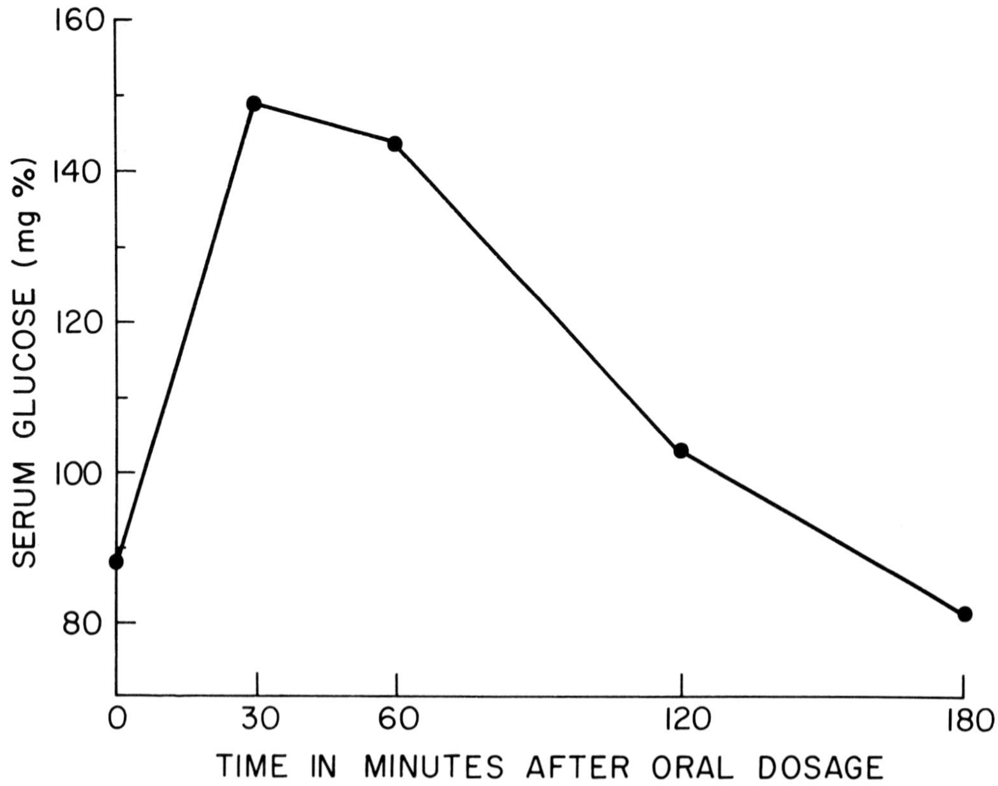

Fig. 13-1. Normal glucose tolerance curve.

with normal fasting blood sugars modest elevations of the two-hour specimens are not specific for diabetes mellitus."

MacDonald and Crossley have also shown that the glucose tolerance level in premenopausal women varies with the menstrual cycle and that the highest glucose level occurs in the middle of the menstrual cycle.[17] They were also able to demonstrate that the rate of gastric emptying increases suddenly in the middle of the menstrual cycle and then gradually and consistently decreases until the middle of the ensuing cycle, when it suddenly increases again. Thus, it was proven that there was a variation in the oral glucose tolerance test which was associated with the menstrual cycle. It was suggested that this variation may be secondary to the influence of hormones on the gastrointestinal tract.

Finally, it is recognized that the interpretation of the results of an oral glucose tolerance test by various criteria such as those of the World Health Organization, the United States Public Health Service, the British Diabetic Association, and Fajans and Conn results in discrepancies.[6,8,18,26] Tests deemed abnormal by one standard may be classified as normal by another. To help solve this problem, Danowski, *et al.* have suggested that the glucose tolerance test be expressed as the glucose tolerance sum for 2 or for 3 hours ($GTS_{0\text{-}2\ hr.}$ and $GTS_{0\text{-}3\ hr.}$).[4]

The $GTS_{0\text{-}2\ hr.}$ value is the sum of the 0, ½, 1 and 2 hr. glucose levels in venous blood when 1.75 Gm. of glucose are administered per kilogram of body weight. Data from more than 1,100 such tolerances indicate that when $GTS_{0\text{-}2\ hr.}$ is 500 or less there is a 98 to 100 percent probability that the test is clearly normal by the standards of the World Health Organization, British Diabetic Association, United States Public Health Service, and Fajans and Conn. On the other hand, when the $GTS_{0\text{-}2\ hr.}$ is 801 or higher the test would meet each of the 4 sets of above-cited criteria for diabetes. Since those values between 501 and 800 are variably classifiable as normal or abnormal by these same 4 standards, this represents the equivocal zone.

The $GTS_{0\text{-}3\ hr.}$ value is based on the sum of 0-, 1-, 2-, and 3-hour blood glucose levels in the above tolerance tests. Using the same criteria, clearly nondiabetic tolerance tests yield $GTS_{0\text{-}3\ hr.}$ values of 450 or less, while those deemed to be diabetic have sums of 701 or higher. Intervening $GTS_{0\text{-}3\ hr.}$ values of 451 to 700 represent the equivocal zone.

Tolerance tests with GTS values in the equivocal zone should be repeated at intervals of months or years. Equivocal tests generally move toward or into the abnormal range, a minority move back into the normal zone and some remain equivocal.

Relationship of Glucose Tolerance to Periodontal Status

There are many contradictory studies in this area. Sheridan and coworkers concluded that there was a positive relationship between impaired glucose tolerance and the presence of alveolar bone resorption.[35] Summers and Oberman, in a study on the relationship between periodontal status and 12 selected variables in 324 dentulous subjects 20 years and older, also showed a significant relationship between the severity of periodontal disease and elevated blood glucose, even though the relationship between age and cigarette consumption was of greater significance.[41] Similarly, Tuckman, *et al.*, studying 54 subjects 25 to 44 years of age who gave no history of systemic disease, noted a statistically significant correlation between the severity of periodontal disease present and results obtained with 3-hour oral glucose tolerance.[43] In brief, they found that those with high 3-hour glucose tolerance scores also had high PI scores indicating a positive correlation between severity of periodontal disease and abnormal glucose metabolism. On the other hand, a majority of publications do not support such a relationship. O'Leary, Shannon and Prigmore carried out conventional 3-hour glucose tolerance tests in 16 patients with advanced periodontal disease and in 15 control patients, and found that the responses were virtually identical for the two groups.[25] There were no significant intergroup differences at any sampling point. They concluded that the oral glucose tolerance test as a "method is suitable only for the diagnosis of established diabetes mellitus and should not be used to study less marked alterations in carbohydrate metabolism." Shannon and Gibson, in a study of 300 males 17 to 22 years of age, found that neither caries experience nor periodontal status was in any way related to carbohydrate metabolism as measured by oral glucose tolerance tests in systemically healthy young adult males.[31] They reported similar findings in a series of more recent studies and thus were able to confirm their earlier work.[31,32,40] Unpublished work in our own laboratory tends to support the findings of these authors that no statistically significant cause and effect relationship could be found between periodontal status and systemic carbohydrate metabolism as determined by the oral glucose tolerance test. Mehrotra, Chawla and Kumar studied blood sugar and the presence of salivary sugar in both diabetics and nondiabetics and correlated these findings with Russell's periodontal index (PI).[21] They came to the conclusion that neither diabetics nor nondiabetics showed any statistically significant correlation between the salivary sugar or blood sugar and the periodontal health status of the patient as determined by the PI.

Rutledge, in 1940, reported in a clinical and roentgenographic study of 20 diabetic children, 5 males and 15 females between the ages of 8 to 18 years, and concluded that "gingival and paradental disturbances are very frequently present."[27] No controls were used, however, and so the significance of his findings have remained in doubt. Sheppard, in 1942, compared 100 patients who were hospitalized for diabetes with a 1,000 normal patients.[33] He found that 80 percent of the normal patients had roentgenographic evidence of periodontal disease. Therefore, he concluded that, "with such a high incidence in the normal patient, pyorrhea is hardly apt to be a pathognomonic symptom of diabetes." In a study at the Mayo clinic, Lovestedt and Austin compared 503 diabetic patients, 316 male and 187 female, with 1,023 control patients, 518 male and 505 female.[16] The control patients consisted of consecutive patients seen in the dental clinic, excluding diabetics. They found a higher incidence of periodontal disease among the diabetic patients. Stahl, in 1948, studied 42 diabetic patients, 14 male and 28 female patients ranging in age from 14 to 55 years, and on the basis of the roentgenographs concluded that "alveolar bone resorption both in amount and severity tended to increase significantly with an increase in the severity of the diabetic condition."[37] The severity of the diabetic condition was assessed by correlating the blood sugar level with the amount of the glycosuria. Stahl, Wisan, and Miller, in an epidemiologic study, compared 200 male patients with various systemic disease (47 had diabetes) with 100 male patients who had only local ailments such as fractures.[38] They concluded that: there was a tendency for increased alveolar resorption with aging, which appeared to be aggravated by the presence of a systemic disease; and that diseases which affected general cellular metabolism seemed to be associated with the more cases of alveolar resorption.

In a somewhat similar study, Sandler and Stahl compared 736 white male patients, 40 of whom had endocrine dysfunction, with a control group of 563 white males, and concluded that: "Inflammation and degenerative gingival symptoms increase with aging but are significantly more widespread in persons with generalized debilitating disease."[28] In addition, they concluded that alveolar bone resorption also increased with aging and tended to be more severe in patients who were suffering from endocrine dysfunctions, malignant neoplasms and cardiovascular disease. In a more recent publication, Sandler and Stahl reported on the prevalence of periodontal disease in a hospitalized population of 3,994 persons.[29] They concluded that the influence of generalized disease upon periodontal health was not remarkable except in patients with relatively severe diabetes and in those with cirrhosis of the liver. Their diabetic patients with a primary diagnosis of diabetes, however, were generally hospitalized because their disease was relatively uncontrolled and ketosis was not uncommon. They felt that the patients with the controlled diabetes did not demonstrate excessive periodontal disease.

Two conflicting reports appeared almost simultaneously in 1967. Benveniste, Bixler and Conneally conducted an investigation on 53 diabetic and 71 nondiabetic individuals, who ranged in age from 5 to 72 years.[2] Multiple regression analysis of the data obtained for tooth by tooth and group by group comparisons for gingivitis, calculus formation and pocket depth failed to show any significant differences between diabetics and nondiabetics. It should be noted that all the diabetics in this study were under insulin and/or dietary regulation. On the other hand, Finestone and Boorujy examined 198 dentulous patients with diabetes and 64 nondiabetic individuals, and came to just the opposite conclusion—that the severity and prevalence of periodontal disease were increased in the diabetic patient.[7] In addition, they found that the periodontal index was related in a positive fashion to age, duration of known diabetes, complications and variations of blood sugar levels.

Belting, Hiniker and Dummett, using the Russell Index, studied the periodontal status of 78 hospitalized patients having diabetes mellitus with 79 other hospitalized patients not having diabetes.[1] Their sample ranged in age from 20 to 89 years. They reported that the severity of periodontal disease was significantly greater among the diabetic group than among the nondiabetic group. They also found that in both groups the severity of periodontal disease increased significantly with age. Therefore, as the degree of diabetes increased, the severity of periodontal disease decreased significantly because of the younger ages of the more severe diabetic patients. Finally, they concluded that the increased severity of periodontal disease found among diabetic patients was another manifestation of the peripheral vascular occlusive disorders associated with diabetes mellitus.

Cohen, *et al.* examined 21 diabetic females and 18 nondiabetic females, ages 18 to 35 years over a 2-year period and found that the diabetic group had significantly more gingival involvement and greater loss of attachment around the teeth than did the nondiabetic group.[3] There was no appreciable difference in the amount of hard deposits observed in the diabetic and nondiabetic group, but the diabetics had significantly more soft deposits. Hove and Stallard, on the other hand, examined 28 diabetic and 16 nondiabetic patients of comparable age and socioeconomic status and reported just opposite results.[12] From the information gathered they concluded that periodontal disease increased with age in both groups, and was directly related to accumulation of plaque and calculus. In a given age group, any increase in periodontal breakdown in the diabetic group could be explained by parallel increase in local etiologic factors. The severity and duration of the diabetes appeared to have little effect upon periodontal disease.

Glavind, Lund and Löe studied the association between the periodontal changes and duration of the diabetes, retinal changes and insulin dosage in 102 dentulous men between the ages of 20 to 40;[10] 51 were young diabetics regularly controlled at a diabetic clinic and 51 were nondiabetic patients. They reached the following conclusions.

1. Up to the age of 40 years the gingival condition of controlled male diabetics is characterized by a chronic inflammatory lesion the severity of which is not different from similar lesions in nondiabetics. The gingival condition is not influenced by the duration of the diabetes or the insulin dosage or with the absence or presence of vascular changes in the retina.
2. The periodontal lesion in diabetics and nondiabetics is characterized by loss of fiber attachment, pocket formation and loss of alveolar bone. Up to 30 years of age the rate of destruction is the same for diabetics and nondiabetics. Between 30 and 40 years of age diabetics show a slight increase in periodontal breakdown as compared with nondiabetics, and patients suffering overt diabetes for more than 10 years show greater loss per periodontal structures than those with a history of less than 10 years. Insulin dosage does not seem to be related to the degree of periodontal destruction. Diabetics with retinal changes have greater loss of attached periodontium than others.

Diabetes and Periodontal Disease

On the basis of present evidence, it is reasonable to conclude that in adult patients who are prone to periodontal disease and who are also uncontrolled diabetics the manifestation of periodontal disease, particularly alveolar bone resorption, would be more severe. In the controlled diabetic, on the other hand, there does not appear to be any uniform results which warrant any conclusion that there is or is not a relationship between diabetes and periodontal disease (i.e., alveolar bone resorption).

In regard to the adolescent with diabetes, the evidence is much better. The relationship has been summed up by Gottsegen who stated that, "Below the age of eighteen there appears to be no premature resorptive bone changes attributable to diabetes."[11]

Histologic Study of Vascular Changes. Almost all studies on the small blood vessels in the gingiva of adult diabetic patients agree that there are significant differences between diabetic and non-diabetic patients.[9,13,14,20,39] Diabetics tend to show an increased positive periodic-acid Schiff reaction (PAS) in the basement membrane area. However, the one study which was done on juvenile diabetics by Löe, Theilade and Glavind showed no apparent difference in the PAS stained reactions between 25 individuals with controlled overt juvenile diabetes and a control group of 7 healthy individuals.[15]

Treatment. In the controlled diabetic patient, periodontal treatment should be undertaken in consultation with the physician. Usually the treatment can proceed in a normal manner without unusual precautions. The response to therapy is generally the same as for a normal non-diabetic patient.

REFERENCES

1. Belting, C. M., Hiniker, J. J., and Dummett, C. O.: Influence of diabetes mellitus on the severity of periodontal disease. J. Periodont., *35:*476, 1964.
2. Benveniste, R., Bixler, D., and Conneally, P. M.: Periodontal disease in diabetics. J. Periodont., *38:*271, 1967.
3. Cohen, D. W., Friedman, L. A., Shapiro, J., Kyle, G. C., and Franklin, S.: Diabetes mellitus and periodontal disease: two-year longitudinal observations. I. J. Periodont., *41:*709, 1970.
4. Danowski, T. S., Aarons, J. H., Hydovitz, J. D., and Wingert, J. P.: Utility of Equivocal glucose tolerances. Diabetes, *19:*524, 1970.
5. Ellenberg, M, and Rifkin, H.: Diabetes Mellitus. New York, McGraw-Hill, 1970.
6. Fajans, S. S., and Conn, J. W.: Early recognition of diabetes mellitus. Ann. N.Y. Acad. Sci., *82:*208, 1959.
7. Finestone, A. J., and Boorujy, S. R.: Diabetes mellitus and periodontal disease. Diabetes, *16:*336, 1967.
8. Fitzgerald, M. G., and Keen, H.: Diagnostic classification of diabetes. Br. Med. J., *1:*1568, 1964.
9. Gellin, M. E., Bautista, A., Haley, J. V., and Mabry, C. C.: Vascular changes in the mandibular alveolar mucosa of diabetic children. Pediatrics, *46:*789, 1970.
10. Glavind, L., Lund, B., and Löe, H.: The relationship between periodontal state and diabetes duration, insulin dosage and retinal changes. J. Periodont. Res., *4:*164, 1969.
11. Gottsegen, R: Dental and oral considerations in diabetes mellitus. New York State J. Med., *62:*389, 1962.
12. Hove, K. A., and Stallard, R. E.: Diabetes and the periodontal patient. J. Periodont., *41:*713, 1970.
13. Keene, J. J., Jr.: Observations of small blood vessels in human non-diabetic and diabetic gingiva. J. Dent. Res., *48:*967, 1969.
14. Keene, J. J.: A histochemical evaluation for small vessel calcification in human non-diabetic and diabetic gingival biopsy specimens. J. Dent. Res., *48:*968, 1969.
15. Löe, H., Theilade, J., and Glavind, L.: Histochemical and electron microscopic investigations of gingiva in controlled juvenile diabetes. J. Periodont. Res., *4:*165, 1969.
16. Lovestedt, S. A., and Austin, L. T.: Periodontoclasia in diabetes mellitus. J.A.D.A., *30:*273, 1943.
17. McDonald, G. W., Hoet, J. P., and Butterfield, W. J. H.: Diabetes mellitus: report of a WHO expert committee. World Health Organization Technical Report Series No. 310, 1965.

18. MacDonald, I., and Crossley, J. N.: Glucose tolerance during the menstrual cycle. Diabetes, *19:*450, 1970.
19. Malina, J.: Clinical Diabetes Mellitus. London. Eyre and Spottswoode, 1968.
20. McMullen, J. A., Legg, M., Gottsegen, R., and Camerini-Davalos, R.: Microangiopathy within the gingival tissues of diabetic subjects with special reference to the prediabetic state. Periodontics, *5:*61, 1967.
21. Mehrotra, K. K., Chawla, T. N., Kumar, A.: Correlation of salivary sugar and blood sugar with periodontal health and oral hygiene status among diabetics and non-diabetics. J. Indian Dent. Assoc., *40:*265, 1968.
22. Mirsky, I. A.: Discussion of paper by Sevringhaus, E. L.: The glucose tolerance test in the diagnosis of diabetes and hyperinsulinism. Proc. Am. Diabetes Assoc., *4:*121, 1944.
23. Mosenthal, H. O., and Barry, E.: Criteria for and interpretation of normal glucose tolerance tests. Ann. Int. Med., *33:*1175, 1950.
24. Myers, G. B., and McKean, R. M.: The oral glucose tolerance test: a review of the literature. Am. J. Clin. Path, *5:*299, 1935.
25. O'Leary, T. J., Shannon, I. L., and Prigmore, J. R.: Clinical correlations and systemic status in periodontal disease. SAM-TDR-61-98, August, 1961.
26. O'Sullivan, J. B., and Mahan, C. M.: Prospective study of 352 young patients with chemical diabetes. N. Eng. J. Med., *278:*1038, 1968.
27. Rutledge, C. E.: Oral and roentgenographic aspects of the teeth and jaws of juvenile diabetics. J.A.D.A., *27:*1740, 1940.
28. Sandler, H. C., and Stahl, S. S.: Influence of generalized diseases on clinical manifestations of periodontal disease. J.A.D.A., *49:*656, 1954.
29. Sandler, H. C., and Stahl, S. S.: Prevalence of periodontal disease in a hospitalized population. J. Dent. Res., *39:*439, 1960.
30. Shannon, I. L., and Gibson, W. A.: Oral glucose tolerance responses in healthy young adult males classified as to caries experience and periodontal status. SAM-TDR-63-87, Nov., 1963.
31. Shannon, I. L., and Gibson, W. A.: Fasting and postprandial serum glucose levels as related to periodontal status and caries experience. SAM-TDR-64-47, Sept., 1964.
32. Shannon, I. L., O'Leary, T. J., Gibson, W. A., and Jenson, R. L.: Glucose tolerance responses in young adults of sharply contrasting periodontal status. SAM-TR-66-9. USAF School of Aerospace Medicine, Brooks Air Force Base, Texas, Feb., 1966.
33. Sheppard, I. M.: Oral manifestations of diabetes mellitus: a study of one hundred cases. J.A.D.A., *29:*1188, 1942.
34. Sheridan, R. C., Jr., Cheraskin, E., Flynn, F. H., and Hutto, A. C.: Epidemiology of diabetes mellitus I. Review of the dental literature. J. Periodont., *30:*242, 1959.
35. Sheridan, R. C., Jr., Cheraskin, E., Flynn, F. H., and Hutto, A. C.: Epidemiology of diabetes mellitus II: A study of 100 dental patients. J. Periodont., *30:*298, 1959.
36. Soskin, S.: Use and abuse of the dextrose tolerance test. Postgrad. Med., *10:*108, 1951.
37. Stahl, S. S.: Roentgenographic and bacteriologic aspects of periodontal changes in diabetics. J. Periodont., *19:*130, 1948.
38. Stahl, S. S., Wisan, J. M., and Miller, S. C.: Influence of systemic diseases on alveolar bone. J.A.D.A., *45:*277, 1952.
39. Stahl, S. S., Witkin, G. J., and Scopp, I. W.: Degenerative vascular changes observed in selected gingival specimens. Oral Surg., *15:*1495, 1962.
40. Stein, G. M., and Shannon, I.: Glucose tolerance and the state of periodontal health. J. Periodont, *41:*520, 1970.
41. Summers, C. J., and Oberman, A.: Association of oral disease with 12 selected variables: I. Periodontal disease. J. Dent. Res., *47:*457, 1968.
42. Traisman. H. S., and Newcomb, A. L.: Management of Juvenile Diabetes Mellitus. St. Louis, C. V. Mosby, 1965.
43. Tuckman, M. A., Kaslick, R. S., Shapiro, W. B., and Chasens, A. I.: The relationship of glucose tolerance to periodontal status. J. Periodont., *41:*27, 1970.
44. Unger, R. H.: The standard two-hour oral glucose tolerance test in the diagnosis of diabetes mellitus in subjects without fasting hyperglycemia. Ann. Int. Med., *47:*1138, 1957.
45. White, P.: Natural course and prognosis of juvenile diabetes. Diabetes, *5:*445, 1956.

14

Management of the Patient with Congenital and Acquired Heart Disease

THE PATIENT WITH CONGENITAL HEART DISEASE

The oral findings in acyanotic patients with congenital heart disease differ little, if at all, from those with normal hearts. Therefore, the descriptions of the oral conditions noted below apply only to those patients with congenital heart disease who are cyanotic. In particular, the most striking changes occur in those patients who have the tetralogy of Fallot. This syndrome consists of pulmonary stenosis, enlargement of the right ventricle with interventricular septal defects, and dextroposition of the aorta so that it receives blood from the right as well as from the left ventricle.

Clinical Characteristics. The teeth, particularly the maxillary incisors, have a peculiar bluish-white hue which has been described as either "paper-white" or the color of "skimmed milk."[13,14] Histologic investigations of the pulp tissue have demonstrated the presence of massive hyperemia with blood vessels of very large diameter.[18,19] For instance, the diameter of the largest blood vessels in the cyanotic patients measured 180 micra as compared to 60 to 80 micra for those found in normal or acyanotic patients with congenital heart disease.[14]

The mucous membranes of the lips, cheeks and tongue have a purplish hue. Fissured tongues, as well as such other abnormalities such as raised prominent, reddened fungiform and filiform papillae and prominent blood vessels on the inferior surface of the tongue, are frequently seen.

The gingiva tends to have a bright bluish-red appearance, the hue corresponding fairly closely to the general degree of cyanosis (Fig. 14-1).[13] Gingivitis is prevalent and therefore clinically the gingivae bleed easily, are edematous and hyperplastic. The high prevalence of gingivitis is associated with poor oral hygiene. This is probably because by and large these patients are not seen too frequently by the dentist because of the special problems which may arise in treating them.[13,14,26] Lack of lip seal, which is common, may play an additional role in the etiology of the gin-

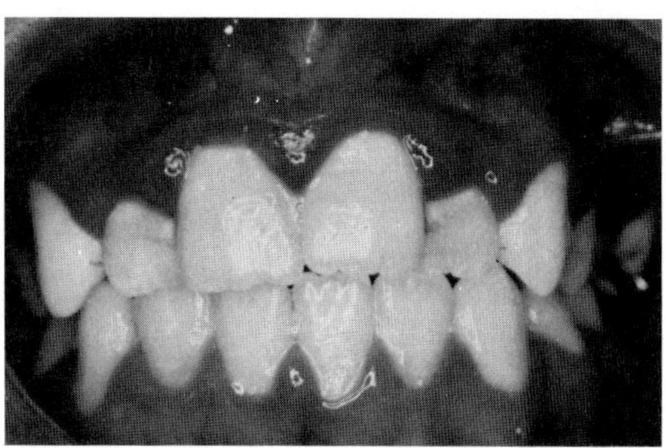

Fig. 14-1. The gingivae in cyanotic patients with congenital heart disease tend to have a bright bluish-red appearance.

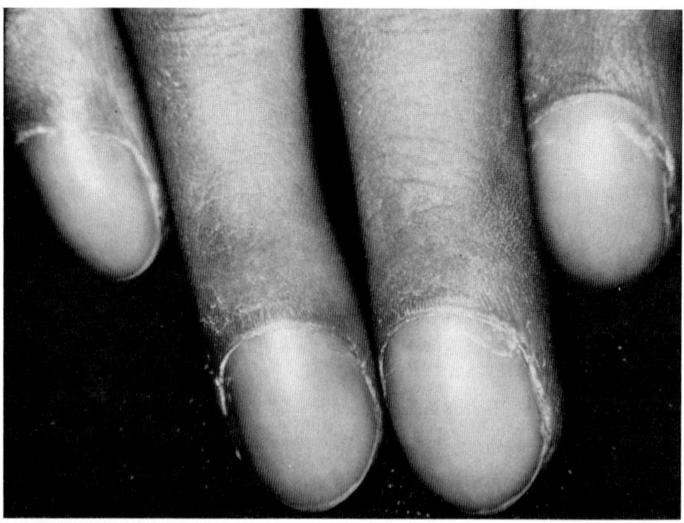

Fig. 14-2. Clubbing and spooning of the fingernails in a patient with congenital heart disease.

gival problem. However, once the valvular and other defects are surgically corrected and the patient is no longer cyanotic, the cyanotic appearance of the lips, buccal mucosa and gingiva disappear and are replaced by more normal coloring. The papillae of the tongue also return to normal and the blood vessels on the inferior surface of the tongue become less prominent.[19]

Roentgenographic Findings. Clubbing and spooning of the fingernails and toenails is an extremely common finding (Fig. 14-2).

Alveolar bone. No obvious changes occur in the alveolar bone. However, other parts of the skeleton reveal changes that are usually associated with the chronic anemias.[13]

Skull. Widening of the diploë, thickening of the tables and the "hair-on-end" striations may be seen.

Long bones. Endosteal cortical defects may occur as well as widening of the medullary canals, loss of diaphyseal tapering and loss of trabeculation in some areas with coarsening in other regions.

Pelvis, spine and ribs. Mottled areas of sclerosis may be seen and/or alteration in trabecular pattern.

TABLE 14-1. SUMMARY OF BACTEREMIA INCIDENCE

	Extraction Series	Periodontal Series
No. cases	34	33
positive	28	29
negative	6	4
With one organism	13	7
With multiple organisms	15	22
Percentage positive	82	88

After Rogosa, *et al.*[25]

TABLE 14-2. GROUPS OF ORGANISMS AND THEIR DISTRIBUTION

Organism	Extraction series		Periodontal series	
	No. organisms	Percent	No. organisms	Percent
Streptococcus	18	38	18	36
Diphtheroid	13	28	16	32
Vibrio	1	2	1	2
Spirillum	2	4	2	4
Tetracoccus	3	6	4	8
Bacteroides	4	8	6	12
Veillonella	0	0	5	10
Fusobacterium	0	0	7	14
Actinomyces	3	6	7	14
Micrococcus	1	2	1	2
"Leptotrichia"	0	0	1	2
Nontypable anaerobes	2	4	2	4
Total	47		70	

After Rogosa, *et al.*[25]

RELATIONSHIP BETWEEN BACTEREMIAS AND DENTAL PROCEDURES

The relationship between various dental procedures and bacterial endocarditis in patients with acquired valvular disease and such congenital lesions as patent ductus arteriosus and ventricular septal defects have been well documented.[10,11,15,20] In one of the early studies on the relationship between transient bacteremias and tooth extraction it was found that bacteremias occurred in 75 percent of patients with obvious septic mouths as compared with 34 percent with no obvious disease.[23] In a more recent study it was reported that transient bacteremias occurred in 82 percent of patients after tooth extraction and in 88 percent after periodontal therapy.[25] Of particular interest in this study was the high percentage of positive blood cultures following such periodontal procedures as curettage and periodontal surgery. Table 14-1 summarizes the incidence of bacteremias in both groups of patients, the instances in which one organism was recovered and those in which two or more different organisms were isolated from the same blood sample. There was no significant difference in the frequency with which streptococci or diphtheroids were recovered after either tooth extraction or periodontal treatment. The large variety of other organism which were recovered represent such genera as Vibrio, Spirillum, Bacteroides, Veillonella, Fusobacterium and Actinomyces. Table 14-2 summarizes the distribution and frequency of occurrence of the various organisms isolated from blood cultures following tooth extraction and periodontal therapy.

Manipulation other than tooth extraction or periodontal therapy may also result in a high number of positive blood cultures. For example, after rocking a single tooth with forceps, 86 percent of 21 patients with marked periodontal disease and 25 percent of 21 patients without obvious disease had positive blood cultures.[9]

Positive blood cultures have also been reported in 24 percent of 305 cases after toothbrushing, 40 percent after oral prophylaxis and in 17 percent of 225 cases after chewing hard candy.[4]

PROPHYLACTIC REGIMEN FOR PATIENTS WITH RHEUMATIC OR CONGENITAL HEART DISEASE

The following regimen as recommended by the American Heart Association may be employed for patients with rheumatic or congenital heart disease.[1]

Penicillin is the drug of choice. While broad-spectrum antibiotics may decrease bacteremia, they cannot be relied upon to eradicate initial bacterial implants and for this reason are not recommended. Sulfonamides are completely unsatisfactory. Optimal dosage and duration of therapy with penicillin are not known. It should be emphasized that good evidence exists that penicillin or sulfonamides in the doses used for prophylaxis against Group A streptococcal infection and consequent recurrence of rheumatic fever are not adequate for prevention of bacterial endocarditis. Larger doses of penicillin are required to prevent implantation of bacteria on heart valves, and a high concentration of penicillin in the blood for several days may well be required to eradicate small bacterial implants should they occur.

Pretreatment Medication. It should also be stressed that there is no disagreement concerning the advisability of using penicillin immediately before and subsequent to dental manipulations. The wisdom of using antibiotics for several days before these procedures are carried out is not yet settled. Some evidence exists that pretreatment may cause sensitive bacteria (e.g., streptococcus viridans and staphylococci), normally present in the oral cavity and upper respiratory tract, to be replaced by penicillin-resistant strains. Bacterial endocarditis resulting from such strains would pose greater therapeutic problems. With the above reservations in mind the following treatment schedules are suggested:

Day of Procedure. Procaine penicillin 600,000 units supplemented by 600,000 units crystalline penicillin IM, 1 to 2 hours before procedure. Although intramuscular penicillin is more reliable, because of practical considerations, some dentists and physicians rely on oral penicillin when the full cooperation of the patient is assured. If oral penicillin is to be employed, 4 doses every 4 to 6 hours of at least 0.25 Gm. of alphaphenoxymethyl penicillin (Penicillin V) or 500,000 units of buffered penicillin G should be given during the day of the procedure. In addition, an extra dose should be taken one hour before the procedure.

After Procedure. Procaine penicillin 600,000 units IM each day for 2 days. In selected instances, 0.25 Gm. Penicillin V or 500,000 units of buffered penicillin G 4 times daily by mouth on each day may be used for those patients in whom full cooperation is anticipated and ingestion is assured. The main contraindication to the above regimen is sensitivity to penicillin. All patients should be carefully questioned for previous history suggesting penicillin sensitivity and even if it is equivocal, penicillin should not be given. Under such circumstances, erythromysin should be used in a dose of 250 mg. by mouth 4 times daily for adults and older children. For small children, a dose of 20 mg. per pound per day divided into 3 or 4 evenly spaced doses may be used. The total dose should not exceed 1 Gm. per day.

PATIENTS WITH A SYSTOLIC CLICK OR A SYSTOLIC MURMUR

It is now known that a systolic click or a late systolic murmur previously diagnosed as "benign sounds" may indeed represent structural changes of the heart valve and may become associated with the subsequent development of endocarditis.

Prophylactic Regimen. The use of prophylatic antibiotics in the manner described above is advised for these persons even when these sounds are considered functional.[16]

PATIENTS WITH PROSTHETIC HEART VALVES

Endocarditis in patients with prosthetic valve replacements, whether dating from the time of operation or occurring in the postoperative period, has almost always proved to be fatal.[8,21] Several reports from the National Heart and Lung Institute have described the clinical and pathological features of this complication.[3,5,24] In each case of endocarditis involving the aortic prosthesis, the infection resulted in detachment of the prosthetic valve and massive, fatal aortic regurgitation. The primary site of infection was found to be the tissues to which the prosthesis had been attached. The sutures had torn through the necrotic aortic annulus and the valve was partially or completely detached. The infectious process also involved the periaortic tissues with acute abscesses and foci of necrosis located between the aorta and the walls of both right and left atria. In some cases, the infection extended into the mitral and tricuspid annulus. In all, secondary operative intervention would have been fruitless because of the extent of the infection and the character of the tissue at the aortic root. In one of the patients, fatal staphylococcal endocarditis followed dental extraction, despite penicillin prophylaxis in doses similar to those recommended by the American Heart Association for patients with valvular rheumatic heart disease. Another patient who received penicillin before and after dental extraction did not contract endocarditis at that time but 6 months later, when he was edentulous, and shortly after he had been fitted with dentures, he developed an ultimately fatal infection caused by beta hemolytic streptococcus.

Prophylactic Regimen. These considerations suggest that a more comprehensive antibiotic regimen be given patients with prosthetic heart valves prior to dental manipulations in order to control bacteremia and to prevent implantation and multiplication of the bacteria in the epithelium of the heart. Multiple extractions or extensive procedures particularly should be avoided in the presence of dental sepsis, because of the increase in intensity of the bacteremia in this situation. The following prophylactic antibiotic coverage is recommended prior to dental manipulation:

On the evening before the procedure, give:
  Penicillin V – 500,000 units orally
One hour before the procedure, give IM:
  Procaine penicillin – 600,000 units, plus
  Streptomycin – 0.5 Gm., plus
  Crystalline penicillin – 600,000 units.
For 3 to 5 days following the procedure,
  Procaine penicillin – 600,000 units IM every 12 hours plus streptomycin – 0.5 Gm. IM every 12 hours.

Alternatively, Penicillin V – 500,000 units orally every 6 hours may be used in the postoperative period rather than the more desirable IM procaine penicillin. If the patient is allergic to penicillin, equivalent doses of an alternate antibiotic (erythromycin – 0.2 Gm. IM or 1.0 Gm. orally or Keflin – 0.5 Gm. IM) should be given. If procedures are of necessity performed in an environment where penicillin-resistant staphylococci are likely contaminants, oxacillin – 1 to 2 Gm. orally every 6 hours may be added to the above program.

Local procedures. Since postoperative bacteremias have been found to occur in a very high percentage of patients following various periodontal procedures, it is

TABLE 14-3. COMPARISON OF POSTEXTRACTION-POSITIVE BLOOD CULTURES

Groups	No. of Patients	Results of Postextraction Blood Cultures	
		Positive	Negative
Antiseptic Mouthwash and Irrigation	67	12 (17.9%)	55 (82.1%)
Saline Mouthwash and Irrigation	67	31 (46.3%)	36 (53.7%)
Control	67	44 (65.7%)	23 (34.3%)

After Jones, Cutcher, Goldberg, and Lilly.[17]

recommended that in addition to the above regimen, the following local procedures be done to further lower the incidence of postoperative bacteremias.[17] Just prior to initiation of therapy have the patient rinse his mouth for 30 seconds with a phenolated mouthwash. The gingival sulci in the involved areas should then be irrigated with 20 ml. of the same phenolated mouthwash solution by means of a syringe fitted with a blunt needle. In an experiment which compared the number of postextraction-positive blood cultures between groups using a phenolated mouthwash solution and sulcus irrigation, with one using a saline mouthwash and irrigation to a normal control group, it was found that those using the phenolated solution had a highly significant reduction in postoperative bacteremias (Table 14-3). Similar results can be obtained by using a providone-iodine solution for rinsing and irrigation.[27]

Dental Evaluation. It is important to point out that a complete dental evaluation with necessary treatment should be performed if possible prior to the prosthetic replacement of heart valves.

Periodontal Treatment. Considering the number of precautions which are necessary in treating these patients, it would appear prudent to accomplish as much as possible each visit. If surgical therapy is required, then in addition to the presurgical use of antibiotics, it is recommended that a zinc bacitracin containing dressing be used postsurgically.[2] Teeth with guarded prognoses should be extracted rather than subjected to extensive periodontal procedures.

Plaque Control. While plaque control is necessary in all patients in order to maintain periodontal health, in these patients, in view of the possible grave systemic complications which could arise from a bacteremia, it is imperative. In all such patients, therefore, preventive programs should be instituted at an early age and maintained scrupulously throughout life.

PATIENTS RECEIVING ANTICOAGULANT DRUGS

In addition to the problem of endocarditis, many cardiac patients undergo dental surgery while being treated with anticoagulant drugs. The administration of the warfarin drugs (e.g., Coumadin) results in a prolongation of the commonly measured one-state prothrombin time by depression factors, II, VII, and X. In addition, it should be pointed out that chronic administration may depress factor IX (Christmas factor or plasma thromboplastin component) which can be missed by the one-stage prothrombin time determination, but may be assessed by its effect in prolonging the partial thromboplastin time. Upon discontinuation of the drug, there is a slow rise of these factors to normal. For the most part, anticoagulation is maintained in virtually all patients and the prothrombin time should be kept in the therapeutic range (approximately twice the control level) until a specific date for the surgery. The anticoagulant is then discontinued for 2 to 3 days prior to operation and the prothrombin time allowed to return to a normal or near normal level. The administration of vitamin K to effect a more rapid restoration of the prothrombin time may induce a hypercoagulable state and use of this drug is inadvisable except as required in a surgical emergency. Although most patients experience little trouble with minor surgery in the presence of anticoagulants, occasional extensive bleeding has followed dental extraction. Thrombosis of a prosthesis or peripheral arterial embolization is extremely unusual in patients when anticoagulation is briefly interrupted. Warfarin administration is usually resumed on the first or second postoperative day and a therapeutic level of anticoagulation is restored as rapidly as possible. It should be emphasized that many drugs affect the anticoagulant action of warfarin and a careful pharmacologic history should be obtained in these patients when administering other drugs.[12]

PATIENTS WITH DYSRHYTHMIAS

A final consideration should be given to the problem of dysrhythmias that may arise under anesthesia. Driscoll, *et al.*[6,7] have called attention to the variety of rhythm problems occurring during outpatient dental procedures.

General Anesthesia. It is desirable to have electrocardiographic monitoring of patients with cardiac disease undergoing dental surgery with general anesthesia. It is also necessary for the cardiologist or monitoring physician to be familiar with the anesthetic agents used as well as to recognize the rapidly changing effects of multiple stimuli upon the heart during anesthesia and operation. The recognition of artifacts also is of great importance. The classical training gained by electrocardiographic interpretation under static conditions must be modified to the dynamic situation of the operating room.

Several precautions should be emphasized when using general anesthesia. The induction and maintenance in extensive operative procedures should be conducted by an anesthesiologist familiar with the management of patients with cardiac disease. Usual premedications are given, but if atropine is utilized the dose should not be one likely to result in tachycardia. Because arrhythmia is most likely to occur during induction and endotracheal intubation, oscilloscopic monitoring of the electrocardiogram is desirable throughout the operation. Frequent ventricular extrasystoles and nodal rhythm most often reflect hypoxia or inadequate muscular relaxation, or both, and may presage the occurrence of ventricular tachycardia or fibrillation. If ventricular irritability persists after control of oxygenation and relaxation, the ectopic focus can usually be suppressed by intermittent doses of lidocaine, 50 to 100 mg. intravenously. An electrical defibrillator, suitable for external application, should, of course, be immediately available. Oxygen administration is continued postoperatively until the patient is fully conscious and electrocardiographic monitoring is desirable during the early postanesthesia period.

Local Anesthesia. The management of the dental patient with heart disease receiving local anesthesia must be individualized. In the majority of instances, this is accomplished without difficulty. Certain patients with advanced conduction disturbances and clinically significant ventricular irritability are best managed in the hospital with electrocardiographic monitoring. A careful history of drug sensitivity is most important. Adeuqate preoperative sedation is most helpful, since the effects of anxiety are probably more stressful to the cardiovascular system than is the local anesthesia. The close cooperation of the physician and the dentist is mandatory and a full discussion of anticipated problems and management should be carried out prior to the operative procedure.

REFERENCES

1. American Heart Association. Statement by the Committee on Prevention of Rheumatic Fever and Bacterial Endocarditis, 1965.
2. Baer, P. N., Sumner, C. F. III, and Miller, G.: Periodontal dressings. Dent. Clin. North Am., *13:*181, 1969.
3. Behrendt, D. M., and Morrow, A. G.: General operative procedures after cardiac valve replacement. Arch. Surg., *98:*824, 1968.
4. Cobe, W.: Transient bacteremia. J. Oral Surg., *7:*609, 1954.
5. Cohen, L. H., Roberts, W. C., Rockoff, S. D., and Morrow, A. G.: Bacterial endocarditis following aortic valve replacement. Circulation, *33:*209, 1966.
6. Driscoll, E. J., Christenson, G. R., and White, C. L.: Physiologic studies in general anesthesia for ambulatory dental patients. Oral Surg., *12:*1496, 1959.
7. Driscoll, E. J., Tanenbaum, H. L., *et al.:* To be published.
8. Effler, D. B., Favaloro, R., and Groves, L. K.: Heart valve replacement. Am. Thor. Surg., *1:*4, 1965.
9. Elliott, S. D.: Bacteremia and oral sepsis. Proc. Roy. Soc. Med., *32:*747, 1939.
10. Ernstene, A. C., McGarvey, C. J., and Ecker, J. A.: Prophylaxis of subacute bacterial endocarditis. Cleveland Clinic Quart., *18:*1, 1951.
11. Favour, C. B., Janeway, C. A., Gibson, J. G., and Levine, S. A.: Progress in the treatment of subacute bacterial endocarditis. N. Engl. J. Med., *234:*71, 1946.
12. Forniller, M., *et al.:* Coumadin and indanedione anticoagulants. Potentiators and antagonists. Am. J. Hosp. Pharm., *26:*574, 1969.
13. Gould, M. S. E., and Picton, D. C. A.: The gingival condition of congenitally cyanotic individuals. Br. Dent. J. *109:*96, 1960.
14. Hakala, P. E.: Dental and oral changes in congenital heart disease. Suom. Hammaslaak. Toim., *63:*284, 1967.
15. Harvey, W. P., Capone, M. A.: Bacterial endocarditis related to cleaning and filling of teeth. Am. J. Cardiol., *7:*793, 1961.
16. Hurst, J. W., and Logue, R. B.: The Heart. ed. 2. New York, McGraw-Hill, 1970.
17. Jones, J. C., Cutcher, J. L., Goldberg, J. R., and Lilly, G. E.: Control of bacteremia associated with extraction of teeth. Oral Surg., *30:*454, 1970.
18. Kaner, A., Losch, P. K., and Green, H.: Oral manifestations of congenital heart disease. J. Pediatr., *29:*269, 1946.
19. Kaner, A., Losch, P. K., and Green, H.: Some postoperative oral observations in congenital heart disease. Oral Surg., *2:*1454, 1949.
20. Lichtman, P., and Master, A. M.: Incidence of valvular heart disease in people over 50 and penicillin prophylaxis of bacterial endocarditis. N.Y. State J. Med., *49:*1693, 1949.
21. Nelson, T. G., and Cooley, D. A.: Prosthetic replacement of the mitral or aortic valves: a preliminary report on 111 cases. Am. J. Cardiol., *14:*148, 1964.
22. Nice, C. M., Daves, M. L., and Wood, G. H.: Changes in bone associated with cyanotic congenital cardiac disease. Am. Heart J., *68:*25, 1964.
23. Okell, C. C., and Elliott, S. D.: Bacteremia and oral sepsis with special reference to aetiology of subacute endocarditis. Lancet, *4:*869, 1935.
24. Roberts, W. C., and Morrow, A. G.: Bacterial endocarditis involving prosthetic mitral valves. Arch. Path., *82:*164, 1966.
25. Rogosa, M., Hampp, E. G., Nevin, T. A., Wagner, H. N., Jr., Driscoll, E. J., and Baer, P. N.: Blood sampling and cultural studies in the detection of postoperative bacteremias. J.A.D.A., *60:*171, 1960.
26. Salloy, C: Periodontal findings in cyanotic individuals. J. Dent. Res., *35:*840, 1956.
27. Scopp, I. W., and Orvieto, L. D.: Gingival degerming by povidone-iodine irrigation: bacteremia reduction in extraction procedures. J.A.D.A., *83:*1194, 1971.

15

Management of Leukemia, Anemias of Dental Interest and Hemophilia

LEUKEMIA

Leukemia is a fatal disease characterized by alterations in the hematopoeitic elements of the body, that is, there is an abnormal multiplication of white cells and their precursors along with an alteration in the number and type of white cells found in the circulating blood.[33] It is the most common fatal disease found between the ages of 1 and 15 years.[17]

Leukemias are broadly classified into acute and chronic types with a further definitive subdivision into the predominating cell types. Until the age of 20 years, 95 percent of all leukemias are acute in nature with acute lymphoblastic leukemia being the predominant form, although chronic lymphocytic leukemia has been reported as well.[7,29,33] Acute lymphoblastic leukemia predominates in childhood until the time of puberty. From then until about the age of 25 years, lymphoblastic leukemia approximately equals the sum of the cases of myeloblastic and monocytic leukemia. After the age of 25 years the latter two forms begin to appear more commonly. Actually the predominant form from ages 20 through 45 years is chronic myelocytic leukemia.[29,33]

Prevalence. In children leukemia occurs at the rate of 3 per 100,000 population with most cases occurring before the child is 5 years of age.[17,26,27] Congenital leukemias have been reported but are rare, only about 45 cases having appeared in the literature.[6,26] The incidence of leukemia begins to elevate during the first 2 years of life, and peaks in the 3- and 4-year age group.[8,9] Leukemia is more frequently observed in males, with the exception of the first years of life.[29] Negroes are less susceptible than Caucasians, and the American Indians have the lowest degree of susceptibility.[29]

Etiology. While the etiology of leukemia remains obscure, several factors have been shown to play a significant role. First, there appears to be considerable evidence of a genetic pattern to the disease. It has been reported in significant numbers in twins and in cases of Down's syndrome (see Chap. 11).[1,13,21,22,24] Also suggestive of a genetic relationship is the demonstration of chromosomal aberrations in some patients with chronic myelocytic leukemia.[31] However, no clear-cut inherited tendency for leukemia has been established, despite the many isolated reports of its occurrence in families.[26,30] Various chemical, environmental, allergic and infectious agents also have been suggested as etiologic factors, but the strongest direct evidence to etiology is linked to irradiation.[9,18,19,28,29] Recently, considerable focus has been placed on the role of viruses in leukemia, owing to the fact that they have been shown to transmit leukemia in experimental animals.[12,15,16] These agents, however, have yet to be identified in man.

Clinical Characteristics. In the early stages, physical findings are essentially normal. The child usually presents with vague generalized aches and pains, malaise and fatigue.[17] Lymph gland enlargement occurs somewhat later. In a study of 322 cases, fatigue was found to be the first symptom in 50 percent of the patients. The most frequent extramedullary involvement is that of the testicles and central nervous system.[17,33] Bilateral enlargement of the salivary and lacrimal glands, called Mikulicz's syndrome, is another common finding.[29] However, a definitive diagnosis is made on the basis of bone marrow studies where one finds 90 percent of the hematopoeitic elements replaced by leukemic cells.[16] This results in the classical signs of the disease: namely, anemia, infection and hemorrhage. Immature leukocytes are generally not found in the circulating blood and circulating leukocytes are usually not elevated in number at the onset of the disease. In fact, at the onset of the disease a leukopenia is often present.

Oral findings. Oral findings vary with the type of leukemia. The most pronounced oral changes occur in monocytic and myelogenous leukemia where extreme hyperplasia of the gingival tissues may occur along with gingival bleeding (Fig. 15-1).[2,32] In severe cases (Fig. 15-2) fulminating necrotic lesions, cancrum oris or nomalike lesions may result from leukemic infiltrate and bacterial infection.[3,4] A differential diagnosis must be made between this disease, agranulocytosis and acute necrotizing gingivitis (Fig. 5-2; see Chap. 3). Since the majority of leukemias in children are not of the monocytic or myelogenous type but of the lymphoblastic type, extreme gingival changes are uncommon. The primary gingival changes noted are related to the anemia and thrombocytopenia, hence bleeding problems are the usual presenting oral symptom. It has been the experience of the authors that the gingival changes in children are not as dramatic as those usually described in the literature, with most publications referring to the more bizarre changes of the uncommon (in children) monocytic and myelogenous forms of the disease.

Radiographic changes. Changes of the maxilla and mandible, while not seen on periapical radiographs, have been reported to occur in 62.9 percent of children with active leukemia when panoramic radiographic techniques are used.[5,10,11] These changes consist of destruction of the apical portion of the most distal developing molar crypt, followed in frequency by the premolar and canine crypts.[10]

Treatment. Chemotherapy and platelet replacement therapy have increased longevity from a median survival time of 3 months for those patients with acute lymphocytic leukemia to approximately 2½ years.[14] Chemotherapy produces long periods of remission during which the child may lead a fully active life.[17] Since the disease is fatal, the oral therapist must think not in long-term success of treatment, but primarily of reducing patient discomfort. This can best be achieved by reducing bacterial plaque at the gingival margin in order to avoid secondary infection during periods of exacerbation. Increased remission time has added to the need for oral management. Therapy should be directed primarily at the reduction of infections and the potential for bleeding. In acute periods where platelet levels are low, normal oral hygiene may cause excessive bleeding. Hence, plaque control must be done carefully. It is suggested that during these periods the sulcus be cleaned by swabbing gently with a rubber stimulator tip, and that toothbrushing be eliminated. An attempt should be made to rid the mouth of local irritating factors during periods of remission so that inflammatory changes in the tissues, particularly increased vascularity, will be kept to a minimum. Plaque control should be meticulous. Secondary oral complications often arise as a result of antimetabolite therapy. Oral ulcerations are common, particularly with methotrexate. Emollients such as Orabase may be used to coat the lesions. Another complicating factor in patients who have received antibiotics and

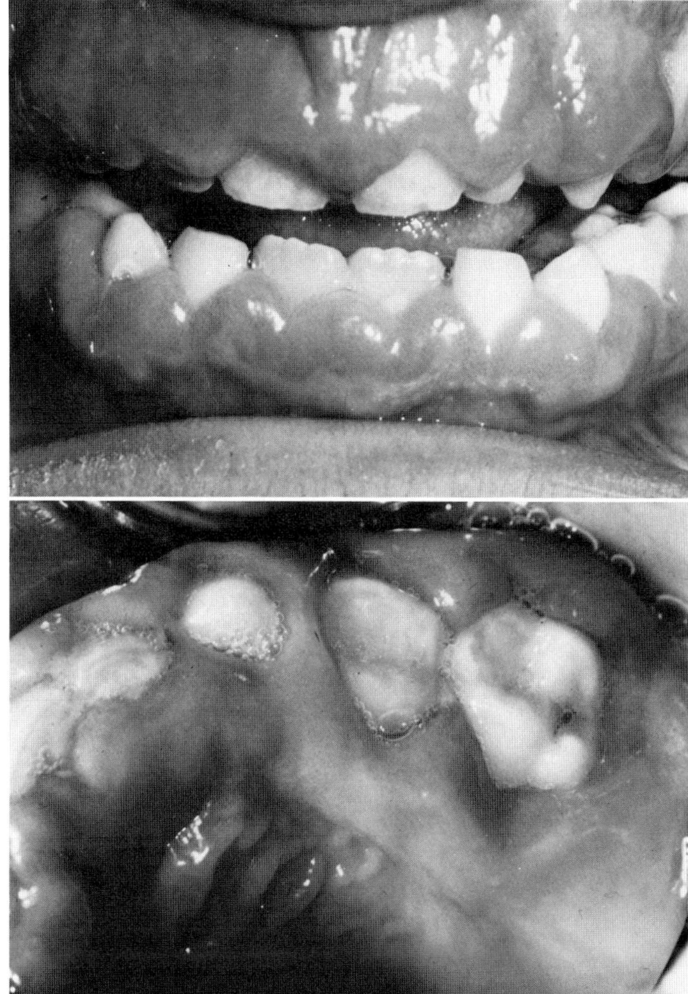

Fig. 15-1. *Top.* A 9-year-old female with chronic monocytic leukemia demonstrating generalized gingival hyperplasia.
Bottom. Gingival enlargement is due to an increased infiltration of abnormal cells.

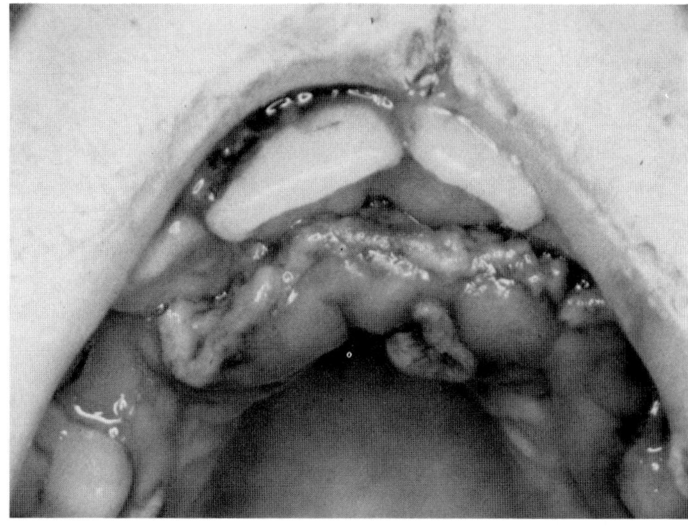

Fig. 15-2. Acute monocytic leukemia in a 13-year-old female. The gingiva is swollen, spongy and bleeds readily. Oral ulcerations and loosening of the teeth are common findings. The oral ulcerations frequently result in a clinical picture resembling acute necrotizing ulcerative gingivitis.

steroids for long periods is moniliasis, which may be treated with mycostatin rinses. In all cases, the oral therapist should be closely coordinated with the attending physician.

SICKLE-CELL ANEMIA

Onset and Prevalence. In approximately half the patients the disease is noted to occur under one year of age. The sickle-cell trait occurs in from 8.5 percent to 13.4 percent of American Negroes while the homozygous form, sickle-cell anemia, occurs in from 0.3 to 1.3 percent of American Negroes.[34,44] It tends to be more common in females than in males.

Etiology. This hereditary from of chronic hemolytic anemia is inherited as an autosomal recessive trait. The anemia is due to a single amino acid abnormality. The glutamic acid normally found in position 6 of the beta chain is replaced by valine.[43] This results in the production of a hemoglobin called hemoglobin S which composes 75 to 100 percent of the hemoglobin and, in turn, results in sickle-shaped red cells as well as signs of excessive blood destruction and active blood formation.

Clinical Characteristics. The disease is characterized by symptoms of anemia, leg ulcers, acute attacks of bone and cardiac failure.

Radiographic findings. There are usually no findings in those individuals with sickle-cell trait. In those with sickle-cell anemia the abnormalities can all be explained as a result of the compensatory hyperplasia of the erythropoietic marrow.

The skull. The most frequent changes noted in the calvarium are a generalized osteoporous and a widening of the diploic space.[40,41,42] Occasionally localized areas of thickening in the skull may also be noted as may the "hair-on-end" pattern which at one time was described as a diagnostic feature of this disease, although it is rarely seen. It is estimated that the "hair-on-end" pattern in the calvarium occurs in 5 percent of the patients at most.[41]

The mandible. The roentgenographic changes seen in sickle-cell anemia are not pathognomonic, since they may also be seen in other anemias and are even observed in the apparently normal patient. Nevertheless, it is felt that the changes seen in the mandible in sickle-cell anemia demonstrate abnormalities with a greater frequency than can be observed in any other bone.[40,41,42] There is generalized osteoporosis and the cortex of the inferior border of the mandible becomes thinned, rarely exceeding 4 mm. in width. Cortical thinning also occurs in the ramus. The marrow spaces are especially prominent and large. While the lamina dura is normal, it gives an illusion of being more prominent against the radiolucent background. The interdental trabeculae between the roots of the mandibular incisors frequently assume a horizontal or "stepladder" arrangement.[38,39] However, it must be emphasized that these roentgenographic features are only suggestive and not diagnostic of the disease. Similar patterns can be observed in perfectly normal individuals.

Treatment. Only palliative management is presently possible.

Dental precautions. Because these patients are highly receptive to infections which can precipitate a "crisis" and death, the major concern is to prevent infections and immediately control them.[36,37] All patients who require surgical procedures should have a medical consultation. It is essential that an adequate hemoglobin level be maintained at all times. If it is too low, transfusions may be necessary to raise the hemoglobin level before surgery. General anesthesia should be avoided because it may further lower the already poor oxygen tension. A resultant hypoxia could precipitate a cerebral or myocardial thrombosis. In general, all surgical procedures, including dental surgery, should be done in a hospital environment so that any emergency which might arise can be properly managed. Antibiotics should be given prophylactically.

Prognosis. There is a high mortality rate in infancy and early childhood. However, those who survive the childhood period demonstrate a remarkable adaptation to their state of anemia and may have few complaints. However, the state of remission of this disease is punctuated at unpredictable intervals by so-called "crisis." This results when intravascular sickling occurs and causes thrombosis and infarctions, which, in turn are responsible for the acute abdominal pain, joint and muscle pain and fever noted clinically. In recent decades the mortality rate has decreased and some patients presently survive beyond the age of 50 years.

Sickle-Cell Hemoglobin C Disease

By the relatively simple techniques of electrophoresis, the various hemoglobins such as hemoglobins S, C, D and E can be easily detected and differentiated from the normal. It is possible, therefore, for an individual to inherit any combination of 2 of these abnormal genes (see Table 15-1). Gene frequency for S and C hemoglobin is relatively high in the Negro population, occurring with about one fourth the frequency of sickle-cell anemia.[44] It now seems probable that the cases which in the past were reported as representing an intermediate form between the asymptomatic sickle-cell trait and the homozygous sickle-cell anemia were actually heterozygous for hemoglobin S and C. These cases are particularly interesting because they may manifest all the signs of sickle-cell anemia in a milder form, with the exception of the cardiac signs. In addition, this disease manifests acute infarctions of the bone marrow, in particular, aseptic necrosis of the humeral and femoral head and pronounced radiographic changes in the mandible,[35,40] which may also represent areas of infarction, are common.

Prognosis. Favorable. However, morbidity and mortality during pregnancy are greater than in nonpregnant women.

GLUCOSE-6-PHOSPHATE-DEHYDROGENASE DEFICIENCY ANEMIA (G6PD)

The importance of this disease lies in the fact that an acute hemolytic anemia may be precipitated by dental infections[46] or by the administration of oxidant drugs which impair glutathione (GSH) synthesis. Common drugs which fall into this category are acetanilid, acetophenetidin (phenacetin), acetylsalicylic acid, sulfanilamide, the sulfones and certain vitamin K derivatives.

Mode of Inheritance and Prevalence. This disease has a sex-linked and incompletely dominant mode of inheritance and occurs in both men and women. It occurs in approximately 13 percent of American Negroes. In addition, however, it is estimated that it affects 100 million or more people of all races throughout the world.[45,47]

Etiology. This disease is due to a deficiency in the enzyme glucose-6-phosphate-dehydrogenase which makes the erythrocyte less able to manufacture glutathione and consequently less able to handle oxidant compounds.[47]

Clinical Characteristics. Under normal circumstances patients with this deficiency have no clinical manifestations.

HOMOZYGOUS BETA THALASSEMIA

Normal Blood Electrophoretic Patterns

The hemoglobin of the normal adult is designated hemoglobin A (HbA) and contains 2 alpha and 2 beta polypeptide chains. The hemoglobin in the fetus and newborn child, called hemoglobin F (HbF), differs from that of the adult and should not persist into adult life in anything but trace amounts. Hemoglobin F contains pairs

TABLE 15-1. COMBINATION OF ABNORMAL HEMOGLOBINS*

	Normal (HbA)			
Normal (HbA)	Normal (A-A)	Sickle (HbS)		
Sickle (Hb-S)	Sickle trait (S-A)	Sickle anemia (S-S)	Hb (C)	
HbC	HbC trait (C-A)	Sickle HbC disease (S-C)	Homozygous HbC disease (C-C)	Beta thalas-semia
Beta thalas-semia	Thalas-semia minor (A-beta Thal)	Sickle-thalas-semia disease (S-beta Thal)	Hb-C thalas-semia disease (C-beta Thal)	Homozygous beta-thalas-semia

* The genetic types are listed in both the horizontal and vertical columns. The resultant hemoglobinopathies appear where the columns cross (Modified after Prowler, and Smith).[40]

of alpha and gamma chains, the latter being replaced by beta chains in the adult. The manner in which the globin chains and their heme groups are bonded together is important since this provides the environment needed for reversible combinations with oxygen under physiologic conditions. If the relationships are disturbed in any way, oxygen binding may be affected and an anemia produced. Disturbances in this system can be detected through hemoglobin electrophoresis studies.[50]

Onset and Inherited Pattern. The onset usually occurs during the first few years of life and is inherited as an autosomal recessive trait. In addition the disease tends to follow a racial pattern, the majority of the patients being of either Greek or Italian stock.[51] However, the disease is widely distributed and is also found along all the countries that lie on the edge of the Mediterranean basin and in southern Asia (i.e., Persia, India, Thailand, China and the Philippines).[51] Carriers of the trait, heterozygous beta thalassemia, are extremely common. In one study it was estimated that one in every 25 adult Italians in the city of Rochester, New York, either carried the trait or suffered from a mild form of the disease.[54]

Etiology. This disease, also known as Cooley's anemia and thalassemia major, is caused by a retardation in the production of the beta chains on the hemoglobin molecule and by the presence of fetal hemoglobin, hemoglobin F, in amounts ranging from 20 to 90 percent, causing a disturbance in the blood morphology. The red cells become hypochromic and microcytic with numerous target and stippled forms and variable numbers of nucleated erythrocytes, polychromatic cells and reticulocytes.

Clinical Characteristics. This disease is in fact the best example of skeletal dwarfism and infantilism caused by chronic anemia.[51] It is characterized by pallor, weakness and marked hyperplasia of the bone marrow with a resulting increase in the volume of active red marrow. This latter pathologic change forms the underlying anatomic basis for the observed skeletal changes.[57] A characteristic "rodent-like" facial expression is another identifying trait, although it does not occur in every case.

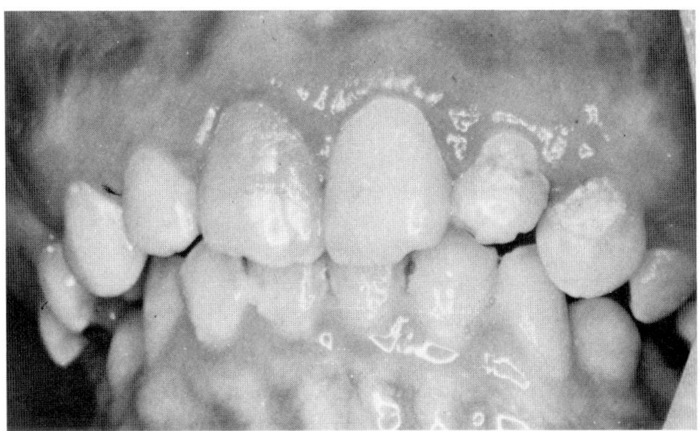

Fig. 15-3. Overgrowth of the maxilla is a prominent feature of homozygous beta thalassemia.

Roentgenographic findings. The skull shows a marked widening of the diploic space and atrophy, particularly of the outer tables. Occasionally, the trabeculae in the diploic spaces become arranged in vertical rows giving the so-called, "hair-on-end" appearance.[49,57] Thickening of the tables alone, however, is much more common. Other prominent features in the skull are failure of pneumatization of the maxillary sinus and considerable overgrowth of the maxilla (Fig. 15-3). This latter feature causes a separation of the orbits and prominence to the maxillary incisors and is responsible for producing the so called "rodent facies"[48,49] also known as the mongoloid facies.[52,53,55]

Oral and dental changes. The most noticeable changes that occur in the oral cavity are:[53]

Maxillary enlargement	64%
Deep overbite	36%
Open bite	15%
Normal occlusion	10%
Some degree of crossbite	8%

The oral mucosa and gingiva may exhibit pallor from the anemia but are often otherwise normal in appearance. If the patient survives adolescence, there is usually some regression of the bony overgrowth and a more normal facial appearance may return.[51] Intra-oral roentgenograms may show nonspecific changes such as irregular enlarged marrow spaces. Occasionally, there is a peculiar thickening to some of the trabeculae. This so-called "pepper and salt" appearance of the trabeculae may indicate a recovery from an abnormally stimulated hematopoiesis.[55]

Comment on Dental Treatment. The patient is weak; appointments should be as short as possible. General anesthetics should be avoided, because of the difficulty caused by low hemoglobin levels and the cardiac problem which frequently is present as a result of anoxia from the anemia. Whenever surgical procedures are indicated, they are best carried out at the time the patient is admitted for a blood transfusion, because at that time the hemoglobin level is at its highest. Since these patients are usually susceptible to infection, antibiotics should be administered prophylactically. Hemorrhage following surgical procedures is generally no problem.[56]

Prognosis. The prognosis depends somewhat on the age of onset. Generally, the earlier in infancy the onset, the more rapidly fatal is the disease. Death is usually due to infection, liver failure or cardiac damage as a result of anoxia from the anemia. When the disease occurs later in childhood, frequent transfusions and appropriate treatment of secondary infections can prolong life.

Variations. In addition to homozygous beta thalassemia, more than one abnormal hemoglobin may be present in a single patient. The combination of thalassemia with abnormal hemoglobins S, C, D and E has been reported. Heterozygous beta thalassemia (thalassemia minor) patients are generally normal or may have a very mild form of the disease.

HEMOPHILIA

Hemophilia is a disease characterized by prolonged and repeated episodes of hemorrhage caused by a coagulation deficiency.

While classical hemophilia is a disease that is caused by a lack of coagulation factor VIII, other bleeding diatheses with similar clinical characteristics have also been identified. These, however, are the result of a lack of other specific coagulation factors. Confusion has arisen over the utilization of the word hemophilia. Wintrobe feels it best that this term be used exclusively to describe classical hemophilia (A) and that the other conditions resembling it be labeled by the appropriate factor deficiency.[96] Over 15 diseases are included in this group of hemorrhagic disorders.[85]

In all, 13 factors have been identified as playing a significant role in coagulation. Wintrobe divides the remaining types of hemophilias, other than lack of factor VIII or IX, into 4 categories:[96]

1. Additional defects in the intrinsic prothrombin activator system (factor XI or XII deficiencies).
2. Defects in the intrinsic prothrombin activator system (factor V, VII and X deficiencies).
3. Abnormalities involving fibrinogen and factor XIII.
4. Circulating anticoagulants.

It is not within the scope of this book to discuss the other deficiencies, since they seldom occur.

Frequency and Severity. The most commonly occurring bleeding problem is true hemophilia (factor VIII deficiency) which accounts for about 80 percent of cases. The second most commonly found bleeding problem is factor IX deficiency (Christmas disease or hemophilia B) accounting for about 20 percent of cases. Hemophilia C (factor XI deficiency) and von Willebrand's disease (a combination of factor VIII and a failure of platelet adhesion) occur at about the same frequency, of 1 percent. The degree of intensity of the disease depends upon the amount of the factor the patient is missing. Thus, in classic hemophilia, factor levels may be less than 1 or 2 percent, while in subhemophilia they may be present at levels of 20 to 30 percent. Normal factor VIII levels may run as high as 65 to 138 percent.[96]

Etiology. Hemophilia is transmitted as a sex-linked recessive to the X chromosome and as such was believed to be transmitted solely to the male. Recently, however, a congenital lack of factor VIII has also been found in females, which would classify them as true hemophiliacs.[64,65,77,86,94] There is some controversy as to whether or not the disease is a result of a lack of production of factor VIII or an immunologic neutralizing of the factor.[67,69,78,92,93] Since the gene is recessive, on a random mixing of the population, one would except the gene to be disseminated so widely as to be insignificant. This does not appear to be true, however, since in one third of all cases no familial antecedents can be demonstrated.[90] Apparently chance mutation is a significant factor in the etiology of the disease. Furthermore, recent findings indicate that the gene may not be entirely recessive, since bleeding tendencies have been found also in female carriers of the disease.[86]

Clinical Characteristics. There is a tendency for marked and prolonged bleeding, particularly into the joints, but other areas may also be affected. However, petechiae are rarely seen. The oral cavity in particular, which is subjected to minor trauma from brushing and exfoliation of teeth, may be the site of bleeding.

Treatment. Prevention must be stressed. This consists of eliminating environmental situations which might lead to trauma to the child. If, however, a bleeding episode is anticipated or occurs, the missing factor must be replaced by either transfusions of whole plasma—the fresh frozen, or lyophilized form—or through cryoprecipitates—frozen crystals containing factor VIII and fibrinogen.[72] Prednisone is sometimes given to reduce inflammation around a hemorrhagic area. Epsilon aminocaproic acid (EACA) (Amicar) blocks the activation of plasminogen to plasma, and thereby prevents the fibrinolytic action from occurring.[73] Thus, a good firm clot will last longer with EACA present. It may also be used to help preserve the blood clot after dental extractions. Estrogen-progesterone therapy may be given to female patients to elevate factor VIII and X levels.[71]

Complications. Aside from the obvious difficulty with hemorrhage, there are two severe management problems. One is the presence of a circulating anticoagulant (a factor VIII inhibitor)[91,92] that renders the factor VIII additive useless; the second is the possibility of hepatitis resulting from a transfusion. It is for these reasons that prophylactic use of plasma to elevate factor VIII levels is not indicated. The use of plasma in those patients with high titer inhibitors is also discouraged, since this would produce an even higher increase in antibody titer.[92] The antibody titer declines if no further exposure to the antigen occurs.[63] Fortunately, this idiosyncrasy is found in only about 5 percent of classic hemophiliacs.

Dental Treatment. The basic thrust in the dental care of the patient must be directed at prevention.[89] Plaque control must consist of meticulous cleaning of the sulcus with a rubber tip or balsa wood stick and brushing with a soft nylon brush. The diet should be low in carbohydrates so as to prevent caries and plaque formation. Fluoride treatments are also recommended.

However, if therapy is necessary, it should be done in consultation with the hematologist in a team approach, preferably in a hospital environment. The dentist should be well versed in the type of bleeding problem with which he is dealing.

Periodontal therapy. If such therapy as scaling and curettage are needed, it should be done on only a few teeth at a time and as atraumatically as possible. Plasma supplementation may be necessary when the factor levels are deemed too low by the physician. Dried thrombin may be placed at the margins or under a periodontal dressing. Surgery and sutures should be avoided at all costs. Local anesthesia should also be avoided but, if necessary, infiltration with a sharp needle is preferable to block injections.[60,70,82,83,87] The anesthetic should be used along with replacement therapy and may be injected into the periodontal ligament to avoid extensive hematoma.[74,89] Some physicians believe that general anesthesia is the solution for treating hemophiliacs, however, hematomas may form from the intubation.[61,74] Restorative procedures should be kept supragingival whenever possible and the isolation done gently with cotton rolls, since the trauma of a rubber dam clamp may be severe.

Endodontic therapy. Use of such therapy is controversial, since some feel that it is safer than a tooth extraction, while others feel that it is hazardous.[70,88] Formocreosote should be used as one of the drugs of choice in pulpotomies, since it controls bleeding extremely well.[58] Zinc-oxide-eugenol cappings have also been used with success.[87]

Tooth extractions. Extractions present a primary hazard for the hemophiliac.[74,75,76,84] If left with no other choice, and an extraction must be performed, it should be done in a hospital situation and as atraumatically as possible. Flaps should be avoided. Postoperatively, dried thrombin should be applied topically along with an acrylic stent or periodontal dressing.[81] Sutures should be avoided. Extractions can also be accomplished by the placement of an orthodontic elastic or rubber band tightly around the neck of the tooth to be extracted.[62] Others recommend using a piece of rubber dam with a small hole punched over the tooth, claiming that this hastens the process of exfoliation.[80] Postoperatively, the use of aspirin or aspirin-containing compounds is to be avoided.[66,95] Analgesics such as acetaminophen should be utilized.

Diagnosis. The diagnosis in about 75 percent of cases is established by 5 years of age, and then the child must learn to live with a series of hemorrhages. The chronicity of the disease, along with overprotection of the child by the parents, creates a difficult psychological problem.[59,68,73,79] The National Hemophilia Foundation in New York provides advice concerning home care for these children.

Differential Diagnosis. The characteristic feature that differentiates hemophilia from other bleeding disorders is the habitual and prolonged bleeding in males, beginning early in life, and the finding of similar symptoms in male siblings or family members. The coagulation time is also prolonged in hemophilia. From the dentist's standpoint, identification of a bleeding problem by history should prompt a referral to a hematologist for a work-up before proceeding with any therapy.

REFERENCES

Leukemia

1. Ager, E. A., Schuman, L. M., Wallace, H. M., *et al.:* An epidemiological study of childhood leukemia. J. Chron. Dis., *18:*113, 1965.
2. Aison, E. I.: Blood dyscrasias: the oral symptoms, their significance and relation to the practice of dental surgery. J.A.D.A., *21:*612, 1934.
3. Amrosin, G. D.: Pathology of Leukemia. New York, Harper & Row (Hoeber Div.), 1968.
4. Baurjea, J. C.: Childhood leukemia. Indiana J. Pediatr., *3:*193, 1936.
5. Bender, I. B.: Roentgenographic significance of the lamina dura in systemic disease. J. Einstein Med. Cent., *9:*82, 1961.
6. Bernard, W. G., Gore, I., and Kilby, R. A.: Congenital leukemia. Blood, *6:*990, 1951.
7. Boggs, S. E., Wintrobe, M. M., and Cartwright, G. E.: The acute leukemias. Am. J. Med., *40:*243, 1966.
8. Cooke, J. V.: The incidence of acute leukemia in children. J.A.M.A., *119:*547, 1942.
9. Court-Brown, W. M., and Doll, R.: Leukemia in childhood and young adult life; trends in mortality in relation to etiology. Br. Med. J., *1:*98, 1961.
10. Curtis, A. B.: Childhood leukemia: initial oral manifestations, J.A.D.A., *83:*159, 1971.
11. Curtis, A. B.: Childhood leukemia: osseous changes in jaws on panoramic dental radiographs. J.A.D.A., *83:*844, 1971.
12. Editorial: Virus and leukemia. Lancet, *1:*1259, 1964.
13. Engel, R. R., Hammond, D., Eitzman, D. V., *et al.*: Transient congenital leukemia in 7 infants with mongolism. J. Pediatr., *65:*303, 1964.
14. Freireich, E. J., Gehan, E. A., Sulman, D., and Boggs, D. R.: The effect of chemotherapy on acute leukemia in the human. J. Chron. Dis., *14:*593, 1961.
15. Gross, L.: Mouse leukemia: an egg-borne virus disease. Acta Haemat., *13:*13, 1955.
16. Gross, L.: Viral etiology of leukemia and lymphomas. Blood, *25:*377, 1965.
17. Hammond, D., Hyman, C. B., Gilchrist, G. S., and Higgins, G.: Leukemia in children. Calif. Med., *114:*31, 1971.
18. Heath, C. W. J., and Moloney, W. C.: Familial leukemia. N. Eng. J. Med., *272:*882, 1965.
19. Heyssel, R., Brill, A. B., Woodbury, L. A., Nishimura, E. T., *et al.:* Leukemia Hiroshima atomic bomb survivors. Blood, *15:*313, 1960.
20. Holowach, J.: Chronic lymphoid leukemia in children. J. Pediatr., *32:*84, 1948.

21. Krivit, W., and Good, R. A.: Simultaneous occurrence of mongolism and leukemia: report of a nationwide survey. A.M.A.J. Dis. Child., *94:*289, 1957.
22. Krivit, W., and Good, R. A.: Simultaneous occurrence of leukemia and mongolism; report of 4 cases. A.M.A.J. Dis. Child., *91:*218, 1956.
23. MacMahon, B.: Prenatal x-ray esposure and childhood cancer. J. Natl. Cancer Inst. *28:*1173, 1962.
24. MacMahon, B.: Prenatal origin of childhood leukemia. N. Eng. J. Med., *270:*1082, 1964.
25. March, H. C.: Leukemia in radiologists. Radiology, *43:*275, 1944.
26. Meighan, S. S.: Leukemia in children. Cancer, *16:*656, 1963.
27. Meighan, S. S.: Leukemia in childhood. Cancer, *18:*811, 1965.
28. Pierce, M. I.: Leukemia in the newborn infant. J. Pediatr., *54:*691, 1959.
29. Smith, C. H.: Blood Diseases of Infancy and Childhood. ed. 2. St. Louis, C. V. Mosby, 1966.
30. Steinberg, A. G.: The genetics of acute leukemia in children. Cancer, *13:*1985, 1960.
31. Tjio, J. H., *et al.:* The Philadelphia chromosome and chronic myelogenous leukemia. J. Natl. Cancer Inst., *36:*567, 1966.
32. Wentz, F. M., Anday, G., and Orban, B.: Histopathologic changes in the gingiva in leukemia. J. Period., *20:*119, 1949.
33. Wintrobe, M. W.: Clinical Hematology. ed. 6. Philadelphia, Lea & Febiger, 1967.

Sickle Cell Anemia

34. Beeson, P. B., and McDermott, W.: Cecil-Loeb Textbook of Medicine. 13 ed., pp. 1501-1503. Philadelphia, W. B. Saunders, 1971.
35. Halstead, C. L.: Oral manifestations of hemoglobinopathies. Oral Med., *30:*615, 1970.
36. Matson, M. S.: Exodontia for a patient with sickle cell anemia: report of case. J.A.D.A., *62:*705, 1961.
37. Michelson, R. K., and Whitmore, R. B.: Sickle-cell anemia in the dental patient: report of two cases. Oral Surg., *23:*19, 1967.
38. Mittleman, G., Bakke, B. F., and Scopp, I. W.: Alveolar bone changes in sickle-cell anemia. J. Periodont, *32:*74, 1961.
39. Morris, A. L., and Stahl, S. S.: Intra-oral roentgenographic changes in sickle-cell anemia. Oral Surg., *7:*787, 1954.
40. Prowler, J. R., and Smith, E. W.: Dental bone changes occurring in sickle-cell disease and abnormal hemoglobin traits. Radiology, *65:*762, 1955.
41. Reynolds, J.: An evaluation of some roentgenographic signs in sickle-cell anemia and its variants. South. Med. J., *55:*1123, 1962.
42. Robinson, I. B., and Sarnat, B. G.: Roentgen studies of the maxilla and mandible in sickle-cell anemia. Radiology, *58:*517, 1952.
43. Scott, R. B.: Sickle-cell anemia. Pediatr. Clin. North Am., *9:*649, 1964.
44. Wintrobe, M. M.: Clinical Hematology. p. 713. Philadelphia, Lea & Febiger, 1967.

Glucose-6-Phosphate-Dehydrogenase Deficiency Anemia (G6PD)

45. Beeson, P. B., and McDermott, W.: Cecil-Loeb Textbook of Medicine. 13 ed., pp. 1488-1490. Philadelphia, W. B. Saunders, 1971.
46. Burket, L. W.: Oral Medicine. 6 ed., p. 315. Philadelphia, J. B. Lippincott, 1971.
47. Wintrobe, M. M.: Clinical Hematology. pp. 656-658. Philadelphia, Lea & Febiger, 1967.

Homozygous Beta Thalassemia

48. Asbell, M. B.: Orthodontic aspects of Cooley's anemia. Ann. N.Y. Acad. Sci., *119:*662, 1964.
49. Baker, D. H.: Roentgen manifestations of Cooley's anemia. Ann. N.Y. Acad. Sci., *119:*641, 1964.
50. Beeson, P. B., and McDermott, H. W.: Cecil-Loeb Textbook of Medicine. 13 ed., pp. 1504-1505. Philadelphia, W. B. Saunders, 1971.
51. Caffey, J.: Cooley's anemia: a review of the roentgenographic findings in the skeleton. Am. J. Roentgenol., *78:*381, 1957.

52. Cohen, M. M., and Baty, J. M.: Oral manifestations of erythroblastic anemia. J.A.D.A., *32:*1396, 1945.
53. Kaplan, R. I., Werther, R., and Castano, F. A.: Dental and oral findings in Cooley's anemia: a study of fifty cases. Ann. N.Y. Acad. Sci., *119:*664, 1964.
54. Neel, J. V., and Valentine, W. H.: Frequency of thalassemia. Am. J. Med. Sci., *209:*568, 1945.
55. Novak, A. J.: The oral manifestations of erythroblastic (Cooley's) anemia. Am. J. Orthodont. Oral Surg., *30:*539, 1944.
56. Parkin, S. F.: Dental treatment for children with thalassemia. Oral Surg., *25:*12, 1968.
57. Powell, J. W., Weens, H. S., and Wenger, N. K.: The skull roentgenogram in iron deficiency anemia and in secondary polycythemia. Am. J. Roentgenol., *95:*143, 1965.

Hemophilia

58. Albert, M.: Management of Pediatric Patients with Bleeding Disorders. M. S. Thesis, University of Southern Calif., 1972.
59. Angle, D. P.: Psychiatric complications of hemophilia. *In* Brinkhous, K. M. (ed.): The Hemophilias. pp. 359-362. Chapel Hill, Univer. of North Carolina Press, 1964.
60. Barrett, K. E.: Cryoprecipitate for oral surgery in factor VIII deficiency. J.Canad. Dent. Assoc., *35:*416, 1969.
61. Cohen, L.: Dental hemorrhage. Oral Surg., *2:*704, 1958.
62. Davidson, C. S., Epstein, P. R., Miller, G. F., and Taylor, F. M.: Hemophilia: a clinical study of 40 patients. Blood, *4:*97, 1949.
63. Feinstein, D. I., Rapaport, S. I., and Chong, M. N. Y.: Immunologic characterization of twelve factor VIII inhibitors. Blood, *34:*85, 1969.
64. Feinstein, D. I., Rapaport, S. I.: Hemophilia polymorphism—the genetic plot thickens. N. Eng. J. Med., *281:*100, 1969.
65. Gilchrist, G. S., Hammond, D., and Melnyk, J.: Hemophilia A in a phenotypically normal female with XX/XO mosaicism. N. Eng. J. Med., *273:*1402, 1965.
66. Heimansohn, H.: Aspirin and hemophilia. J.A.D.A., *83:*975, 1971.
67. Hoyer, L. W., and Breckenridge, R. T.: Immunologic studies of anti hemophiliac factor: cross reacting material in a genetic variant of hemophilia A. Blood, *32:*962, 1968.
68. Hurt, C.: Psychosocial problems of hemophilia. J. Am. Physical Ther. Assoc., *46:* 1282, 1966.
69. Hynes, H. E., Owens, C. A., Jr., Bowie, E. J., *et al.:* Development of the present concept of hemophilia. Mayo Clinic Proc., *44:*193, 1969.
70. Kaplan, R. I., Werther, R., Carson, I. H., and Wolman, I.: Dental care of hemophiliac patient. Dent. Clin. North Am., *4:*491, 1960.
71. Kasper, C.: Transfusion therapy in hemophilia. Unpublished data. Lectures Orthopedic Hospital, Los Angeles, May, 1970.
72. Kasper, C.: Personal communication. Oct.-Nov., 1971.
73. Kontras, J. B.: Use of epsilon aminocaproic acid in hemophiliacs for dental extractions. Ohio State Med. J., *65:*391, 1969.
74. Leatherdale, R.: Anesthesia for dental extractions in hemophiliacs. Anesthesia (London), *13:*27, 1958.
75. Linenberg, W. B., Harpole, H. J.: Full-mouth extractions in a hemophiliac patient. Oral surg., *14:*782, 1961.
76. Linz, A. M.: The true hemophiliac as a problem in oral surgery. A critical review of the literature. New York J. Dent., *21:*9, 1951.
77. Lusher, J. M., *et al.:* Hemophilia A in chromosomal female subjects. J. Pediatr., *74:*265, Feb. 1969.
78. McDonald, R.: Dentistry for the Child and Adolescent. p. 416. St. Louis, C. V. Mosby, 1969.
79. McIntyre, H., Nour-Elden, F., Israels, M. E., and Wilkinson, J. F.: Dental extractions in patients with hemophilia and Christmas disease. Lancet, *2:*642, 1959.
80. Mammen, E. F., Inhibitors and factor VIII. *In* Brinkhous, K. M.: The Hemophiliac. Chapel Hill, Univ. North Carolina Press, 1964.
81. Mattsson, A., and Gross, S.: Adaptational and defensive behavior in young hemophiliacs and their parents. Paper read at one hundred twenty-first annual meeting of the Am. Psychiat. Assoc., New York, May 1965.

82. Nazif, M.: Local anesthesia for patients with hemophilia. J. Dent. Child., *37:*79, 1970.
83. Parnell, A. G.: Danger to hemophilia of local anesthesia. Br. Dent. J., *116:*183, 1964.
84. Pertarshy, R. L.: Oral surgery and the hemophiliac. New York State Dent. J., *21:*205, 1955.
85. Quick, A. J.: Bleeding Problems in Clinical Medicine. pp. 5, 133. Philadelphia, W. B. Saunders, 1970.
86. Rapaport, S. I., Patch, M. J., and Moore, F. J.: Anti-hemophilic globulin levels in carriers of hemophilia. A. J. Clin. Invest., *39:*1619, 1960.
87. Rubin, B., Levine, P., and Rosenthal, M. C.: Complete dental care of the hemophiliac. Oral Surg., *12:*665, 1959.
88. Simpson, W. R.: Management of pulpa disease in hemophiliac patients. Dent. Digest., *69:*407, 1963.
89. Snyder, D. T., and Penner, J. A.: Preventive and restorative dental care for the hemophiliac. J. Michigan Dent. Assoc., *52:*6, 1970.
90. Soulier, J. P.: Etude genetique des syndromes hemorrhagiques. Sang, *25:*335, 1954.
91. Strauss, H. S.: Acquired circulating anticoagulants in hemophilia A. N. Eng. J. Med., *281:*866, 1969.
92. Strauss, H. S., and Merler, E.: Characterization and properties of an inhibitor of factor VIII in the plasma of patients with hemophilia A following repeated transfusions. Blood, *30:*137, 1967.
93. Tocantins, L. M.: Symposium: What is hemophilia? Hemophilic syndromes and hemophilia. Blood, *9:*281, 1954.
94. Whissell, D. Y., Hoag, M. S., Aggeler, P. M., *et al.:* Hemophilia in a woman. Am. J. Med., *38:*119, 1965.
95. Wilson, C.: Dental care of the hemophiliac. Wisconsin State Dent. Soc. J., *41:*167, 1965.
96. Wintrobe, M. M.: Clinical Hematology, ed. 6, pp. 866-883, 935-971. Philadelphia, Lea & Febiger, 1968.

16

Dentistry for Handicapped Children

Dental treatment of the handicapped child lies well within the province of every general practitioner and specialist who is willing to contribute understanding, patience and ingenuity. These children should be thought of as patients with dental and oral problems who have an additional handicap or illness.

Even though the chronically ill or handicapped do not constitute a large portion of a dentist's practice, it is important that he be psychologically and technically prepared to work with these patients. Treatment planning may have to be altered somewhat on a basis of the physical and mental aspects of the handicapping conditions, but the principles of good dentistry do not have to be altered. The problem with the handicapped and chronically ill is more one of management than of the actual dental procedure involved. The development of the oral structures basically does not vary from that of the normal mouth.[22,44,49] There are a few rare and bizarre diseases or syndromes that influence growth and development, but they are more the exception than the rule.

How may chronic illness be defined? In one community study the chronically ill person was defined as one who had been ill for three or more months and had difficulty moving about outside his place of residence; or a person who lived in a nursing home. Prominent among chronic illnesses are diseases of the nervous system (e.g., multiple sclerosis, cerebral vascular accidents or strokes), arthritis and rheumatism, traumatic accidents (e.g., those leading to paraplegia or quadraplegia), tumors and malignant neoplasms, cardiac disease and tuberculosis. It has been estimated that there are 1,700,000 long-term chronically ill or handicapped persons in the United States.

Massler has been a bit more general in defining a handicapped child as "any child in whom there exists a physical, mental or emotional defect which interferes with his ability to meet with and solve life's problems and which prevent him from integrating into normal daily activity."[27]

The National Institute of Neurological Diseases and Blindness says that 1 in every 16 children born will have a congenital defect, such as blindness, mental retardation or a form of cerebral palsy. Based upon available statistics, it is estimated that for every practicing dentist in the United States there are 200 chronically ill patients who need dental care.

Etiology of Dental Disease. The main cause of dental disease in the handicapped child is the same as in the normal patient, that is the accumulation of bacterial plaque.[37] However, in the handicapped there are some significant modifying influences that must be considered: (1) Inability to perform plaque control, (2) abnormal muscular influences, (3) side effects of drug therapy, (4) loss of functional stimulation, (5) nutritional disturbances, (6) genetic influences.

TABLE 16-1. SUGGESTED INITIAL DOSAGES OF SEDATIVE AGENTS THAT MAY BE USED IN DENTISTRY FOR CHILDREN.*

BARBITURATES (Short-acting)

Effect
1. Sedative
2. Hypnotic

Type of Patient
1. Apprehensive
2. Behavior problem
3. Mentally and physically handicapped
4. Brain damaged

Dosage Form (Seconal Sodium and Nembutal Sodium)
1. Parenteral (3/4 gr./cc.)
2. Capsule (1/2, 3/4 and 1 1/2 gr.)
3. Suppository (1/2, 1, 2 and 3 gr.)

Dosage (Seconal, Nembutal)

Age (yrs.)	Weight (lbs.)	Mg./dose (oral)	Gr./dose
2	27	60	1
4	35	90	1 1/2
6	45	100	1 1/2
8	55	120	2
10	65	150	2 1/2
12	85	150	2 1/2

Note: Dosage based on 2 1/2 mg./lb. of body wt. (not exceeding 150 mg.).

CHLORAL HYDRATE (Noctec, Somnos)

Effect
1. Sedative
2. Hypnotic
3. Does not despress respiration

Type of Patient
1. Anxious and apprehensive
2. Behavior problem (the very young)
3. Mentally and physically handicapped
4. Brain damaged

Dosage Form
1. Capsule
   250 mg. (3 3/4 gr.)
   500 mg. (7 1/2 gr.)
2. Syrup
   7 1/2 gr./5 cc.

Dosage

Age (yrs.)	Gr./hypnotic dose
Up to 6	15-20
6 and over	20-30

Note: Dosage based on 20-22 mg. per pound of body wt. Give medication 1/2 hr. before appointment: Somnos (1 cap. = 4 gr.) (1 tsp. = 7 1/2 gr.); Noctec (syrup, 1 tsp. – 7 1/2 gr.) (1 cap. = 3 3/4 gr.)

NARCOTICS – Meperidine – HCl (Demerol HCl)

Effect
1. Analgesic
2. Antispasmodic
3. Sedative

Type of Patient
(Comedication with sedatives and ataractics)

Dosage Form
1. Tablet (50 and 100 mg.)
2. Syrup (50 mg./5cc.)
3. Parenteral (50 and 100 mg./cc.)

Dosage

Age (yrs.)	Mg./dose
2-3	12.5-5.25
3-4	25.0-50
5-6	37.5-60
7-8	40.0-60
9-12	60.0-75
13 plus	75.0

* Statements regarding dosages of these drugs for the medication of children, which have been published in the medical, dental, and pharmaceutical literature have been reevaluated for dental usage. The dosages are modified toward higher levels, since they are not proportionate to age or weight or other dosage formulae in general use.

ATARACTICS

Phenothiazine Derivatives

Promethazine (Phenergan)

Effect
1. Antihistaminic
2. Anti-emetic
3. Potentiates CNS depressants

Type of Patient
1. Normal, but apprehensive and fearful
2. Mentally handicapped

Dosage Form
1. Tablet (12.5 and 25 mg.)
2. Syrup (6.25 and 25 mg./5cc.)
3. Parenteral (25 and 50 mg./cc.)
4. Suppository (25 mg. and 50 mg.)

Dosage Age (yrs.)	Weight (lbs.)	Mg./dose (oral—tablet or syrup)
2-5	27-40	12.5-25 mg. h.s. and 1 hr. before appointment
6-8	43-60	15 mg. h.s. and 1 hr. before appointment
9-12	60-80	37.5 mg. h.s. and 1 hr. before appointment Meperidine (12.5-25 mg.)
12-14	80-100	50 mg. as above and same for Meperidine

Note: The use of promethazine and meperidine is suggested for those problem patients who may require extensive treatment in a prolonged appointment.

Carbamate Derivatives

Meprobamate (Equanil, Miltown)

Effect CNS
1. CNS relaxanat
2. Anticonvulsant
3. Potentiates barbiturates

Type of Patient
1. Anxious and tense, gagger
2. Physically handicapped

Dosage Form
1. Tablet (200 and 400 mg.)

Dosage of Meprobamate (Equanil, Miltown)

Age	mg./dose (tab.)
3-5	200 mg. 2-3 times daily before appointment; 1 tablet 1 hr. before dental appointment
5-12	200-400 mg. t.i.d. and at bedtime, night before appointment; 1 dose 1 hr. before appointment.
Over 12	400 mg. as described above.

Note: The tablets may be crushed and mixed with jam or taken in flavored syrups. In severe cases of neuromuscular tensions, the dosages should be started 48 hrs. before dental appointment.

BENZODIAZEPINE DERIVATIVES

*Diazepam (Valium)**

Type of Patient
1. Athetoid cerebral palsy
2. Mentally retarded
3. Extremely fearful

* Do not exceed 20 mg.

Dosage Age	Mg./dose (tablet)
Small children	2-5 mg. t.i.d. before dental appointment
Larger children	5-10 mg. t.i.d. before dental appointment

TABLE 16-1. *Continued.*

DIPHENYLMETHANE DERIVATIVES

Hydroxyzine Dihydrochloride (Atarax, Vistaril)

Effect
1. Antihistaminic
2. Tranquilizer
3. Potentiates

Type of Patient
1. Emotionally disturbed and behavior problem
2. "High strung," extreme apprehension

Dosage Form

Atarax	*Vistaril*
1. Tablet (10 and 25 mg.)	1. Capsule (25, 50 and 100 mg.)
2. Syrup (10 mg./5cc.)	2. Suspension (25 mg./tsp.)
3. Parenteral (25 and 50 mg./cc.)	3. Parenteral (25 and 50 mg./cc.)

Dosage
Generally determined according to the apparent individual requirements. Nervous, anxious children can be given 3-5 tsps. (30-50 mg.) or two 25 mg. tab. 2 hours before the appointment and then repeat the dose 1 hour before appointment.

For the hyperkinetic child, whether normal or emotionally disturbed. The dosage may be started t.i.d. and at bedtime on the day before the appointment with 25 mg. each time. The 50 mg. dosage can be started as above 2 hrs. before the appointment and repeated 1 hr. before.

For extensive operative work, an initial dose of 25 mg. of Demerol is suggested. If a low threshold of pain is found, increase the dose to 50 mg.

Atarax is available in 10 and 25 mg. tab. and in a syrup form with 10 mg./tsp.

Vistaril is available in a 25 mg. cap. and a syrup with 25 mg./tsp.

FIXED COMBINATIONS

Phenergan and Demerol (Mepergan)®

Mepergan (combination of Promethazine and Meperidine)

Dosage Form
1. Capsule (50 mg. of Meperidine, 12½ mg. of Promethazine)
2. Mepergan Fortis (50 mg. of Meperidine, 25 mg. of Promethazine)
3. IM parenteral (25 mg. Meperidine, 25 mg. Promethazine)

Oral Dosage

Weight (lbs.)	Mg./dose
25	25 mg. Demerol + 25 Phenergan
35	25 mg. Demerol + 25 Phenergan
50	50 mg. Demerol + 25 Phenergan

Injectable Dosage

Age (yrs.)	Mg./dose
3-5	0.5 per lb. of body wt.
6-8	1.0 per lb. of body wt.

Chloral Hydrate and Phenergan

Dosage

Age (yrs.)	gr./dose
3-6	7½ gr. Chloral hydrate + 12.5 mg. Phenergan
6 plus	15 gr. Chloral hydrate + 25 mg. Phenergan

Chloral Hydrate (syrup) and Hydroxyzine Vistaril
30 cc. of each mixed together: 3-4 tsps. 1 hr. before appointment.

D.P.T. or Lytic Cocktail (Injectable)

For severe management problems; combine into 1 cc.:

Demerol 25 mg.
Phenergan 6.25 mg.
Thorazine 6.25 mg.

Dosage
1 mg. per 2.2. lb. body wt.

Treatment. In dealing with the handicapped the clinician needs to be technically equipped, emotionally understanding and have a thorough knowledge of the conditions with which he deals. In treatment planning for the handicapped one must consider the following.[26]

1. The physical condition of the patient. Can the patient sit unsupported? Can he hold his head erect in a stationary position? Can he expectorate? Are there systemic contraindications to the use of local anesthetics? Is he on any type of drug therapy which must be considered?

2. The mental capacity of the patient for understanding the dental situation. Does the patient possess a high enough IQ to permit the dentist to gain some rapport? Does the patient appreciate dental care?

3. The emotional background of the patient. Is the patient adjusted to his handicap? What is the attitude of parents and family toward him? As a group, handicapped children are overprotected. The children do not have the usual childhood associations and therefore may be very apprehensive toward another doctor in a dental office. The basic decision in dealing with the handicapped is whether or not to treat the patient in the office or under general anesthesia in the hospital. Considerations in making the determination for the use of general anesthesia are: Severity of physical handicap, severity of damage to the intellect, extent of the dental pathology, current physical health, distance to the office, failure to obtain adequate premedication at the office. In order to treat patients at the office, one must be versed in the use of balanced premedication in order to allay fear, elevate the pain threshold, control excessive secretions and gagging and reduce neuromuscular activity. (See Table 16-1 for dosage schedule.) In addition to premedication such additional adjuncts are necessary as various types of restraints, both extra-oral and intra-oral (i.e, seat belts, hand restraints) as well as mouth props and finger guards (Figs. 16-1 through 16-7).

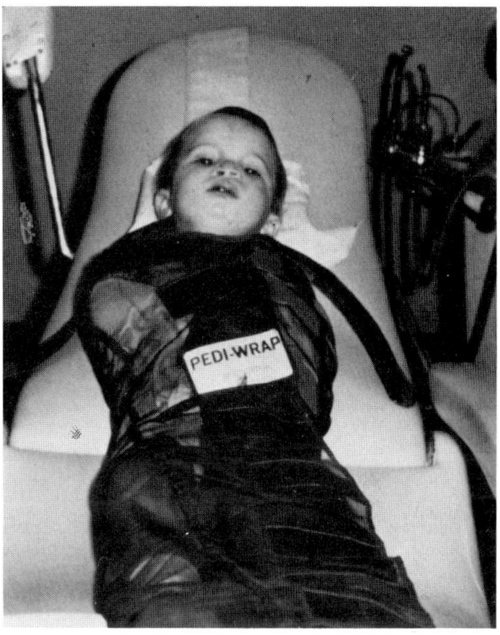

Fig. 16-1. The Pedi-Wrap frees the dental assistant from holding the arms and legs of the patient. This restraining device provides a sense of comfort and security for the physically handicapped and mentally retarded patient. (Courtesy of Dr. Harvey A. Beaver, Harper Woods, Mich.)

NEUROMUSCULAR DISABILITIES

Such neuromuscular disease as cerebral palsy, multiple sclerosis, Parkinson's disease, muscular dystrophy and arthritis have certain common problems in the management of the patient for dental treatment—postural positioning, abnormal skeletal, oral and facial muscular tensions, and uncontrolled or involuntary movements of the patient. In cerebral palsy there also may be a certain percentage of mental retardation present. The oral health of the majority of the disabilities in this category will be usually poor, since many of these patients are homebound and oral hygiene is difficult to maintain and often completely neglected.

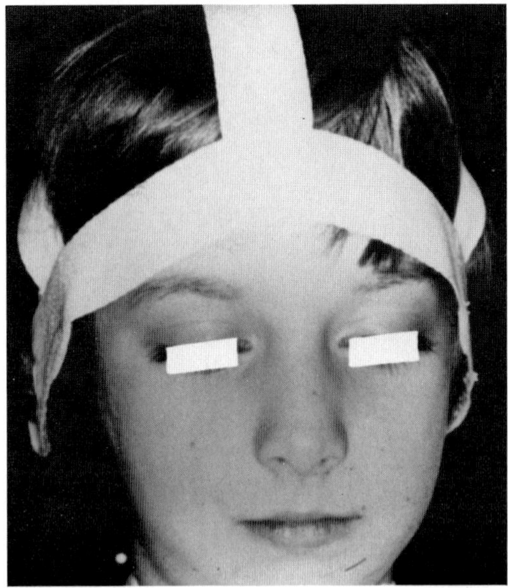

Fig. 16-2. Head restraint on an 8-year-old cerebral palsy patient. (Courtesy of Dr. Harvey A. Beaver, Harper Woods, Mich.)

Cerebral Palsy

Cerebral palsy is a term used to designate any paralysis, weakness, incoordination, or functional aberration of the motor system resulting from a pathological condition which has damaged the motor centers of the brain and usually originates prenatally or in early infancy. More frequently, the damage to the brain is diffuse and may cause convulsions, reduced intellectual inability, defects of speech, behavioral disturbances and sensory losses of variant degrees, particularly of hearing and vision. It is estimated that about 10,000 babies are born each year with cerebral palsy or about 6 per 1000 live births.

The life expectancy of those afflicted is considered somewhat shorter than that of a group without known handicaps. Because of the wide range of the brain damage, children with cerebral palsy seldom have the same type of loss. One may be physically helpless but mentally alert, whereas another with only slight muscular deficit may have severe mental or psychological impairment. Some cannot hear, while others cannot recognize what they hear. Others may have minor to severe trouble with vision and still be able to ambulate with or without orthopedic appliances.

The dentist who treats these patients should ascertain the type of neuromuscular disorders present, since each may present a different problem in management. The diagnosis is based on the presence of a definite motor deficit, and classification is according to the type of motor abnormality. The motor pattern that becomes apparent is related to localization of the fixed motor lesion. If it is in the motor cortex, there will be long tract signs of an upper motor neuron lesion including hypertonicity, Babinski sign, and clonus. This is the spastic form seen in about 50 percent of cases. If the lesion is primarily in the basal ganglia, the motor pattern is the athetoid form of cerebral palsy in which there is uncontrollable, rhythmic movement, frequently associated with ten-

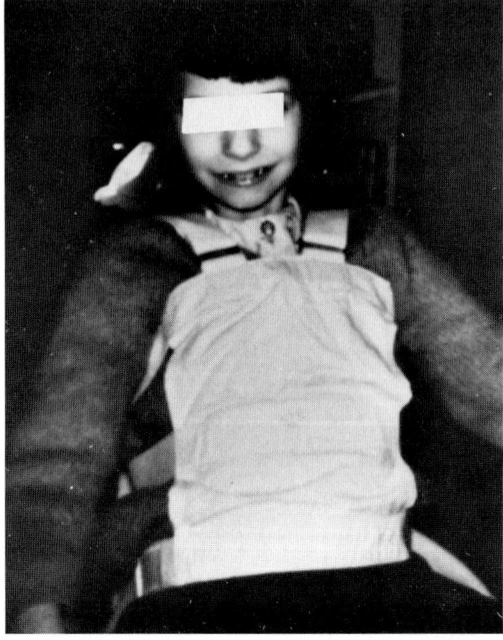

Fig. 16-3. Restraining strap for 7-year-old mentally retarded patient. (Courtesy of Dr. Harvey A. Beaver, Harper Woods, Mich.)

sion. This form comprises about 20 percent of cerebral palsy cases. The ataxic form of cerebral palsy, which makes up about 10 percent of the cases, is due to a fixed cerebellar lesion. Rigidity, referring to decerebrate rigidity, involves total brain abnormality with severe opisthotonos. It is seen in about 1 percent of the cases.

The spastic, athetoid, and the ataxic forms may be seen individually, but are also noted rather frequently in mixed patterns. These include a combination of athetosis and spasticity or ataxia with spasticity.[34a] The reader is urged to consult appropriate textbooks and journal articles for more details.

It can readily be seen from this brief description that obstacles may be present in providing dental treatment for these handicapped patients. A discussion of some associated symptoms found in cerebral palsy should prove to be helpful, since many of these same symptoms are present in other handicapping diseases.

Associated symptoms that may be found in cerebral palsy are:

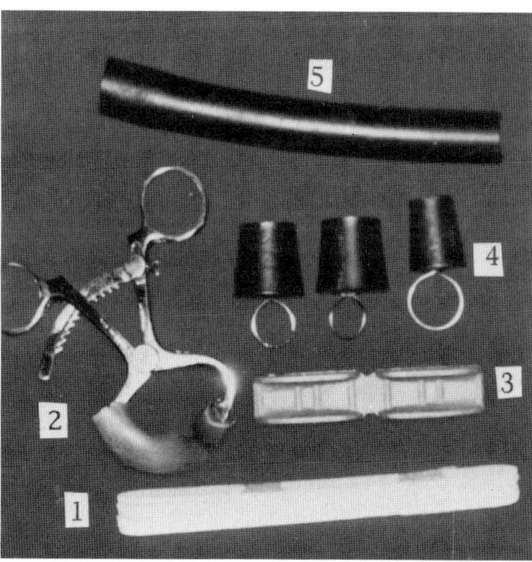

Fig. 16-4. Mouth props: (1) taped tongue blades; (2) small, adjustable Molt mouth prop; (3) flexible rubber prop; (4) Mizzy variable size rubber props; and (5) rubber garden hose which also can be used as a finger protector. (Courtesy of Dr. Harvey A. Beaver, Harper Woods, Mich.)

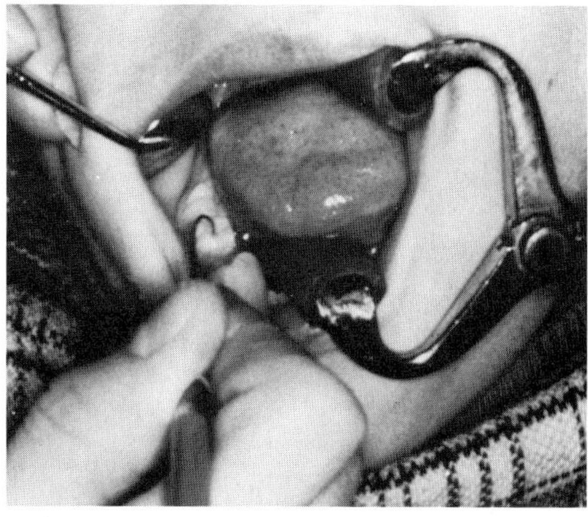

Fig. 16-5. Adjustable Molt mouth prop. (Courtesy of Dr. Harvey A. Beaver, Harper Woods, Mich.)

1. Convulsions. Convulsions occur in about 0.5 percent of the total population. In contradistinction, they occur in approximately 40 percent of the cerebral palsied. It is generally thought to be three times as great in the spastics as in the athetoids. The incidence of convulsion seems to increase with age.

2. Feeding difficulties. Because of reverse tongue movements, there is difficulty in swallowing and this is associated with persistent vomiting. Unusual chewing movements result in improper mastication

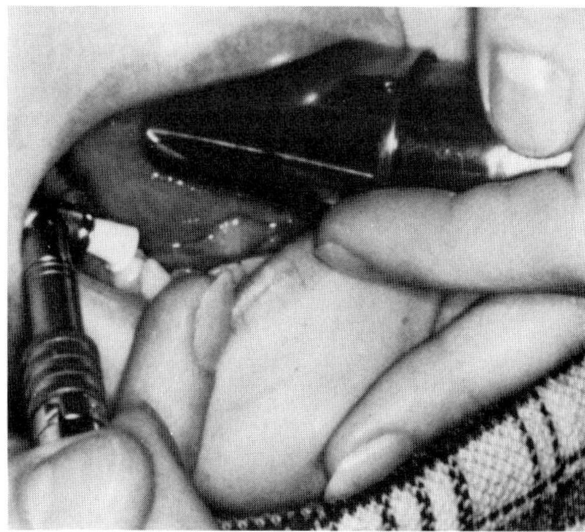

Fig. 16-6. Flexible finger protector. (Courtesy of Dr. Harvey A. Beaver, Harper Woods, Mich.)

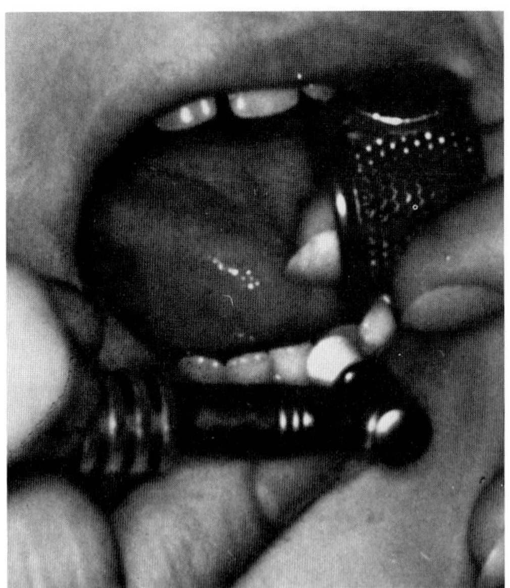

Fig. 16-7. Metal sewing thimble used as a finger protector. (Courtesy of Dr. Harvey A. Beaver, Harper Woods, Mich.)

of food and therefore the swallowing of uneven food bolus size. The feeding difficulties eventually may bring about a highly hypertonic child who is very irritable and exhibits excessive spells of crying, arching of the back and drawing up of the legs.

3. Drooling. Excessive drooling is characteristic of most cerebral palsy patients. Impaired neurological reflex, difficulty in keeping the mouth closed, reversed tongue movements, and unusual low head positions are factors which contribute to the tongue protrusion and drooling.[21]

4. Delayed or imperfect speech may result in failure of communication and in frustration. Speech defects may lead to a false impression of mental defectiveness. Although impaired intelligence is very frequently found among children with cerebral palsy, there are degrees of mental impairment. The dentist should be aware that though some of these children cannot relate to the dental situation, they are trying to cooperate within their physical limitations. The dentist must also differentiate between sudden motions caused by pain from those due to uncontrolled movements.

Because these children cannot communicate their complaints or feelings, it is often difficult for the dentist to know when he has established rapport with the child, since sudden jerking motions can easily be misinterpreted. The noise and/or vibrations of the dental handpieces may start uncontrolled crying or tremors even though the child is not particularly uncomfortable. The absence or presence of an overindulgent parent or familar face in the operatory may also set up negative behavior.

The practitioner who is interested in treating the handicapped should be aware of the oral and dental conditions expected. There is an increased amount of dental disease in these patients as a result of poor oral hygiene and the failure on the part of the dental profession to provide care, but there is no dental disease that is unique to cerebral palsy.[48] Modifications in the prevalence of the disease are a result of the altered dentofacial patterns of development.[13,8]

Growth and Development of the Teeth. In only one report has mention been made of eruption abnormalities.[36] In a 2- to 5-year age group of cerebral palsied children, 18 percent had patterns of a delayed eruption of their primary teeth which might have been attributed to a hypometabolism. Magnuson stated that cerebral palsied children exhibit a high incidence of premature loss of the primary teeth and earlier eruption of the permanent premolars and cuspids.[28] However, it should be pointed out that early loss of primary teeth due to extensive caries may hasten the eruption of the permanent teeth. Significant differences in the incidence of supernumerary teeth or congenitally missing teeth have not been found.

Tooth Defect. Hypocalcified or hypoplastic defects have been noted, being highest when Rh factor incompatibility is associated with the cerebral disorder.[7,31,45,46,47]

Occlusal Problems. It has been a common assumption that because of the abnormal muscle forces present in the dental/facial areas of the cerebral palsied, malocclusions, narrow maxillary dental arches, protrusion of the maxillary anterior teeth and high arched palates are almost universal. Several investigators have reported a high incidence of Class II division I occlusions, crossbites, open bites, premature loss of primary teeth, abnormal contractions and pernicious oral habits, such as tongue thrusting, lip biting and bruxism.[1,2,17,18,19,23,36] However, more recent and extensive studies have not corroborated these earlier reports. It is now believed that the cerebral palsied group have skeletal and denture patterns which are well within normal limits as seen in cephalometric analyses.[14] Malocclusions and factors affecting occlusion are not found with greater frequency in cerebral palsied children. Bruxism, however, is prevalent and has been confirmed by all investigators.[29,33]

Dental Caries. Early investigators reported a high incidence of dental caries.[1,6,35] However, more recent findings indicate that the caries prevalence is similar between cerebral palsied and normal children with no statistical difference in the number of caries found in the various types of cerebral palsied patients.[18,28,38,39,42] There is also no difference in the pattern of the caries attack within or between any of the groups and normal controls.[34,37] The greater number of missing teeth found in the cerebral palsied population merely reflects the type of treatment received (i.e., fewer teeth filled and more extracted).

Gingival and Periodontal Conditions. The incidence of gingival disease in children with cerebral palsy has been reported to be 3 times greater than in normal children. In one study of 253 cerebral palsied patients, aged 6 to 8 years, the incidence of gingivitis was found to be 80 percent, with the spastic group having the greatest involvement, approximately 90 percent, and the athetoid the least.[38] In another study, it was reported that 65 percent of 75 cerebral palsied patients had some form of gingivitis compared to 20 percent in a control group, and that a more severe hyperplastic type of gingivae was noted in the cerebral palsied group. The type of cerebral palsy did not influence the degree of gingivitis.[1] Other investigators, on the other hand, have reported completely different findings (i.e., that gingivitis, as measured by the P.M.A. index, compared favorably to a group of normal children). Calculus and materia alba were found to be within normal range. The differences in the findings of the various investigators may be due to several factors—whether the patients studied were institutionalized or living at home; the degree of their physical and/or mental handicap; the amount and type of dental care they received.[10]

Treatment. The only satisfactory method of dealing with dental disease in children with cerebral palsy is to institute prevention as early as possible. The first therapeutic procedure is to initiate dietary supplements of a fluoride along with multivitamin therapy. For the very young child, it is wise to provide the fluoride in the form of drops. Later, with the development of the dentition, the child should be able to masticate a fluoride tablet. This method of administration provides a topical as well as a systemic effect and can be used until the child is about 10 years of age.

Parental counseling. Parental counseling as to proper dietary regime for their child, one which limits the intake of refined carbohydrates, is also advised.[1,48] It is important to make the parent realize that the frequent ingestion of refined carbohydrates not only contributes to dental disease but also does not provide proper nutrition. Parental counseling is also desirable before instituting a plaque control program. In some instances specially designed tooth-

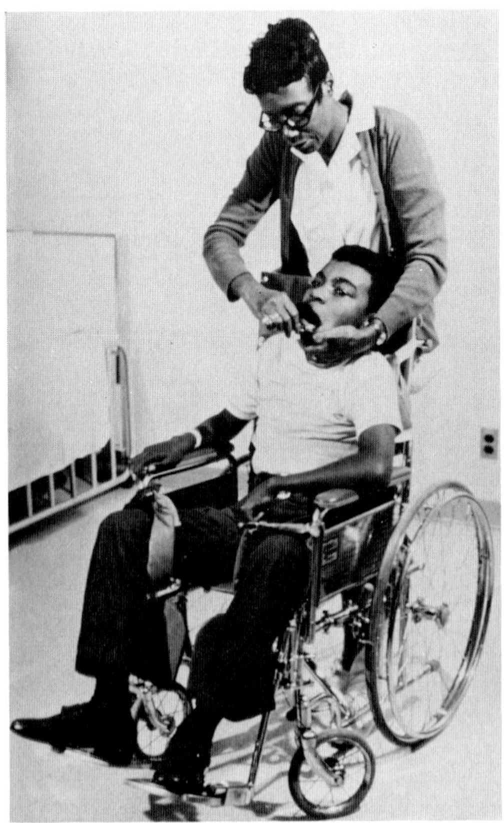

Fig. 16-8. For the patient who has the capability to cooperate, the parent can stand behind the child and cradle his head in her arms to stabilize it. (Courtesy of Dr. Ronald Johnson, Martin Luther King, Jr., General Hospital, Los Angeles, Calif.)

brush handles will aid the patient. Some authors have reported on favorable results with the electric toothbrush, used by the patient or parent. The electric toothbrush should be considered particularly in a preventive program for patients with limited manual dexterity, regardless of whether they use it themselves or are assisted in its use by responsible adults.[9,11,30,39] The dentist can demonstrate to the parents how to prop open the patient's mouth.

Parental assistance. When communications and cooperation can be obtained, the parent can stand behind the child and stabilize his head by cradling it in her arm (Fig. 16-8). In cases where the child's movements are more difficult to control, the child can be placed supine on a bed and the parent can lean across the child's body to restrain the uncontrolled arm movements (Fig. 16-9); or the child may lie on a couch and place his head on the parent's lap (Fig. 16-10). In some situations, two persons may be needed to provide sufficient control (Fig. 16-11). If the child cannot sufficiently open his mouth, a tongue blade may be slid along the inside of the cheek back to the anterior border of the ramus and gentle pressure applied there.[20] A mouth prop can then be inserted between the child's teeth to stabilize the jaws and allow sufficient access and visibility (Fig. 16-12). Probably the easiest mouth prop for the parent to use is made by placing 4 or 5 tongue blades together and wrapping gauze and adhesive tape around one end.

MENTAL RETARDATION

The American Association of Mental Deficiency defines mental retardation as subaverage general intellectual functioning which originates during the developmental period and is associated with impairment in adaptive behavior. Mental retardation, then, is a condition in which the brain, either through insult while in utero, during the birth process, or through hereditary defects or disease, is prevented from obtaining its full intellectual capacity. This limitation usually prevents these individuals from leading a normal life.

In addition many mentally retarded patients have associated medical and surgical conditions. In one study 92 percent of the children examined were found to have one or more medical problems distinct from their mental retardation.[39] Neurological problems, of course, were the most common finding in 45 percent of these children. Multiple handicapping conditions were noted in up to 54 percent of all children examined. Other associated

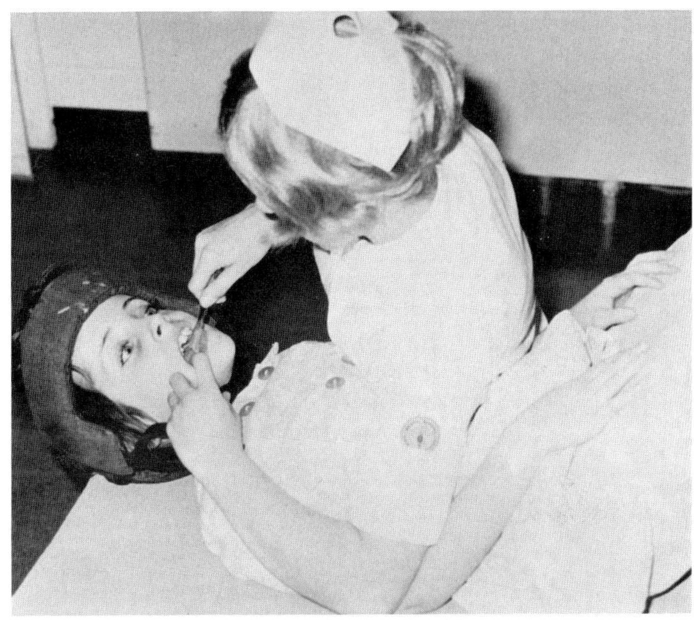

Fig. 16-9. Child supine in bed. Assistant shows how a parent can lean across the child's body to restrain possible uncontrolled arm movements. (Courtesy of Dr. Ronald Johnson, Martin Luther King, Jr., General Hospital, Los Angeles, Calif.)

problems commonly observed were orthopedic handicaps, behavioral disorders, vision and eye problems and respiratory disease. Such severe mental and behavioral problems as aggressiveness, self-mutilation, extreme hyperactivity and destructiveness are also common in retarded children and can cause severe problems in the dental environment.

Certain physical abnormalities appear more frequently in the mentally retarded than in children of normal intelligence—skull anomalies such as microcephaly, macrocephaly and otherwise asymmetrical cranial shapes; asymmetries of the face; malformations and abnormal positioning of the ears; and anomalies of the eyes. The shape and structure of the hands of suspected or indicated mental retardates should also be considered in assembling a history leading to a definitive diagnosis. It should be emphasized that this definitive diagnosis is very important for the dentist, since it is possible that certain abnormalities in the physical make-up of the child will preclude or modify certain dental procedures (i.e., premedicant drugs, anesthesia).

Prevalence. It is commonly estimated that 3 percent of the population in the United States are mentally retarded. It is further estimated that there are more than 2 million retarded children under the age of 21 in this group. Others have stated

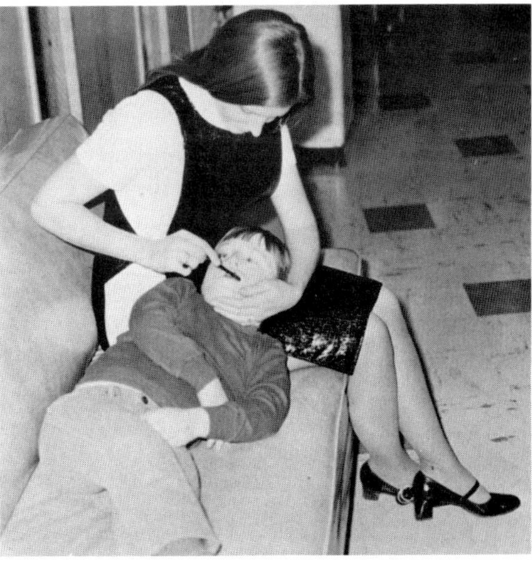

Fig. 16-10. The child is positioned on the couch with his head on the assistant's (parent's) lap. (Courtesy of Dr. Ronald Johnson, Martin Luther King, Jr., General Hospital, Los Angeles, Calif.)

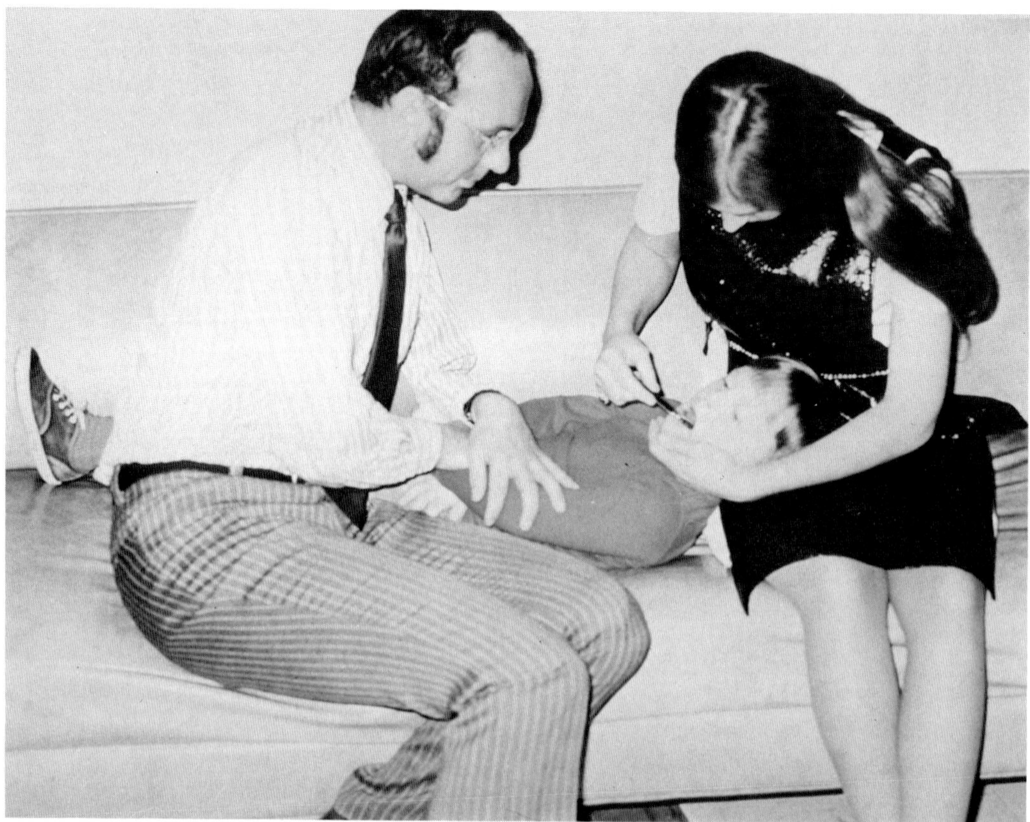

Fig. 16-11. In some situations two persons may be needed to provide sufficient control. (Courtesy of Dr. Ronald Johnson, Martin Luthur King, Jr., General Hospital, Los Angeles, Calif.)

that 3 out of every 100 children born are retarded or about 128,000 babies each year. Mental retardation shows no racial, social, economic or educational prevalence.

Classification. Mentally subnormal children may be generally divided into 2 major groups:[4] mental defectives and mental retardates. The mental defective is one who is mentally subnormal from birth or shortly after birth and a basic central nervous system defect may be assumed. The mental retardate may be categorized as an individual who is intellectually inadequate in his society. Mentally retarded children are generally classified according to their educational capacity as slow learners, educable, trainable or totally dependent. The terms mental retardation and mental deficiency are often used interchangeably. However, mental deficiency is generally used to designate children whose ultimate potential would still be below normal because of limited or structural defects of brain tissue. In contrast, a mentally retarded child might have the possibility, with optimal training and treatment, to achieve a lower range of normal intelligence. Though there has been some confusion in classifiying mental retardates according to IQ levels, one thing agreed upon by all is the discouragement of such terms as feeble-minded, moron, imbecile and idiot. The American Association of Mental Deficiency recognizes a classification of mild retardation, IQ 53 to 68; moderate retardation, IQ 36 to 52; severe retardation, IQ 20 to 36 and profound retardation, IQ 0-20. For purposes of

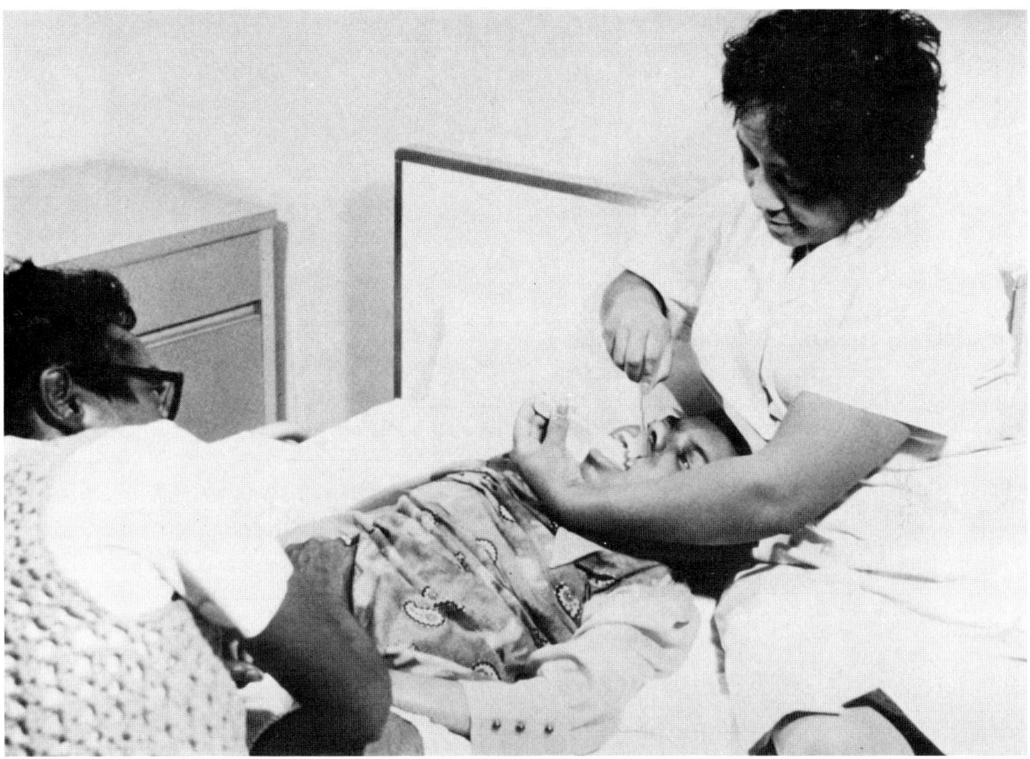

Fig. 16-12. In some patients a tongue blade may have to be used to gain access to the mouth and a mouth prop made of padded tongue blades needed to obtain visibility. (Courtesy of Dr. Ronald Johnson, Martin Luther King, Jr., General Hospital, Los Angeles, Calif.)

dental mangement of these children, the practitioner might want to think in terms of the current educational classification: Slow learner, IQ 85; educable mentally retarded, IQ 50 to 75; treatable mentally retarded, IQ 25 to 50 and totally dependent, IQ 0 to 20.

Etiology. The causes of mental retardation are complex. Although over 100 causes of mental retardation are known, in any given case the etiology remains obscure. Some etiological classifications have made use of the growth and development of the human life cycle—prenatal, natal and postnatal. Other classifications usually include as a basis heredity and environmental and congenital factors. Since mental retardation represents an associated symptom in well over 200 different human physical and mental deviations, it is extremely difficult to pinpoint exact causes. For the dentist a precise classification of the etiology may be only of academic interest, unless the etiological factors affect the actual dental management. Many of these children are readily identified as mentally retarded. However, mental retardation may not be suspected if the child appears normal and has good physical attributes. Holmes stated "the causes of mental retardation are many. The largest portion, 75% to 90% represent the mildly familial or physiologically retarded whose intelligence tests usually vary between 50 and 70. The majority of these individuals do not demonstrate and do not have demonstrable brain pathology. It can be said that 89 percent of mild mental retardates cannot be distinguished from their normal peers."[16]

Biomedical causes. Approximately 25 percent of mental retardation may be attributed to biomedical causes and it is in this group that we find clear-cut dental manifestations. For purposes of convenience we may divide these patients into 5 groups: The encephalopathies, the endocrinopathies, the inborn errors of metabolism, the neurocutaneous disorders and the chromosomal aberrations.

Oral Conditions. In the retarded a higher incidence of oral developmental malformations has been observed, some specifically associated with peculiar syndromes or conditions, such as Down's syndrome (mongolism, trisomy-21). This syndrome probably represents the greatest number of mental retardates who seek private office dental care because of the high percentage of live human births and survival of these children. The incidence and description of oral anomalies, therefore, excludes the unique oral conditions of the trisomy-21 children as these are discussed in Chapter 11 but includes problems resulting from metabolic disorders, infectious diseases, birth traumas and congenital disorders.

Anomalies of the dentition. A marked association has been found between the occurrence of multiple dental abnormalities and mental retardation in such disorders as phenylketonuria and maternal rubella.[12,13,22,25,40,43] Enamel hypoplasia seems to be the primary defect, with the first molar followed by the lateral incisor as the teeth most frequently affected.[15,45]

Caries. A study of the DMF or def rates in handicapped children presents some misleading data, simply because a much lower percentage of handicapped children receive dental treatment. Therefore, to discover whether the retarded have higher or lower caries rates, only the D (number of carious teeth) should be considered. Even this might be misleading because of the poor oral hygiene, and dietary, physical and mental limitations of these children. One must also consider whether the studies were conducted in institutions with controlled diets or with noninstitutionalized children who have a greater freedom of dietary habits. It has been substantiated that institutionalization lowers the caries rate in the mentally subnormal.[4]

Results of caries studies in mentally retarded patients are, therefore, conflicting.[6,24,34,41,43] However, in one excellent controlled study, no significant difference in caries rates was found to exist when the retarded group was compared to their control group but, when separated into component categories of severe, moderate and mild, it was discovered that the caries of the severe type were significantly higher in the mentally retarded group.[32] It is hypothesized that 3 factors are responsible for this difference: Oral hygiene, diet and defective development.

Periodontal disease (excluding the Down's syndrome patient). Studies show a higher rate of inflammatory periodontal disease in mentally retarded patients than in normal patients.[5,13,40] However, in all of these studies many of the patients were on anticonvulsant drugs, thus making the results difficult to interpret. The higher prevalence and severity of periodontal disease is in proportion to the debris score.

Emphasis must be placed on the necessity for guardians and parents to perform the plaque control procedures and dental care in mentally retarded children. There is a tendency for mentally retarded children to consume soft, high carbohydrate foods and to have unusual eating habits (i.e., many of these children eat large quantities of baby foods, which contributes to the formation of abundant plaque and concomitant inflammatory changes in the gingival tissues), and therefore dietary counseling for the parents is advisable.

REFERENCES

1. Album, M. M.: The effect of vitamins on the gingival tissues of handicapped children. Oral Surg., *10:*148, 1957.

2. Album, M. M., Krogman, W. M., Baker, D., and Colwell, F. H.: An evaluation of the dental profile of neuromuscular deficit patients. J. Dent. Child., *31*:204, 1964.
3. Brown, R. V., and Sharma, P. S.: Facial growth of cerebral palsy subjects. Cerebral Palsy J., *26*:3, 1967.
4. Cohen, M. M.: Periodontal disturbances in the mentally handicapped. Dent. Clin. North Am., *4*:483, 1960.
5. Cohen, M. M., Wexler, R. A., and Shklar, G.: Periodontal disease on a group of mentally abnormal children. J. Dent. Res., *39*:745, 1960.
6. Eisenfeldt, I., and Friedman, E.: Observations on dental treatment of cerebral palsied children. A.D.A.J., *47*:538, 1953.
7. Forrester, R. M., and Miller, J.: Dental changes associated with kernicterus. Arch. Dis. Child. *30*:224, 1955.
8. Gellis, S. S., and Fersgold, M.: Atlas of mental retardation syndromes. Washington, D. C., U. S. Dept. of Health Education and Welfare, Division of Mental Retardation. pp. 118-19, 1968.
9. Gertenrich, R. L., and Lewis A. J.: A study of automatic and hand tooth brushing as used with retarded or handicapped patients. J. Dent. Child. *34*:145, 1967.
10. Goyings, E. D., and Riekse, D. M.: Periodontal condition of institutionalized children; improvement through oral hygiene. J. Public Health Dept., *28*:5, 1968.
11. Green, A., Rosenstein, S. N., Park, S., and Kutscher, A. H.: The electric toothbrush as an adjunct in maintaining oral hygiene in handicapped patients. J. Dent. Child., *29*:169, 1962.
12. Guggenheimer, J., Novak, A. J., and Michaels, R. H.: Dental manifestations of the rubella syndrome. Oral Surg., *32*:30, 1971.
13. Gullikson, J. S.: Oral findings of mentally retarded children. J. Dent. Child, *36*:59, 1969.
14. Gum, S.: Roentgenographic cephalometric survey of skeletal and dental patterns of the cerebral palsied. Am. J. Orthod., *48*:66, 1962.
15. Herman, S. C., and McDonald, R. E.: Enamel hypoplasia in cerebral palsied children. J. Dent. Child., *30*:46, 1962.
16. Holmes, L. B.: Mental Retardation: An Atlas of Diseases with Associated Physical Abnormalities. p. 1. New York, Macmillan. 1972.
17. Isshiki, Y.: Caries incidence among cerebral palsied children. Bull. Tokyo Med. Dent. Univ., *9*:29, 1968.
18. Isshiki, Y.: Occlusion of cerebral palsied children. Bull. Tokyo Med. Dent. Univ., *9*:163, 1968.
19. Jackson, G. E.: A systematic analysis and classification of the dento-facial abnormalities shown in cerebral palsy. Am. J. Orthod., *42*:310, 1956.
20. Johnson, R., and Albertson, D.: Plaque control for handicapped children. A.D.A.J., *84*:824, 1972.
21. Kastern, S.: Oral, dental, and orthodontic problems of speech in cerebral palsy. J. Dent. Child., *24*:247, 1957.
22. King, W. C.: Oral characteristics of phenylketonuric children. J. Dent., *36*:61, 1969.
23. Kopel, H. M.: Dentistry and the child with cerebral palsy. Cerebral Palsy Rev., *15*: June-July, 1954.
24. Koster, S.: Diagnosis of disorders of occlusion in children with cerebral palsy. J. Dent. Child., *23*:81, 1956.
25. Kraus, B. S., Clark, G. R., and Oka, S. W.: Mental retardation and abnormalities of the dentition. Am. J. Mental Def., *72*:905, 1968.
26. Lyons, D. C.: The dental problem of the spastic or the athetoid child. Am. J. Orthod., *37*:129, 1951.
27. Magnusson, B., and DeVal, R.: Oral conditions in a group of children with cerebral palsy. I. General survey. Odontol. Rev., *14*:385, 1963.
28. Magnusson, B., and DeVal, R.: Oral conditions in a group of children with cerebral palsy. II. Orthodontic aspects. Odontol. Rev., *15*:41, 1954.
29. Massler, M.: Review of the problems in dealing with the handicapped. J. Dent. Educ., *21*:62, 1957.
30. Oldenberg, T. R.: The effectiveness of the electric toothbrush in reducing oral debris in handicapped children. J. North Carolina Dent. Soc., *49*:39, 1966.
31. Perlstein, M. A., and Massler, M.: Prenatal dental enamel dysplasia with special reference to its occurrence in kernicterus. Am. J. Phys. Med., *35*:324, 1956.

32. Pollack, B. R., and Shapiro, S.: Comparison of caries experience in mentally retarded and normal children. J. Dent. Res., *50:*1364, 1971.

33. Rosenbaum, E. H., McDonald, R. E., and Levitt, E. E.: Occlusion of cerebral palsied children. J. Dent. Res., *45:*1696, 1966.

34. Rosenstein, S. N., Bush, C. R., Jr., and Gorelick, J.: Dental and oral conditions in a group of mental retardates attending occupation day care centers. N.Y. State Dent. J., *37:*416, 1971.

34A. Scherzer, A. L.: Current concepts and classification of cerebral palsy. Clin. Proc. Child. Hosp. Nat. Med. Ctr., *29:*143, 1973.

35. Shmarak, K. L., and Bernstein, J. E.: Caries incidence among cerebral palsied children. J. Dent. Child., *28:*154, 1961.

36. Siegel, J. C.: Dental findings in cerebral palsy. J. Dent. Child., *27:*233, 1960.

37. Smith, B. H.: Gingival and caries interrelationship of noninstitutionalized cerebral palsy patients. Am. Acad. Pedodontics Research Report. Aug., 1970.

38. Smith, D. C., Decker, H. A., and Herberg, E. N.: Medical needs of children in institutions for the mentally retarded. Am. J. Public Health, *59:*1376, 1969.

39. Smith, J. E., and Blankenship, J.: Improving oral hygiene in handicapped children by use of an electric toothbrush. J. Dent. Child., *31:*198, 1964.

40. Snyder, J. R., Knopp, J. J., and Jordan, W. A.: Dental problems of noninstitutionalized mentally retarded children. North-West Dent. J., *39:*123, 1960.

41. Steinberg, A. D., and Zimmerman, S.: The Lincoln dental caries study. I. The incidence of dental caries in persons with various mental disorders. J.A.D.A., *74:* 1002, 1967.

42. Swallow, J. H.: Dental disease in cerebral palsied children. Develop. Med. Child. Neurol., *10:*180, 1968.

43. Tannenbaum, K. A., and Miller, J. W.: Oral conditions of the mentally retarded patient. J. Dent. Child., *27:*227, 1960.

44. Trausch, G. S.: Morphologic change in the oral cavity induced by eccentric muscular activity in cerebral palsy children. M. S. Thesis, Northwestern University School of Dentistry, Nov., 1954.

45. Vea, W. F., and Churchill, J. A.: Relationship of cerebral disorders and faults in the enamel. Am. J. Dis. Child., *94:*137, 1957.

46. Watson, A. O.: Infantile cerebral palsy. D. J. Australia, *27:*6, 1955.

47. Watson, A. O., Massler, M., and Perlstein, M. A.: Tooth analysis in cerebral palsy. Am. J. Dis. Child., *107:*370, 1964.

48. Weisman, E. J.: Diagnosis and treatment of gingival and periodontal disease in children with cerebral palsy. J. Dent. Child., *23:*73, 1956.

49. Wessels, K. E.: Oral conditions in cerebral palsy. Dent. Clin. N. A., *4:*455, 1960.

17

Adolescent Nutrition

Adolescence is characterized by a rapid increase in physical size. The rate at which growth occurs is exceeded, on a relative basis, only by the first few weeks following birth, when the normal infant doubles its birth weight. Satisfying the nutritional requirements during adolescence is complicated by the fact that adolescents, concomitantly, are undergoing profound physiological and psychological changes. The latter often loom so large and important in the adolescent's mind that food intake and nutrient requirements become of minor significance.

The adolescent may overindulge in food as a means of relieving anxiety, inevitably becoming obese and aggravating the physiological, psychological and nutrutional problems. Obesity which develops and becomes established during adolescence is frequently very difficult to treat, since it involves coping with many factors. At the other extreme, is the development of anorexia nervosa, which, although a relatively rare disturbance, first appears in adolescence. Treatment of this condition also is very discouraging for essentially the same reasons that little success is attained with treating adolescent obesity.

Obesity among adolescents in the United States is and will continue to be one of our major nutritional problems, since our economy favors replacing physical activity and labor with mechanical devices, appetizing food in superabundance is available at all times in the remotest of places, and advertising by food purveyors has become so widespread that considerable will power is required to resist their claims. Finally, all the factors that encourage the development of obesity become very real obstacles to the attainment of a slim figure, since, in many cases, the adolescent has sufficient money with which to indulge his temptations.

The term adolescence has come to be associated with teenager which, by definition, refers to the age group between 12 and 20 years of age. Although that approximately encompasses the group under consideration, it may be advisable to review the accepted definition of adolescence as given in an unabridged dictionary.

Prevalence. The number of persons in the age range 11 to 20 years in the United States was 39,068,240 according to the 1970 census.[56] That represents an increase during the preceding decade of almost 9 million in this age group, although the increase in the number of adolescents is occurring at a slower rate than was anticipated, as evidenced by the fact that the actual figure is 732,000 less than the value predicted in 1962. Although there is only about a 2 percent difference between the actual and predicted values, it would seem reasonable to expect a closer approximation. Theoretically, it should have been possible to predict the increase in this age group with considerable accuracy, since all adolescents included in the 1970 figure were alive in 1962 or thereabouts when the prediction was made. At the moment, there is no explanation for the smaller than anticipated number of adolescents listed in the 1970 census. There are about 3 percent more males than females in this age group according to the 1970 census, this sex differential existing for all ages until 18 years, at which time the crossover begins to become apparent.[56] In the nineteenth year, the number of females exceeds the number of males and in the twentieth year, females exceed males by 8.3 percent. A trend similar to this but perhaps on a slightly greater percentage basis existed in the data recorded in the 1960 census.[55] The differences for all adolescents are reflected among the Negroes except for an indication of a deviation among the 11- and 12-year-olds. Whether the changes in the relative sex ratio of adolescents has any nutritional significance is difficult to determine. When the values for the numbers of males and females listed in the 1970 census are plotted against age, a sharp drop in the number of males starts following the eighteenth year. No comparable change occurs among the females. A possible explanation for this difference may be that there is an increase in accidents among males; and for those who survive the accidents, varied problems may be associated with both the general and facial trauma following such an experience. On this basis, older adolescents may pose a special problem in both orthodontics and periodontics. Nevertheless, the number of adolescents is sufficiently large to merit considerable attention from the dental profession, especially in the area of periodontal care, since it appears to be required, at least in some patients, following a psychologically traumatic experience. Adolescence is a period when such experiences are probably more common than at any other time.

Growth and Development. Growth does not occur at a unifrom rate for the different parts of the body, as vividly illustrated in a diagram by Scammon that indicates that the brain and head during the first few years of life rapidly increase in size and are essentially completed before adolescence starts.[44] At that time the reproductive system is still in an infantile state, but beginning with puberty, the genital organs rapidly increase in size until the end of adolescence. Concurrently, there is a rapid development of the changes which are grouped as the secondary sexual characteristics. The spurt in physical development at adolescence extends to practically all parts of the body except the head as evidenced in the measurements made by Reynolds and Schoen of 8-year-old triplet boys recorded over a 10-year period.[42] For them, there was a marked acceleration in the rate of increase for most anthropometric measurements when the boys were 11 years old. This accelerated rate increase included body weight, height, hand length and bi-iliac diameter; head circumference showed no such dramatic change. Although these changes take place in a short period of time, they do not occur simultaneously. According to Tanner the feet and then the legs are the first to show a peak in the rate at which they increase in length.[53] Hip width (bi-iliac diameter) and chest breadth show maximum rates of change some 4 months after the legs. A few months thereafter, shoulder breadth increases at a maximum rate; trunk length and chest depth appear to be the last to exhibit their maximum rate changes. These changes involve primarily the skeletal system. Muscle mass increases at a rapid rate about 3 months after maximum acceleration in height has occurred. These combine to produce the greatest rate of increase in body weight about 6 months after the maximum rate of height increase.

Genetic factor. Obviously, the magnitude and course of these physical changes during adolescence are influenced by many factors, one of the more important being the genetic factor. One of the more dramatic illustrations indicating this fact was provided by Garn and Rohmann.[15] Data from the children in the Fels Longitudinal Study showed that a girl whose parents averaged 180 cm. in height increased in height at a linear rate through her eighteenth year. On the other hand, the daughter of parents whose average height was 156 cm. increased at a slower rate and practically ceased growing at 12 years. At 12 years of age, the tall and short girl differed by almost 20 cm. in height. This difference became greater with the passing years so that when both girls were 16 years of age, there was more than 30 cm. difference in their heights. A similar effect is seen, according to Garn and Rohmann insofar as muscle development is concerned.[15] For that body component, the genetic contribution of the father seems to predominate.

Height and weight increase. The physical changes during the adolescent spurt may result in a linear increase in height of 0.25 mm. per day with the skeleton increasing in weight by 1.2 Gm. of dry matter.[16] Although these changes are very dramatic, the end of adolescence does not necessarily signal the termination of the growth phase. The standard height-weight tables suggest that as both men and women age, an increase in body weight occurs. After the age of 20 years that increase is associated primarily with an accumulation of adipose tissue. There is reported to be an increase in muscle mass in the years from 17 to 30 which may add an extra 5 percent to the size of that tissue. For many people who were tall adolescents, there is an increase in height, at a slow rate into the mid-twenties.[16] This increase is usually accompanied by an increase in ossification of the skeleton which may proceed into the fortieth year; after adolescence, it involves principally a thickening of the cortical bone.

High nutrient requirements. These observations suggest that the nutrient requirements of the adolescent are necessarily very high in order to provide for the rapid changes in over-all size occurring at that time. Since some of these changes extend into early and perhaps even later adulthood, it becomes extremely important that the nutrient intake in that period be as complete as possible. Furthermore, the eating patterns established at that time may carry over into early adulthood during which time many females become pregnant. Pregnancy may prolong any nutritional disturbance that may have existed during adolescence and markedly increases the nutritional requirements. The significance of this becomes apparent when it is realized that 31 percent of all firstborn children in the United States in 1955 had mothers who were less than 20 years of age.[50] Each year 800 unwed girls in a city of 900,000 inhabitants drop out of school because of pregnancy.[49] This figure does not include all pregnancies among teenagers, since many of them are married; furthermore, it does not include abortions, stillbirths or births among girls who left the city prior to parturition. "More pregnancies are reported among adolescent girls living in the United States than for this age in any other western nation. In 1965 in the United States there were more than 196,000 live births to girls 17 years of age or younger."[46]

Fat reduction. The energy needed for the rapid body changes occurring during adolescence exceeds that which the individual can consume.[50] Partly for that reason, the adolescent spurt, especially for boys who are growing at a very rapid rate, is associated with a reduction in both percentage and absolute amount of fat.

Secular Changes in Maturation. The growth spurt has resulted in an increasingly larger percentage of tall people. Information from medical examinations of entering college students, indicates that from 1948 to 1950, a fourth of the 18- to 19-year-old males were at least 6 feet tall in their stocking feet, while one sixth of the female students were at least 67 inches tall.[32] Compared to a period 20 years earlier, the percentage of tall young men doubled and the percentage of tall young women increased one and a half times. This increased stature among American young men and women has been attributed primarily to better nutrition, advances in medicine and public health and higher standards of living.[32] These changes in adolescent size are not unique to the United States. Changes among the Japanese children have received a great deal of study, because the changes in Japan have been very dramatic since World War II. During the 15 years after World War II, Japanese 14-year-old boys increased in height by 11.1 cm. and 12-year-old girls by 8.9 cm.[36,37] Obviously, genetics could not be responsible for this rapid and startling increase in stature. This change in stature involved primarily the long bones in the legs, since prior to World War II the Japanese children had torsos that were as long as those of American children of comparable age.[37] According to Mitchell, the increased height reflects not only an overall increase in caloric intake but, perhaps of greater importance, an increased protein intake with a marked increase in animal protein.[37]

However, the increase in height of Japanese children is not uniform throughout the country. In the rural areas of Japan, 10- to 13-year-olds are approximately 2 cm. shorter than the urban children.[23] The increased caloric intake of the children, especially in the urban centers, has resulted in the emergence of obesity as a major health hazard. Now about 5 percent of the children in the central areas of Japan's major cities are obese.[23]

For the United States and northern European countries, the increase in height and weight of adolescent children is not a new phenomenon. Evidence from the regions where records are available indicates that this trend existed more than 50 years ago. Records for English schoolchildren show that 12-year-old boys and girls progressively increased in height from 1911, the first year of general records, through 1955, with temporary cessations in the trend during both world wars.[3] These 12-year-old English boys increased in height by 7.5 cm. during that period, while their weights increased by 5.2 kg. The secular increase in body weight was proportionately greater than the increase in height. An acceleration in this rate of change set in about 1945.[3] These data again emphasize the fact that in many areas where the nutritional condition is improving, the development of obesity appears to be one of the penalties that accompanies better living.

That a progressive increase in height and weight in United States children is also occurring is suggested by observations of 7-year-old children in Philadelphia. There public school children in both the wealthier and poorer areas showed a gradual increase in height and weight from 1920 to 1950 with no indication that the trend had come to an end.[22] While these trends were apparent for children as a whole, the data indicated that children in the wealthier areas were taller and heavier for their age than those in the poorer areas. However, over that 30-year-period, the weight of children in the higher income areas when adjusted to the same height decreased slightly over the years, whereas comparable data for children in the poorer areas indicated an increase in weight over the years.[32] These changes in weight were evident in both boys and girls.

Seasonal Changes in Growth. Beside the secular changes in height and weight that have and are occurring among adolescents, there are also seasonal changes which have received only a modicum of attention, despite the fact that they were well documented by various investigators as far back as 1880.[11] These data indicate that the most rapid changes in weight occur in the fall, with the greatest increase in height appearing in the spring. For large numbers of children measured each month, the average changes throughout the year and from year to year are very dramatic.[40] The maximum increase in weight for adolescent boys (13 to 14 years old) may exceed 0.9 kg. (2 lb.) per month in October to November (for the Northern Hemisphere) with a sharp reduction thereafter in the rate, so that by late spring or summer there may be no monthly increments or an actual loss of weight. The changes in rate of height increase with the seasons is less dramatic than the weight gains. Beginning at adolescence, these seasonal rate changes are smaller for girls than for boys. Although these average changes appear to be very dramatic when averaged for large numbers of children, they may not be too apparent in the individual child. Actually, it has been claimed that "relatively few individual children have curves which coincide with them; the time of year at which different individuals have their seasonal peak varies considerably. . . , and so also does the degree to which seasonal peaking occurs at all."[51] Many attempts have been made to elucidate the factors responsible for the seasonal changes in growth rates. A number of these have involved measurements of the activity of a variety of endocrine systems but no acceptable explanation has emanated from that work.[51] A more naive suggestion proposed that during the spring and summer the children accumulated in their bodies a reserve of nutrients as a result of the availability of fresh fruits and vegetables. That reserve might permit the body in the fall more effectively to conserve the surplus energy associated with the reduced physical activity when school started. The combination of extra nutrients and energy should enhance body tissue synthesis, resulting in an accelerated rate of weight gain. Theoretically this spurt should deplete the body's nutrient reserves and with a concomitant reduction in food intake as the school year progresses, there should follow a decrease in the rate of weight gain. To test this theory, a large group of children in a Georgia orphanage were given daily multivitamin supplements, whereas a comparable group of children received placebos. Both groups of children showed similar changes in their monthly weight gains. The vitamin supplements neither accelerated the initiation of the spurt in weight gain nor was it prolonged beyond that of the placebo group.[33]

Temporary Growth Retardation. In discussing height and weight changes, it is important to consider the effect of a temporary cessation in these changes. Obviously, the factor(s) responsible for the cessation of growth, the age at which the stress was initiated and the duration of the stress determines whether recovery therefrom can take place. There are practically no studies bearing on that point. Indirect information is available from the height-weight records of Stuttgart schoolchildren. These records dating back to 1911 indicate an actual reduction in the average height of the younger adolescents during World War I with a rapid increase in height during the 1920's.[20] During the economic depression of the 1930's that upward trend ceased. At that time the children were as tall as children of comparable age 10 years earlier. The situation became worse during World War II when the children were actually shorter for their age than children of comparable age during the depression of the 1930's. Despite the poor growth during the war, the rate increased very markedly when Germany was provided with large amounts of food from abroad. As emphasized by Howe and Schiller, these data do not provide a definite answer to the question "Does the child retarded by an inadequate food supply make up the growth that was restricted during the period of food shortage?"[20] These data only suggest that the retardation in height gains experienced by the German children were made up as soon as a plentiful food supply became available. Similar records from World Wars I and II indicate that both adolescents and preadolescents who had been retarded in growth as a result of the ravages of war gained an average of 3.2 kg. in weight and 2.8 cm. in height within periods of 6 to 8 weeks.[26] Such phenomenal growth rates were possible only with very large food intakes. Wherever that occurred it was concluded "That the food crises of the 1940's . . . , if they were not of too long duration, will probably have no permanent harmful effect on the generation of growing children."[26]

Sexual Maturation. Closely allied to the secular change in height and weight seen among adolescents is the reduction in the age when sexual maturation is initiated. The latter is frequently a more vividly remembered date than the beginning of a period of rapid growth. An accelerated growth rate does become apparent when children outgrow their clothes more rapidly than usual. With increasing affluence and the pace with which styles change, especially those for young people, there is an ever-decreasing segment of the population in which children outgrow their clothes.

Longitudinal studies. A number of longitudinal studies have indicated a correlation coefficient of +0.84 or better between the beginning of the growth spurt and the first appearance of secondary sexual characteristics.[51] For this reason it may be advisable to assess the start of adolescence on the basis of the changes in sexual characteristics rather than on an accelerated rate of height increase.

Sexual development. Just as height is ultimately controlled by genetic factors but subject to alteration by environmental forces, so is the age at which sexual development occurs. The latter changes have been recorded more extensively for girls than for boys and for the girls most attention has been given to age at which menarche started, although that is not an accurate index of the beginning of sexual maturity, since "in the girl the first signs of puberty (pubic hair growth and breast development) precede menarche by about two years."[8] The action of a genetic factor influencing menarchial age is suggested by the similarity in the ages when menses first appeared in mothers and their daughters as well as among sisters, the similarity in ages being slightly greater for twins and highest for identical twins. However, the genetic factors involved in this pheomenon are either very complex or readily influenced by environmental conditions, since for large numbers of mothers and daughters the correlation coefficient is only 0.4.[51] Concomitant with the greater growth in stature that has occurred during the past century, there has been a reduction in the age at which sexual maturity occurs. For northern European girls, the data compiled by Tanner indicates an almost linear reduction in the age at which menarche appears.[51] That age has gone from 17 years in 1840 to 14 years in 1950. A similar trend was reported for women entering the University of North Carolina; over a 35-year-period, there was a one-year reduction in the age at which menses started.[35] This rate of change is the same as that observed in the northern European countires over a longer period. Due to the scarcity of records in other parts of the world, it is not known whether a comparable reduction has occurred elsewhere. Similar changes may have occurred, especially in the regions where the accouterments of increasing economic prosperity are appearing.

Oral Contraceptives. A problem closely allied to the development of sexual maturation among females is the nutritional effect that may be associated with the use of oral contraceptives. Such contraceptives are being used by ever younger girls for protracted periods of their lives. One of the first areas to be studied was the effect of oral contraceptives on bone growth and development, since estrogens reportedly have been used to inhibit bone growth of adolescent girls who might otherwise have become too tall.[59,60] Controlled studies were performed with female rats which were fed a normal ration containing the active ingredients of a widely used contraceptive agent. The levels of steroid compounds added to the ration were such that the rats received the same amount of the pill ingredients per kilogram of body weight as that recommended for women. In the skeleton of the rat which was still increasing in size, the estrogenic compounds inhibited longitudinal growth of the bones, whereas in the adult rat in which long bones normally do not increase in length, the normal increase in cross-sectional area of the bone was inhibited.

With these histologic changes, there were reductions in the amounts of calcium, phophorus and magnesium absorbed and retained by female rats receiving the "pill."[60] A small percentage of women who have been taking oral contraceptives show increase in their fasting blood sugar levels.[27] When an oral glucose tolerance is administered to these women, the resulting blood sugar levels begin to resemble those seen in a typical diabetic glucose tolerance curve.[47] With that alteration goes an increased blood insulin level.[48] These facts explain why the literature accompanying these pills stipulates that they should not be used by diabetic women. Studies with rats in our laboratory confirm the increase in fasting blood glucose level when oral contraceptives are fed. However, the increase in blood insulin level so far has been insignificant.[27] When only the estrogenic hormone was administered to adolescent girls there was a reduction in calcium retention which is associated with an increased excretion of calcium in both urine and feces.[24] However, estrogen action in the postmenopausal woman appears to reverse a calcium deficiency.[24] Beside its effect on calcium, estrogen administration is reported to have had an anabolic action on protein in 3 of 5 girls so treated. These actions of estrogens were duplicated by Stilbestrol.[24] The physiological alterations alone that occur in the adolescent are sufficient to cause psychological problems. The situation is compounded by the fact that our mores, especially as they relate to the sexual behavior of the young, are becoming less rigid. Combined therewith is the increased financial independence, mobility and freedom available to many adolescents. These changes make that period of life a most distressing time not only for the adolescent but for his parents as well, and for all those responsible for his health care. The rapid changes occurring both within and about him may aggravate his psychological and emotional state to such an extend that, if periodontal disturbances have any psychosomatic components, adolescence is the time when that may be most important.[2]

Nutritional Requirements. The exact nutritional requirements of the adolescent are characterized by a hiatus stemming from the fact that his growth and development are changing so rapidly and are so different for individual adolescents that any metabolic study would provide, at best, only inconclusive answers. Furthermore, the adolescent is not very amenable tò the kinds of restrictions essential for any meaningful balance study, since they necessitate his willingness to consume only those foods included in the prescribed menu. For such measurements to be accurate, levels of nutrients must be fed for a sufficient length of time to establish the minimal amounts compatible with good nutritional status and that frequently requires that some of the subjects he maintained on a diet that provides what may be an inadequate amount of the nutrient being studied. Information on nutrient requirements depends on records of food intakes secured from adolescents. Presumably, the lowest value for each nutrient recorded by healthy adolescents should approach the requirement. However, in an opulent society where there is abundance of food, the lowest value for any nutrient intake may still be far greater than the minimum required for good nutritional health. The situation is further complicated by the fact that there is no universally accepted means of designating the various stages of the adolescent growth spurt. Most available records are based on chronological age and do not indicate the rate at which the adolescent was increasing in weight or height when the dietary information was secured. Furthermore, there are certain problems involved in compiling such information. For instance, the variation in food intake throughout the week, especially when holidays, parties or weekends enter in, makes the choice of days for dietary records a difficult decision. A day must be established that will provide nutrient intake information representative of the subject's average intake. How to collect information about the adolescent's food intake poses another problem. Reliance is frequently put on a 24-hour dietary recall; thus obviating any change in eating patterns the subject may make when he is forewarned that a dietary survey will be carried out. There are questions not only as to the accuracy with which the subject can recall the items of food consumed throughout the previous day but also about the amounts of the foods consumed. There is the problem of translating the estimates of food consumed into quantities of specific nutrients. This is difficult enough for such relatively standard foods—an apple, orange and other raw fruits and vegetables—but when the food is cooked questions arise concerning the nutrient content of the raw foods, which vary from season to season, ripeness of the fruit or vegetable when harvested, and conditions and time of storage. Also to be considered are a list of other substances with which the food was cooked (e.g., butter added to the vegetables during cooking) and the effect that cooking and possible storage after preparation had on the content of such relatively unstable nutrients as thiamin, ascorbic acid and vitamin A.

Nutrient Intakes. The results of a number of dietary surveys compiled by Heald and coworkers indicate surprisingly little variation in the mean caloric intakes of large numbers of children in the same age group, despite the fact that the groups examined were in different parts of the United States and were studied by different investigators.[18] Where there were marked variations they were the average for only a very few subjects. These deviant values (all of them very low) may indicate something about the range of the individual values that made up the means. For none of the figures is any indication given as to the range of the values within any age group. Practically all of the diet surveys were carried out in the 1940's or early 1950's, and since then some changes may have developed in the food patterns of adolescents. The data indicated that food consumption of boys steadily increased from the time they were 7 years of age when the caloric intake averaged 1788 kcal to 16 years when it was 3470 kcal. Thereafter, it decreased to about 3000 kcal at 19 years of age. The changes for girls were somewhat similar, with the 7-year-olds averaging an intake of 1670 kcal. Girls showed a peak intake at 12 years when they consumed 2556 kcal which was about three fourths of the peak intake of boys. After 12 years, there was a progressive reduction in food intake to 1918 kcal for the 19-year-olds. Most of the average caloric intakes listed by Heald are below the values listed in the 1963 edition of the Recommended Dietary Allowances.[13,18] For younger children, the average recorded intakes are below the RDA's by as much as 1000 kcal whereas for adolescents, the differences are closer to 100 kcal. The magnitude of the latter differences are anticipated since the RDA's were developed and modified to provide for the nutritional needs of practically all people in the United States.

These values for caloric intake provide only an indication of the amounts of food the average adolescent can consume. Unfortunately, most reports and compilations provide no indication as to whether the subjects studied were of normal weight or is any mention made of their physical activity.[18] At best, it can be stated that the energy requirement of adolescents is that caloric intake which permits a normal increase in height and weight without the accumulation of an excessive amount of body fat. To set limits for the latter may be difficult. The importance of considering the deposition of body fat in estimating caloric requirements becomes apparent when it is realized that the initiation of obesity in adolescence makes it very difficult to reverse that situation as adulthood progresses.

Age of growth spurt. A further problem involved in estimating the caloric requirements of adolescents is the variability in the age when the growth spurt starts. Wait and Roberts observed a spread from 1649 to 2925 kcal in the daily food intake of 12-year-old girls.[58] The large spread in intake values was rationalized only when the developmental stage of each girl, based on the age when menses started and the appearance of the "growth spurt," was related to her caloric intake. When the caloric intake was plotted against the stage of development regardless of chronological age, there was a peak in intake at the period of most rapid weight gain. Using this charting system did not completely eliminate the reported spread in caloric intakes. The average for girls who had not reached the first development stage (no growth spurt and no menses) was 2100 kcal, while the intake of the girls growing most rapidly was 2469 kcal. Unfortunately no other attempts have been made to explore this method of evaluating individual caloric intakes. When that is done, attention should also be given to the accumulation of body fat by the adolescent subjects.

Protein intake. The amount of protein consumed by children of various ages in the United States ranges from a mean of 74 Gm. per day for 8-year-old boys to 117 Gm. for the 13-year-olds.[18] A comparable spread in protein intakes is seen among girls where it increases from a mean of 60 Gm. per day for 7-year-olds to 80 Gm. for 12-year-olds. Despite this large variability, the protein intakes are closely related to the caloric intakes. When expressed in terms of the energy content of the ration, the protein intake ranges from 29 to 39 Gm. per 1000 kcal with most of the values clustered from 30 to 34 Gm. per 1000 kcal. On that basis, protein contributes about 12 to 14 percent of the daily caloric intake, the same as the average for the entire United States. Almost all surveys of teenage diets suggest that protein intakes are adequate or at least that there are very few if any indications of a protein deficiency among them. In all such cases, the protein intake is frequently expressed as the mean for an age and sex group; that value is then compared with the most recent level proposed in the Recommended Dietary Allowances, the result is that the average intake often exceeds the RDA for protein. Admittedly, that method of expressing results gives no indication as to whether there are any adolescents with extremely low or deficient protein intakes. However, if there had been any such values, it is likely that specific attention would have been given to them. There is a possibility that these surveys do not provide an accurate indication of the nutritional situation among all adolescents. Frequently, the subjects chosen for the survey are "healthy" adolescents attending a school where all the students are "normal." Furthermore, when 70 percent of the population volunteer to participate in the survey, the response rate is considered to be very good. Unfortunately, no indication is given as to the nutritional condition of the 30 percent of the students who refused to volunteer. Finally, it should be reemphasized that the RDA's for most nutrients include a wide margin of safety which for protein may represent at least a twofold increase over the minimum requirement. One reason for this large safety margin was the fact that when the RDA's were first established a large proportion of the protein intake came from plant sources that were considered inferior to animal proteins on the basis of essential amino acid content.[12] A recent survey of Canadian teenagers indicates that almost twice as much protein from animal as from plant sources appears in their diets.[59]

Fat intake. The fat content of the diets of teenagers has received relatively little attention and for many dietary surveys is not even mentioned. The compilation by Heald indicates that for adolescents as well as for the rest of the United States population, there is a close relation between the amount of fat in the diet and the total caloric intake.[18] For adolescents, from 40 to 43 percent of the calories come from fat for which there is no indication as to its makeup.

Vitamin C intake. Of the other nutrients listed in the dietary surveys, the one most frequently receiving attention is vitamin C. According to a summary of the dietary surveys made in the United States from 1947 through 1958,[38] the nutrient intakes of 13- to 20-year-old males were adequate except for vitamin C. That nutrient plus calcium, iron and thiamin were "seriously low" in the diets of the females in the same age category. Such conclusions invariably are based on a comparison of recorded nutrient intake with the Recommended Dietary Allowances. When such comparisons have been made at different time periods, different conclusions may be secured for the same nutrient intake. This stems from the fact that the values listed in the RDA's for almost every nutrient and for most age and sex groups have been changed since the first edition appeared in 1943.

Changes in the Recommended Dietary Allowances. The Food and Nutrition Board which is responsible for establishing Recommended Dietary Allowances prepares a new set every five years. Of the nutrients listed in the RDA's, calories have probably posed the greatest problem. The first edition suggested that 16- to 20-year-old males should receive 3800 kcal per day; the next three editions retained that figure. In the last three editions, the caloric intake for that age group was rapidly lowered to 3000 kcal. There it has remained and is listed as such in the current version for the 14- to 18-year-old males. Although the reduction in caloric allowances for females was not as great, it did go from 2800 kcal in 1943 for 13- to 15-year-olds to 2400 kcal in the most recent edition.[14]

Reduction in vitamin C intake. These changes are even more dramatic for vitamin C. The recommended intake of that nutrient in the 1943 edition for 16- to 20-year-old boys was 100 mg. per day. That level was retained almost unchanged until recently when it was precipitously dropped to 55 mg. for 14- to 18-year-old males. The 1968 Recommended Dietary Allowances provides no explanation for this dramatic change in the listed levels for vitamin C.[14] It does state the "evidence indicates that the minimal daily intake of ascorbic acid needed to prevent scurvy is about 10 mg." and that "in man, efforts to demonstrate beneficial effects resulting from large doses of ascorbic acid have been unproductive." The reduction in the RDA for vitamin C came just before that nutrient was subjected to a great deal of popular publicity brought about by Pauling's claim that man's requirement for vitamin C is far greater than was recognized previously.[41] He maintained that amounts of vitamin C in gram doses (as much as 10 Gm. per day) were needed by the average person to protect against and to abort such infections as the common cold. Pauling's statements were based partly on his calculated vitamin C intake by subhuman primates in their natural environment. These animals, like man, depend upon a dietary source for this nutrient. In addition, Pauling criticized all previous studies which had been interpreted by the original investigators as demonstrating no beneficial effect from the ingestion of large doses of vitamin C by persons consuming their ordinary diets. The supplemental vitamin C (in amounts ranging up to 1 Gm. per person per day) had no statistical effect on either the number or duration of colds experienced by those subjects when compared with a comparable group receiving placebos.

Effects of vitamin C on colds. No definitive answer is available insofar as it concerns the effects of vitamin C supplementation on the incidence and severity of colds. A recent, carefully controlled study in Toronto indicated that a significantly larger percentage of 407 adults who received 1 Gm. of vitamin C as a daily supplement remained free of colds as compared with the 411 who received placebos.[1] Of greater statistical significance ($P < 0.001$) was the smaller number of illness days among the vitamin C subjects compared to the placebo group which required confinement to the house. All subjects, regardless of whether they received placebos or vitamins, were requested to increase their intake of capsules the first day symptoms of a cold were noted. The vitamin C intake for the subjects in that group was raised to 4 Gm. per day for the duration of the cold. Despite that high intake, essentially the same number of subjects in both the placebo and vitamin groups reported disturbing but relatively mild side effects. The nature and severity of these side reactions were similar among those who experienced them regardless of the group they were in.

Hazards of long-term vitamin C intake. The hazards of the long-term ingestion of large amounts of vitamin C have not been completely established. Rhead and Schrauzer in reviewing one type of such hazard mention a number of reports that describe a dependence on the high intakes of this vitamin which appeared to develop after prolonged intakes of vitamin C supplements ranging upward from 250 mg. per day.[43] When these persons were no longer able to secure their daily supplement they developed symptoms of scurvy on levels of the vitamin that should have been adequate or developed scurvy earlier than the rest of the population, as in the case of the Russians during the seige of Leningrad.

Nutritional Problems of Adolescents

Obesity. Results of a study performed a few years ago among adolescents in the Seattle area showed that one of the major health problems as perceived by adolescents is their body weight. In replying to a questionnaire, 48 percent of the girls and 28 percent of the boys "felt they had a weight problem."[6] Among those students, only 8 percent believed their weight problem "was related to eating." Despite the large percentage of adolescents who were concerned about their weight, Deischer and Mills devoted little attention to that problem and concentrated on the more popular sexual concerns, real or imagined, that are common to all adolescents.[16] The widespread interest in body weight is confirmed by another of secondary school children in Berkeley, California. Over 50 percent of these boys and girls "were keenly interested in the size and shape of their developing bodies."[21] An earlier study in the state of Washington indicated a real basis for the adolescents' concerns about body weight—21 percent of the adolescent girls and 14 percent of the boys in a county near Yakima were 10 percent or more "overweight," while in an adjacent county, 30 percent of the girls and 16 percent of the boys were "overweight."[17]

Only a few studies have been made to secure an accurate estimate of the incidence of obesity on the basis of body fat content and these have been limited to an evaluation of the thickness of the fat pad in specific areas of the body. That type of measurement provides an indication of total body fat content since, under ordinary circumstances, about 50 percent of the body fat is in the subcutaneous regions.

Skinfold study. One study of adolescents that involved a measure of skinfold thicknesses was carried out in Burlington, Vermont among 12- to 15-year-olds.[31] That study indicated an incidence of obesity which was as high as that reported for the state of Washington. An even greater incidence of obesity was recorded in Ten-State Nutrition Survey carried out from 1968 to 1970.[52] The incidence of obesity was based on triceps skinfold thicknesses, although skinfolds in other areas of the body were measured. The surveys in each state were limited to the regions where the largest pockets of poverty were thought to exist. Any adolescents in those areas who had incomes above the poverty limit were included in the survey. The results of that survey indicated that 18 percent of the 12-year-old white boys in the higher income groups were considered obese; that value increased to 39 percent among the 16-year-olds. For the lower income groups, 14 percent of the 13-year-old boys were listed as obese and that increased to 28 percent among the 15-year-olds. There was a lower percentage of white girls than boys in both economic groups who were characterized as being obese. Among the blacks in the higher economic groups, the frequency of obesity increased very rapidly with age with 4.5 percent of the 12-year-olds in that category and 33.3 percent of the 17-year-olds. The rapidly increasing incidence among the high-income blacks contrasts with the more uniform and lower rate among the lower income blacks in which obesity was reported to occur in from 9 to 12 percent of the boys. Far more black girls than boys were obese in each economic group, with 13 percent of the black girls in each age category listed as being obese.

Extent of adolescent obesity. The figures in the report of the National Nutrition Survey (1972) for the number of obese adolescents are startling in both the magnitude of the numbers and the fact that more boys than girls are reported to be obese. These values are so large as to suggest that if the data are confirmed by more extensive and, hopefully, additional information on the estimated amount of fat in the bodies of the subjects, then obesity among the adolescents is far more prevalent than had previously been suspected. It is unfortunate that this information which will be quoted extensively is based on such small numbers of subjects. For the adolescents, the largest group included 137 low-income 12-year-old black boys while most of the other age and income groups had less than 100 subjects; the smallest group being 9 black 17-year-old boys in the high-income group. A reevaluation of the extent of obesity among adolescents would be desirable. If that were done, additional skinfold measurements should be used in estimating body fat content. Such estimates can be made from the tables developed by Seltzer and Mayer and Durnin and Rahaman.[9,45] Obesity in adolescents occurs when body fat exceeds about 20 percent in boys and 25 percent in girls.[21] The amount of body fat in secondary school boys and girls in Berkeley, California was determined by a variety of techniques. The results of the tests indicated that about 14 percent of the boys as well as the girls in the ninth through twelfth grades were obese. An additional difference in the results of the Berkeley study and the report of the Ten-State Nutrition Survey was the higher incidence of obese subjects among the Negroes than among the Caucasians or Orientals.[52]

Factors affecting obesity. Although the development of obesity in the adolescent involves an intake of calories greater than what is needed for normal growth and development, more subtle factors may be associated with their excessive food consumption. Frequently, the obese adolescent is experiencing or has experienced some psychological or emotional disturbance which initiated the excessive eating pattern.[5] The emotional disturbance may have resulted from interpersonal relations generated by a difficult family situation as suggested by Bruch and others.[4,7,10,36] When the periodontist treats obese adolescents he may have to refer the patient to a psychiatrist before any periodontal work is started, since emotional trauma may have a profound effect on the development and course of periodontal disease.

Anemia. The reported prevalence of incipient anemia, especially among adolescents, has led to an increase in the current level of iron in the Recommended Dietary Allowances (1968). From the first edition of these allowances to the present, the recommended daily intake of iron was 15 mg. for both adolescent boys and girls. The 1968 edition of the RDA raised the iron level of 18 mg. since a "borderline stage of iron balance is indicated by the greatly reduced or absent iron stores in two-thirds of menstruating women. . . ." Although only one publication is listed in support of this claim, others have appeared since then. These reports provide sufficient evidence to support both sides of an argument about the need for increasing the iron intake of the people in the United States. The results of the Ten-State Nutrition Survey will be quoted to bolster the efforts to secure greater and wider fortification of our foods with iron compounds.[53] That report concluded that there was "a high prevalence of 'deficient' and 'low' hemoglobin values in all population subgroups and particularly in the black population in both the low-income-ratio and high-income-ratio states. There was a general trend toward higher dietary iron intakes among groups of persons with higher hemoglobin levels and a low but positive coefficient of correlation between hemoglobin and iron intake of individuals." The results of the Ten-State Nutrition Survey raise a number of questions to be considered before any attempt is made to drastically alter the nature of our food supply. Although the survey included more than 33,000 blood samples that were analyzed for hemoglobin, there may be a basis for concern about the reliability of the results. To most biochemists, the hemoglobin determination is considered to be a very simple procedure under most laboratory conditions. However, when it is performed in field surveys various unforeseen difficulties may arise, such as partial or complete change in some of the reagents required for the determination when these reagents are frozen for even a very short time.[34] Reagents may freeze when stored in a vehicle overnight, especially when the temperature at night drops below freezing. When that happens, low hemoglobin values will be recorded for individuals who by another evaluation have normal levels. That this may be one explanation for some of the low hemoglobin values observed in the Ten-State Nutrition Survey has not been ruled out, since the survey teams operated throughout the year traveling from one region to another in each state. Another problem that has not been resolved is the disparity in hemoglobin levels between Caucasians and Negroes. Studies have repeatedly indicated that the hemoglobin levels among Negroes are about 1 Gm. per 100 ml. of blood less than among Caucasians of the same age and sex.[57] Finally, the physiological significance of low iron stores in the body as revealed by low levels of blood siderophilin, or transferrin, should be evaluated before these parameters can be accepted as valid indicators of nutritional difficulties.

Iodine Deficiency. In the past, one of the major nutritional problems, especially among adolescent girls, was the presence of enlarged thyroid glands associated with an inadequate iodine intake. That problem was more acute and prevalent in certain areas than others; for instance, the region around the Great Lakes was known in medical circles as the Goiter Belt. The high incidence of goiter among the schoolchildren in that area led to the introduction of iodized salt in May 1924.[25] Despite continuing public health efforts, only about 60 percent of the table salt sold in the states bordering the Great Lakes is iodized. On that basis, some concern has been expressed about the current extent of iodine deficiency, especially among adolescent girls who are most vulnerable to that deficiency. One study among girls in the Detroit area indicated that about 20 percent had basal metabolic rates that were 10 percent below standard values.[25] Since a large proportion of these girls were adolescents, the results of that study were used to indicate the "need for continuous promotion of iodized salt."[25] Unfortunately, that study made no reference to the presence of enlarged thyroid glands among the girls with the low basal metabolic rates. Another survey of the inhabitants of a small semirural community in southern Michigan appeared to support the existence of a fairly high incidence of iodine deficiency goiters.[29]

Endemic goiter. Increasing evidence suggests that much of what is being diagnosed as endemic goiter may be caused by something other than a deficient intake of iodine. Some of that evidence involves the reported increase in the iodine content of foods indigenous to the goiter belt. Milk produced on Illinois farms contains fairly large amounts of iodine.[19] Oddie and collaborators emphasized a concern for the high levels of iodine intake reported throughout the United States after studying the uptake of radioactive iodine by the thyroid glands of some 34,000 subjects.[39] Their evidence indicated an intake of iodine fivefold greater than that required to prevent endemic goiter. Support for that conclusion was provided by the Ten-State Nutrition Survey which suggested that most of the enlarged thyroids observed in the ten states were not related to the "occurrence of 'deficient' and 'low' urinary iodine values."[53] Even in the groups where the mean urinary iodine values were low, these values were still ten times greater than those seen "in areas where endemic goiter is prevalent." The primary significance of the questions raised as to the existence of endemic goiter among adolescents is that any enlargement of the thyroid gland requires a careful examination to determine the nature of the goiter and its etiology. Only after an unequivocal diagnosis should therapy be instituted.

Caries and Periodontal Disease

Although refined carbohydrates, as discussed in Chapter 18, are important etiologic factors in dental caries, no nutritional factors, by themselves, can cause gingivitis or periodontitis. Local factors are essential for the initiation of these diseases.

A diet that requires vigorous mastication and chewing fibrous foods is not as effective in plaque control or in the prevention of periodontal disease as proper oral hygiene procedures.[1a,27a,57a]

REFERENCES

1. Anderson, T. W., Reid, D. B. W., and Beaton, G. H.: Vitamin C and the common cold: a double blind trial. Can. Med. Assoc. J., *23:*503, 1972.

1a. Baer, P.: The relation of the physical character of the diet to the periodontium and periodontal disease. Oral Surg., *9:*839, 1956.

2. Baer, P.: The case for periodontosis as a clinical entity. J. Periodont., *42:*516, 1971.

3. Boyne, A. W., Aitken, F. C., and Laitch, I.: Secular changes in height and weight of British children, including an analysis of measurements of English children in primary schools 1911-1953. Nutr. Abst. Rev., *27:*1, 1957.

4. Bruch, H.: The Importance of Overweight. Norton & Co., New York, 1957.

5. Bruch, H.: Juvenile obesity, its course and outcome. Inst. Psychiatr. Clin., *7:*231, 1970.

6. Deischer, R. W., and Mills, C. A.: The adolescent looks at his health and medical care. Am. J. Public Health., *53:*1928, 1963.

7. Deri, S. K.: A problem in obesity. *In* Burton, A., and Harris, R. F.: Clinical Studies in Personality. p. 525. New York, Harper & Row, 1955.

8. Donovan, B. T., and van der Werff Ten Bosch, J. J.: Physiology of Puberty. London, Edward Arnold, 1965.

9. Durnin, J. V. G. A., and Rahaman, M. M.: The assessment of the amount of fat in the human body from measurements of skinfold thickness. Br. J. Nutr., *21:*681, 1967.

10. Fenichel, O.: The Psychoanalytic Theory of Neurosis. New York, Norton & Co., 1945.

11. Fitt, A. B.: Seasonal influence on growth, function and inheritance. Wellington, New Zealand Council for Educational Research, 1941.

12. Food and Nutrition Board: Recommended Dietary Allowances. Nat. Research Council, Washington, D.C., 1943.

13. Food and Nutrition Board: Recommended Dietary Allowances. Nat. Research Council, Washington, D.C., 1963.
14. Food and Nutrition Board: Recommended Dietary Allowances. Nat. Research Council, Washington, D.C. 1968.
15. Garn, S. M., and Rohmann, C. G.: Interaction of nutrition and genetics in timing of growth and development. Pediatr. Clin. North Am., *13:*353, 1966.
16. Garn, S. M., and Wagner, B.: The adolescent growth of the skeletal mass and its implications to mineral requirements. *In* Heald, F. P. (ed.): Adolescent Nutrition and Growth. New York, Appleton-Century-Crofts, 1969.
17. Hard, M. McG., and Esselbaugh, N. C.: Nutritional status of selected adolescent children. I. Description of subjects and dietary findings. Am. J. Clin. Nutr., *4:*261, 1956.
18. Heald, F. P., Remmell, P. A., and Mayer, J.: Caloric protein and fat intakes in children and adolescents. *In* Heald, F. (ed.): Adolescent Nutrition and Growth. New York, Appleton-Century-Crofts, 1969.
19. Hemken, R. W., Vandersaal, J. H., Oskarsson, M. A., and Fryman, L. R.: Iodine intake related to milk iodine and performance of dairy cattle. J. Dairy Sci., *55:*931. 1972.
20. Howe, P. E., and Schiller, M.: Growth responses of the school child to changes in diet and environmental factors. J. Appl. Physiol., *5:*51, 1952.
21. Huenemann, R. L., Hampton, M. C., and Shapiro, L. R.: Adolescent food practices associated with obesity. Fed. Proc., *25:*4, 1966.
22. Hundley, J. M., Mickelsen, O., Matel, N., Weaver, R. N., and Taber, R. C.: Height and weight of first grade children as a potential index of nutritional status. Am. J. Public Health, *45:*1454, 1955.
23. Innami, S., and Mickelsen, O.: Nutritional status—Japan. Nutr. Rev., *27:*275, 1969.
24. Johnston, J. A.: Nutritional Studies in Adolescent Girls and Their Relation to Tuberculosis. Springfield, Ill., Charles C Thomas, 1953.
25. Kenyon, F., Kelly, H. J., and Macy, I. G.: Basal metabolism of girls in the Great Lakes region; need for continuous promotion of iodized salt. J. Am. Diet. Assoc., *30:*987, 1954.
26. Keys, A., Brozek, J., Henschel, A., Mickelsen, O., and Taylor, H. L.: The Biology of Human Starvation. vol 2. Minneapolis, University of Minnesota Press. 1950.
27. Lei, K. Y., and Yang, M. G.: Oral contraceptives, norethynodrel and mestranol: effects on glucose tolerance, tissue uptake of glucose-U-^{14}C and insulin sensitivity. Proc. Soc. Exp. Biol. Med., *141:*130, 1972.

27a. Lindhe, J.: Effect of nutritional hyperparathyroidism on experimental periodontitis in the dog. Scand. J. Dent. Res., *81:* 155, 1973.

28. Manoharan, K., Yang, M. G., and Mickelsen, O.: Oral contraceptive steroids: effects on various nutrient balances and body composition in adult female rats. Proc. Soc. Exp. Biol. Med., *133:*774, 1970.
29. Matovinovic, J., Hayner, N. S., Epstein, F. H., and Kjelsberg, M. O.: Goiter and other thyroid diseases in Tecumseh, Michigan. JAMA, *192:*234, 1965.
30. Mayer, J.: Physical activity and anthropometric measurements of obese adolescents. Fed. Proc., *25:*11, 1966.
31. Merrow, S. B.: Triceps skinfold thicknesses of Vermont adolescents. Am. J. Clin. Nutr., *20:*978, 1967.
32. Metropolitan Life Insurance Co.: Growth trends in the teen ages. Statistical Bull., *41:*3, 1960.
33. Mickelsen, O., and Spiers, M.: Unpublished of Vermont adolescents. Am. J. Clin. Nutr.,
34. Mickelsen, O., Woolard, H., and Ness, A. T.: Decolonization on freezing of ferricyanide-cyanide solution used for hemoglobin determinations. Clin. Chem., *10:*611, 1964.
35. Mills, C. A.: Temperature influence over human growth and development. Human Biol., *2:*71, 1950.
36. Mitchell, H. S.: Nutrition in relation to stature. J. Am. Diet. Assoc., *40:*521, 1962.
37. Mitchell, H. S.: Japanese youth are growing taller—but why? Nutrition News, National Dairy Council, Chicago, *28:*5, 1965.
38. Morgan, A. F.: Nutritional Status, U.S.A. California Agricultural Experimental Station Bull., No. 769, 1959.
39. Oddie, T. H., Fisher, D. A., McConahey, W. M., and Thompson, C. S.: Iodine intake in the United States: a reassessment. J. Clin. Endocrinol. Metab., *30:*659, 1970.

40. Palmer, C. E.: Seasonal variation of average growth in weight of elementary school children. Pub. Health Report, *48*:211, 1933.
41. Pauling, C. C.: Vitamin C and the Common Cold. San Francisco, W. H. Freeman, 1970.
42. Reynolds, E. L., and Schoen, G.: Growth patterns of identical triplets from 8 through 18 years. Child Dev., *18*:130, 1947.
43. Rhead, W. J., and Schrauzer, G. N.: Risks of long-term ascorbic acid overdosage. Nutr. Rev., *29*:262, 1971.
44. Scammon, R. E.: The measurement of the body in childhood. *In* Harris, J. A., *et al.*, The Measurement of Man. Minneapolis, University of Minnesota Press, 1930.
45. Seltzer, C. C., and Mayer, J.: A simple criterion of obesity. Postgrad. Med., *38*: A101, 1965.
46. Shank, R. E.: The role of nutrition in the course of human pregnancy. Nutrition News, National Dairy Council, Chicago, *33*:11, 1970.
47. Spellacy, W. N.: A review of carbohydrate metabolism and the oral contraceptives. Am. J. Obstet. Gynecol., *104*:448, 1969.
48. Spellacy, W. N., Buhl, W. C., Birk, S. A., and McCreary, S. A.: Studies of ethynodioldiacetate and mestranol on blood glucose and plasma insulin. I. Six month oral glucose tolerance test. Int. J. Fertil., *16*:55, 1971.
49. Stine, O. C., Rider, R. V., and Sweenly, E.: School leaving due to pregnancy in an urban adolescent population. Am. J. Public Health, *54*:1, 1964.
50. Storvick, C. A., and Fincke, M. L.: Adolescents and young adults. *In* Food, the Agriculture Yearbook. p. 303, U.S. Department of Agriculture, Washington, U.S. Government Printing Office, 1959.
51. Tanner, J. M.: Growth at Adolescence. Oxford, Blackwell Scientific Pub., 1962.
52. Ten-State Nutrition Survey 1968-1970. vol. II. Clinical Anthropometry, Dental. Center for Disease Control, Health Services and Mental Health Administration, Dept. Health, Education, and Welfare, 1972.
53. Ten-State Nutrition Survey 1968-1970. vol. IV. Biochemical. Center for Disease Control, Health Services and Mental Health Administration, Dept. Health, Education, and Welfare, 1972.
54. Trenholme, M., and Milne, H.: Studies of teenage eating in Ontario. Canad. J. Pub. Health, *54*:455, 1967.
55. U.S. Bureau of the Census: U.S. Census of Populations: 1960. vol. 1. Characteristics of the Population; Part 1, United States Summary. Department of Commerce, Washington, U.S. Government Printing Office, 1964.
56. U.S. Bureau of the Census: General Population Characteristics. United States Summary. Department of Commerce, Washington, U.S. Government Printing Office, 1972.
57. U.S. Public Health Service, Nutrition and Progress Analysis Branches: The nutritional status of Negroes. J. Negro Educ. *18*:291, 1949.
57a. Wade, A. B.: Effect on dental plaque of chewing apples. Dent. Pract., *21*:194, 1971.
58. Wait, B., and Roberts, L. J.: Studies in the food requirement of adolescent girls: The energy intake of well-nourished girls 10 to 16 years of age. J. Am. Diet. Assoc., *8*:209, 1932.
59. Yang, M. G., Sanger, V. L., and Mickelsen, O.: Feeding norethynodrel and mestranol to immature and adult female rats; cross-section and length of long bones. Proc. Soc. Exp. Biol. Med., *130*:1146, 1969.
60. Yang, M. G., and Mickelsen, O.: Functional and compositional bone changes of rats fed the oral contraceptive steroids, mestranol and norethynodrel. Nutr. Reps. Int., *3*:247, 1971.

18

Prevention of Periodontal Disease

Inflammatory periodontal disease and dental caries are to a large extent the result of dental plaque. Dental plaque may be defined as an adherent structured mass that forms on the tooth surfaces, composed primarily of microorganisms. As microorganisms colonize, they grow and produce products destructive to the underlying tissues.

As a result of the importance of plaque as an etiologic agent, a considerable portion of dental therapy is aimed at the removal of plaque and the prevention of its reformation. Control of the growth and formation of the plaque is essential to the control of dental disease.

Plaque control consists of more than the mere techniques of removal. It also includes an educational approach whereby the patient is presented the cause, nature and consequences of dental disease as well as a motivational aspect to encourage him to follow the prescribed programs.

Because it is a harder task to break old habits than instil new ones, childhood is the time to start teaching effective home oral care. Children's Dental Health Week (first week in February) can be a time for promoting it by appealing to the parents to help the children learn how to care for their own teeth. Since children practice dental habits observed in parents, instruction on proper oral home care is productive only if parents practice proper habits.[3,6] Since home care for the very young child must be performed by the parent[1] it is the best time to establish good dental care habits. When the child develops his own capabilities, the parent can act in a supervisory capacity.

Plaque Control Program

To teach plaque control to younger children, the program should include the entire family. In adolescents this may be less necessary, since the need for independence from the family may be a factor in motivation.

The development of an effective home care plaque control program requires a great deal of time and patience. Generally, four or more instruction appointments at the dentist's office are necessary before the patient is capable of properly removing most of the bacterial plaque from the tooth surfaces. Since recent findings show that the average patient retains only 25 percent of what is shown to him at each oral hygiene demonstration, constant reinforcement is essential to insure that the patient achieves minimal levels of technical competence in the procedures taught.

Audiovisual material is essential in the educational phase. Many companies produce films of excellent quality which offer a graphic presentation of the recommended techniques for a plaque control program or the dentist or his control therapist can devise their own visual aids, if they prefer. A verbal discussion after the presentation should reinforce the material presented, and the patient should be given a printed pamphlet illustrating what has been shown. A verbal explanation may be used, although this method is inferior. In brief, let the patient know that he, as almost everyone else, is susceptible to caries and periodontal disease which unless treated can result in loss of teeth. The patient should also be informed that the etiology of periodontal

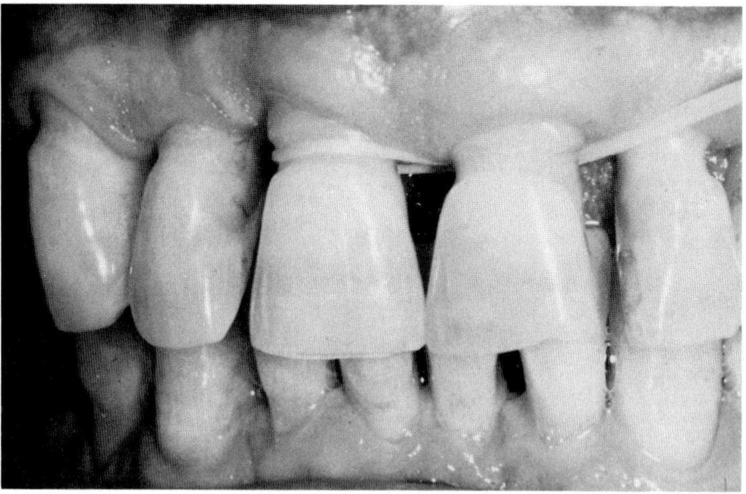

Fig. 18-1. Floss improperly used, as shown in this illustration, can be harmful.

diseases are largely known and that most of them are preventable. Obviously, to prevent disease it is necessary to remove the cause.

Initial Visit. The first instruction session on plaque control should consist of audiovisual material or a verbal explanation of the nature of the disease. A disclosing solution should be used and the location and amount of the plaque shown to the patient with a mirror. A phase contrast microscope may be used to illustrate the microorganisms to the patient. A brushing demonstration is then given on a model and the patient shown how to carry out the same procedure in the mouth. Disclosing tablets, a toothbrush and a pamphlet are given to reinforce the material covered. The specific technique taught for brushing is of minimal importance. Of utmost importance is the review of the technique with the patient demonstrating and the doctor or nurse making certain that the patient completely understands what is to be accomplished by the procedure. The most popular method and perhaps one of the easier methods to learn is the Bass, or modified Bass technique of brushing.[2,5] In this method a nylon brush of soft bristles, with polished ends is placed at the gingival

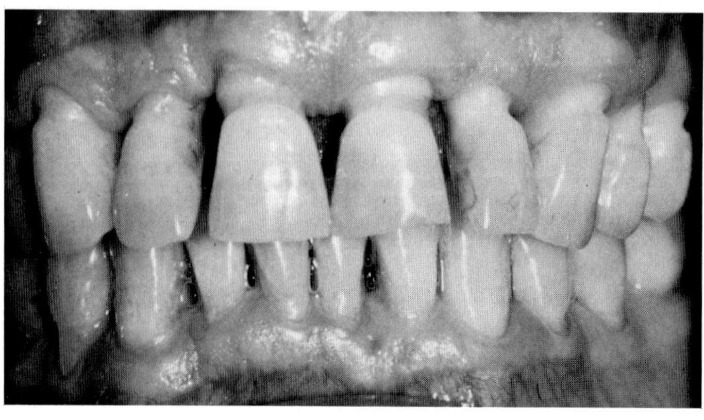

Fig. 18-2. Same patient shown in Figure 17-1 showing cervical abrasions resulting from improper flossing technique.

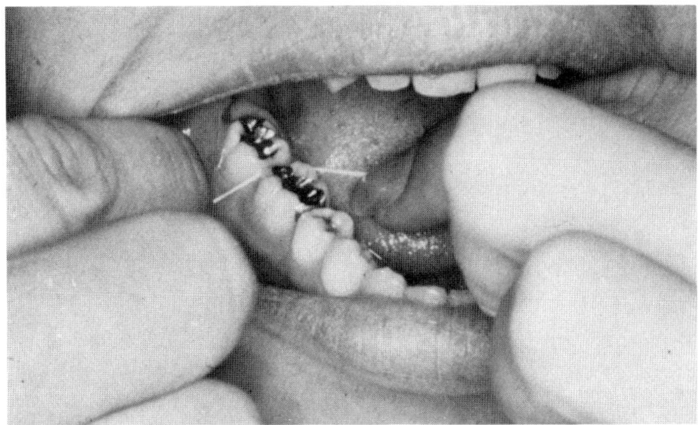

Fig. 18-3. The floss is passed through the contacts of the teeth with a back-and-forth motion to minimize gingival injury.

margin at an angle of 45° to the long axis of the tooth and is moved in a horizontal or scrub motion.

Second Visit. The second visit follows one or two days after the initial visit. The patient is given a disclosing tablet and asked to demonstrate the toothbrushing technique. Corrections are made as necessary. The use of floss is then demonstrated by film or on a model and the patient is asked to demonstrate. In children the primary means of plaque removal should be the toothbrush. Flossing is a fairly difficult procedure to learn, and if not properly mastered can result in harm through traumatic injury (Figs. 18-1, and 18-2). Therefore, its routine use as a preventive procedure in young children is not recommended. In late adolescence a flossing technique is added to the preventive program in order to better clean the interproximal surfaces of the teeth. It is unimportant whether the floss is waxed or unwaxed, the only important thing is that it be used properly and without causing injury.[4] The floss should be passed through the contacts between the teeth with a back-and-forth motion to minimize gingival injury (Fig. 18-3). Once through the contact, the floss is placed against the tooth and drawn apically as far as the gingiva permits (Fig. 18-4). The floss is then moved up and down holding it firmly against the side of one tooth 6 or 7 times; this is repeated on the side of the adjacent tooth. This procedure is repeated until all the interproximal surfaces of all the teeth have been cleaned. In

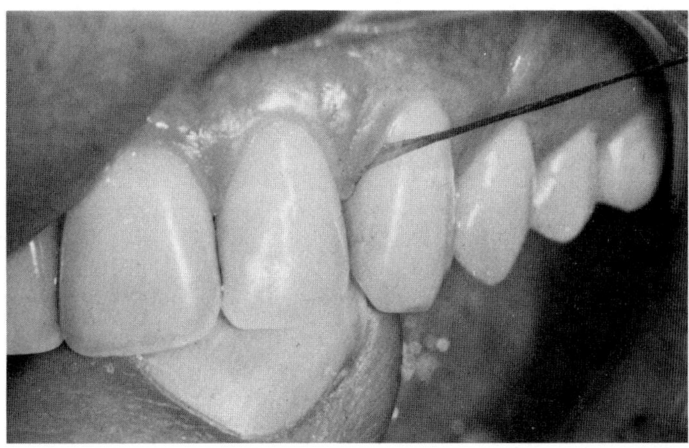

Fig. 18-4. The floss is placed against the tooth and drawn apically as far as the gingiva permits. It is then moved up and down while being held firmly against the side of one tooth six to seven times. This motion is repeated on the side of the adjacent tooth.

addition, particularly in patients who have orthodontic appliances, the use of an oral irrigation device is recommended. Although use of the irrigation devices does not remove bacterial plaque, it does remove some bacteria and bacterial products and aids in gross removal of retained food particles. The irrigation devices should be used with warm water and with minimal pressure to prevent tissue injury. The tip of the irrigator is placed perpendicular to the tooth at the junction of the gingival margin and the tooth. The tip is moved quite slowly from tooth to tooth with a sufficient pause in the interproximal areas to obtain full benefit from the water irrigation device. The lingual as well as the facial aspects of the teeth are to be cleansed in this manner. During the early phases of learning procedures, a disclosing tablet should be first used to identify the location of the bacterial plaque and a mirror used by the patient to insure the correct placement of the device and that the plaque has been thoroughly removed. The complete sequence of brushing, oral irrigation and flossing should be done at least once daily and preferably at night before retiring. Recent studies have shown that complete once-a-day removal of the bacterial plaque is sufficient to prevent it from accumulating to a degree in which it will prove to be harmful to the teeth or gingiva.

Third Visit. The third visit should come within the same week as the initial visit where possible and should consist of a review of the previously taught techniques with a critique by the control nurse. Additional cleaning aids may be added if necessary.

Fourth Visit. The final visit should be one week following the preceding visit and should consist of demonstration by the patient with a critique by the control nurse. The patient is scheduled for further checks, weekly or monthly, as deemed necessary by his progress. Considerable variation exists in the response to the control program. The dexterity and motivation is quite diverse. It is up to the control nurse to judge the progress and apply the necessary reenforcement. However, patients who, despite all attempts at motivation, do not appear to be sincerely interested in preventing future dental disease, should not be badgered. Their refusal to follow the program is entered on the record, and they are given a warning that the best dental service will fail in mouths that do not receive proper plaque control.

Diet Control

Cariogenic bacteria may colonize in pits and fissures or on smooth surfaces of teeth where they form an adherent and difficult-to-remove bacterial plaque. Although there are many varieties of cariogenic microorganisms, all are characterized by their requirement of a sucrose substrate for rapid growth. Thus, one of the most effective but difficult-to-implement methods of caries control and prevention is to reduce the intake of refined sugars, particularly those which are consumed in large quantities between meals. Effective diet control requires intelligent understanding by the parents but often fails due to lack of cooperation and understanding from the child. Nonetheless, if diet control can be instituted, it is an effective means of drastically lowering the caries attack rate. Almost total withdrawal of sugar, however, as must be practiced by the diabetic child, is neither feasible, nor desirable. Instead, acceptable noncariogenic foods and between-meal snacks should be substituted (see Table 18-1).

Fluoride. The use of fluorides in the drinking water and topical applications twice a year as well as their daily use in a dentifrice are also recommended. The daily use of a fluoride rinse after brushing, 15 drops of a 2 percent solution of sodium fluoride to one third glass of warm water, has also been shown to reduce the caries attack rate in children.[7] However, it must be remembered that fluorides only make the tooth surface more resistant to disease and do not in any way eliminate the cause.

TABLE 18-1. CARIOGENIC FOODS AND NONCARIOGENIC SUBSTITUTES

Cariogenic	Noncariogenic
Sucrose (table sugar)	Saccharin and sorbitol
Caramels and milk chocolates	Potato chips and corn chips
Jellies, jams, honey	Raw vegetables, cabbage, lettuce, fresh strawberries and cherries
Dried fruits (sugared; figs, raisins, dates)	Fresh fruits (oranges and apples)
Candies, cookies and cakes	Popcorn, peanuts
Chewing gum and mints	Sugarless gum and mints
Malted and sweet chocolate drinks	Whole and skim milk
Synthetic orange drinks	Orange juice (whole orange is best)
Colas and other beverages sweetened with sucrose	Diet colas and other diet drinks
White and raisin bread	Whole wheat bread
Peanut butter and jelly on white bread	Hamburgers, cold cuts and cheese on whole wheat bread

SUMMARY

Periodontal diseases (and dental caries) are diseases wherein colonization by bacteria on the tooth surface (plaques) are a primary factor in the progress and severity of the diseases. Local mechanical irritants and tissue health and resistance are also important determinants in periodontal diseases but both experimental and clinical observations indicate that bacterial plaque accumulations appear to be more important in the progress of these diseases if not their initiation. Because these bacterial plaques form quickly (within 3 to 6 days), removal by the dentist is not enough. Oral hygiene by the patient or his parent to prevent new accumulations of plaque is essential to the control and prevention of periodontal diseases (and caries).

The prevalence of both caries and acute gingivitis reach their peaks during the adolescent period. Preventive practices must therefore begin early—no later than adolescence—if it is to succeed.

REFERENCES

1. Arnim, S.: Prevention of dental disease. Pediatr. Clin., N. Amer., *10:*275, 1963.
2. Bass, C. C.: An effective method of personal oral hygiene. J. Louisiana State Med. Soc., *106:*57, and 101, 1954.
3. Cohen, L., and Lucye, H.: A position on dental health education. J. Sch. Health, *40:*361, 1970.[4]
4. Hill, C. H., Levi, P. A. and Glickman, I.: The effects of waxed and unwaxed dental floss on interdental plaque accumulation and interdental gingival health. J. Periodont., *44:* 411, 1973.
5. Masters, D.: Oral hygiene procedures for the periodontal patient. Dent. Clin. North Am., *16:*3, 1969.
6. Rayner, J.: Socioeconomic status and factors influencing the dental health practices of mothers. Am. J. Public Health, *60:*1250, 1970.
7. Torell, P., and Ericsson, Y.: The value in caries prevention methods for applying fluorides topically to the teeth. Int. Dent. J., *17:*564, 1967.

19

Psychophysiologic Aspects of Periodontal and Stomato-Gingival Disorders

This chapter is in essence a review of the psychophysiologic literature and represents an attempt to develop from this literature a more understandable, comprehensive and usable theory of the psychophysiologic aspects of periodontal disease.

Psychophysiological Theories

It is well known that emotional factors play a significant role in most body tissue reactions. The role may be direct in cases of self-mutilation or indirect, in cases where the emotions affect the patient's ability to properly care for himself. A deeper and less easily seen aspect is the effect of the emotions on the vascular, endocrine and exocrine systems, and eventually on the cellular levels where acid base balance, enzymatic processes and so forth respond to various emotional states. Much has been written to try to develop and substantiate valid theories which might explain the unfolding process of interaction between emotions and body states. Methods have been described by which subcortical centers in the central nervous system control visceral activity and integrate functioning at all levels down to the cellular in order to maintain the interior milieu. The following are some attempts to understand the powerful role feelings play in the genesis of illness. Jurgen Reusch proposed that the psychosomatically ill patient cannot communicate verbally in an adult manner, has regressed, and uses his body as a means of symbolic communication.[17] Psychiatrists had long proposed a conversion theory, similar to that of conversion reaction in hysteria, where emotional conflict at an unconscious level could be converted to a disease which symbolically expressed the conflict (i.e., anger being expressed through diarrhea when other means of expression were forbidden and leading to ulcerative colitis). Flanders Dunbar discarded the conversion theory of psychophysiological illness and attempted to correlate specific personality profiles with each disease such as the driving, aggressive executive personality of those suffering from peptic ulcer.[4] Margaret Gerard and Rene Spitz emphasized the predisposing factors of the mother/child relationship and the importance of the character and behavior of the mother in the genesis of psychosomatic disorders in the child.[9,19,20] Franz Alexander developed a specificity hypothesis emphasizing not superficial behavior but a nuclear emotional conflict enduring in time with prolonged specific physiological determinants eventually resulting in structural changes in the involved organ, because of chronic excessive innervation.[1] Psychological determinants included the aggressive facade of the peptic ulcer patient which concealed a hungry, yearning, profoundly dependent person whose physiologic response was to secrete hydrochloric acid and pepsin in readiness for nurturing and its accompanying warmth and affection. Alexander's theory was criticized by Grinker and others who felt psychosomatic illness represented a psychologic and physiologic regression and return to earlier undifferentiated states of organization.[13] The adult's physiology was seen as unable to stand the wide homeostatic swings that are characteristic of infancy and the result was a psychosomatic illness. H. G. Wolff suggested (as a predisposition) a specificity based on a genetically determined response pattern to a stressor (i.e., a precipating event) situation.[22] This response pattern serves a protective adaptive function but when maintained beyond tolerable limits results in tissue damage. McLean theorizing on the relationship between the brain, emotional state and physiological changes stated "the phylogenetically old brain," (the rhinencephalon) or the "visceral brain" is largely concerned with visceral and emotional functions, which brings into association all of the sensations from the eye, ear, nose, throat, and viscera as well as the genitals.[14] There are many and strong connections with the hypothalamus for discharging its impressions but this part of the brain is quite separate though connected with the neopallium, or new brain, where our intellectual functions are carried out. McLean points out that this is a clue to understanding the difference between what we "feel" and what we "know." He also points out that the psychosomatic patient, therefore, needs to be approached more on a feeling level before one can effectively reach his "animalistic and illiterate" visceral brain.

Psychoanalytic studies reveal that patients with duodenal ulcer, irrespective of their "personality type" or overt behavior, show persistence of strong infantile oral dependency wishes, marked immaturity, tendency to please and placate and tend to have problems revolving around the management of oral incorporative impulses by passivity and hostility. Weisman's feeling is that the nuclear conflict of the patient with duodenal ulcer is between both "active seeking and passive yielding" and that the conflict about oral dependent wishes is a special aspect of a passivity-activity conflict.[21] Environmental factors which induce immobilization of unconscious oral receptive incorporative wishes or serve as a threat to dependent relationships are associated with a significant but transient increase in the rate of pepsinogen excretion in apparently healthy subjects.

The work of I. A. Mirsky is particularly significant.[15] In a study of the essential determinants in the precipitation of nine cases of peptic ulcer in a group of 2073 army inductees he found the following: (1) a physiological parameter which determined the susceptibility of the duodenum to ulceration: a high rate of gastric secretion as measured by blood pepsinogen levels; (2) a psychological parameter which determined the relatively specific psychic conflict which induces psychic tensions: major unresolved and persistent conflict in the area of dependency and oral gratification as measured by Rorschach tests, Blacky tests, Draw-a-person, Cornell Medical Index and Saslow tests; and (3) a social parameter which determines the environmental event which will prove noxious to the particular individual: basic training in the army over a 16-week period.

In further support of his theory he did a long-term study of 1600 children from several months to 16 years of age and 4460 adult men and women from various socioeconomic strata. As was predicted a fairly large number of these patients developed duodenal ulcers. A fairly high rate of duodenal ulcer in children from 4 to 6 years of age and 10 to 14 years was also reported. He concluded that a duodenal ulcer should develop when an individual with a sustained rate of gastric hypersecretion is exposed to an environmental situation which mobilizes the aforementioned psychic conflict and induces psychic tensions.

Psychophysiologic disorders are different from psychogenic disorders in that they are not brought about by psychologic factors alone. An example of a psychogenic disorder is that of a conversion reaction with paralysis of a limb, blindness or abdominal pain caused by an unconscious conflict; or the sweating, trembling and weakness because of an anxiety neurosis, again directly attributable to an unconscious conflict emerging in partial fulfillment of the conflict as a physical disability. These are compromises by the ego between unacceptable impulses that strongly press for gratification and equally strong pressure denying gratification from conscience or society.

Psychophysiologic disorders, on the other hand, are those requiring certain predisposing factors along with certain precipitating social, psychologic and physiologic factors.

All illness has emotional concomitants, but in some emotions seem to play a more significant role than in others. There is an individual variation in psychophysiologic illness as to the degree that each of the determinants acts in bringing about the onset of the disease and in the course of the disease process.

Let us look at peptic ulcer from this viewpoint. The infant who has a high circulating blood pepsinogen, according to Mirsky's study, has a high secretor of stomach pepsin and acid—the predisposing physiologic determinant.[15] Beside this high level of secretion, this infant is likely to be hungry more frequently than the normal child and cry earlier and more frequently for food. If the mother of this child feeds rigidly on schedule without concern for her infant's early hunger, is frequently absent at feeding times or is particularly erratic in her feeding habits, these could be seen as the predisposing social determinant.

The psychologic determinants are the anger the baby experiences and the feelings he gets of being deprived. The baby can express his discomfort only by crying and kicking and when in addition he experiences hunger impulses from the stomach, the crying and the urgency are intensified.

Later in life a social stress situation, such as that due to loss of a job, can trigger in this person a psychological conflict around oral dependency, deprivation and anger. The high pepsinogen level, meanwhile, is present with all the determinants functioning and with no immediate response to the problem and this can result in an ulcer. The therapy for this condition requires frequent feedings and care from a significant number of people. This, in turn, partly helps to solve the problem and helps with the cure.

Periodontal and Stomato-Gingival Tissues

Several studies, notably those of Belting, *et al.* have indicated that there is an increased incidence of certain types of periodontal disease in emotionally disturbed persons.[3] Belting's findings clearly indicate that mental disturbances and periodontal disease are associated because of some unknown intrinsic factor over and above the existence of possible poor oral hygiene habits, excessive calculus or bruxism and clenching. He also felt that the severity of periodontal disease increased significantly as the degree of anxiety increased. This unknown intrinsic factor is apparently closely associated with the degree of anxiety manifested by the patient and therefore probably is under the control of the autonomic nervous system. The close relationship between the central and autonomic nervous systems is well known. Vascular changes, tissue metabolism, and endocrine function are all influenced by the autonomic system. It is, therefore, reasonable to assume that the periodontal changes seen in the psychiatric patient are mediated through one or more of these same processes.

Psychosomatic factors may also interfere with periodontal health by other means such as: (1) by reducing local nutrition through vasospasm; (2) developing objective habits which are antagonistic to the health of the periodontal tissues, such as, pencil biting and fingernail biting; (3) by inducing excessive chewing, clenching and grinding, creating excessive wear and excessive pressures; (4) by creating taste perversions causing the ingestion of foods which are locally and systemically harmful to periodontal health, such as extremely spicy or acid foods or excessive carbohydrates which create direct effects on the teeth structures; (5) by permitting insufficient food intake through limitation of gastrointestinal function, anorexia nervosa, intestinal spasm, ulcers, gall-bladder symptoms; (6) by producing neglect of oral sanitation; (7) by evolving subjective habits which are harmful to the periodontal structures, that is lip biting, cheek biting, tongue thrusting and tapping teeth together; and (8) by causing body conditions inimical to the health of the periodontal tissue.

The psychologic characteristics of patients with periodontal disease has been studied by some investigators and shown to vary according to the type of periodontal disease present (i.e., whether acute necrotizing ulcerative gingivitis, periodontitis or periodontosis.[16] A striking psychologic characteristic found as a whole in all patients with periodontal disease was the marked prevalence of oral dependency as a central life problem. As for the specific disease entities, it was found that patients with acute necrotizing ulcerative gingivitis (ANUG) tended to be either adolescents or young adults and in all instances the onset of the disease was precipitated by an acute anxiety arising from a life situation of conflict about dependency or sexual need; local factors were minimal. The patients with chronic destructive periodontitis, on the other hand, had a background of long-standing less acute conflicts mainly involving dependency needs. They tended to have considerable marital conflicts and many psychosomatic symptoms involving the gastric area, the head and neck. Bleeding gums were often noted at a time of greatest anxiety and bruxism was an extremely frequent habit. In contrast, those patients with periodontosis had much less evidence of either neurotic trends or destructive oral habits. This result suggested that degenerative oral processes were less correlated with acute emotional conflict than inflammatory processes involving primarily the soft tissues.

Therefore, it can be seen how emotional tension can create oral disease through a disturbance of the oral physiology (i.e., bruxism resulting from unrealized aggression or a change in the salivary composition caused by emotional disturbances when combined with other factors can cause oral disease). On the other hand oral deformity owing to loss of teeth, cleft palate or harelip can cause mental disturbance.

Periodontal disease, therefore, will be considered from three areas or determinants of psychophysiologic disorders, namely, psychologic, physiologic and social. These three factors will be considered from a predisposing and a precipitating viewpoint.

The predisposing aspect of the psychophysiologic condition, in the case of periodontal disease, may have occurred very early in life and in a latent state may continue to operate throughout the life of the individual. Precipitating factors are the specific psychologic, physiologic and social factors that bring about the chronic or acute symptomatic response of disturbed functioning. In each of these factors around periodontal disease we might see the predisposing psychologic factor as an old underlying fear of abandonment that developed in the course of the early parent-child interaction. Predisposing physiologic factors could be early or progressing, primitive homeostatic reactions along the line of early physical traumatic experience, general systemic stress factors and local or topical stress reactions. The predisposing social factors would be actual, geographical or emotional separation from significant figures early in the child's development significant enough to bring about the psychologic and physiologic reactions. The physiologic predisposing factors also include the genetic endowment of the child, his reactibility or lack of sensivity to stress and stimuli. It would also include his various levels of excretion both endocrine and exocrine, his available level of energy and the acuteness of his sensory system, as well as other factors of the central nervous system and body in general. Precipitating factors in the psychologic area would be emotional conflict and activation of the old underlying fear of abandonment, in the physiologic area infection or local trauma sufficient to set up a local or topical stress reaction or sufficiently widespread to set up a general systemic stress reaction. Social determinants would be the actual interpersonal interaction that set up the psychologic and physiologic stress factors. This could be a break in a relationship where one person needs another but is angry with the other person. There may be a bind in that they cannot actually escape from the situation because of fear of abandonment. Faced with no active way out the person evokes psychologic, and physiologic responses that lead to a type of escape or a potential end of the difficulty through disability. In this way the precipitating social determinant may be seemingly separate but is actually connected with the physiologic and psychologic determinants.

Predisposing Physiologic Determinants. The literature is rich in suggesting possible predisposing physiologic determinants in relation to acute necrotizing ulcerative gingivitis. The autonomic nervous system, adrenal cortical hormones, salivary changes and local neurovascular reactions have all been implicated and any or all of these mechanisms could play a part as predisposing physiologic determinants in periodontal disease. We know that the infant, in preparation for pleasurable activities in the early months of life, responds to the mother with facial animation, smiling, and that the tissues infuse with blood and the gastrointestinal tract responds as if the child were preparing to be fed. The close connection between attention of mother and feeding brings about a physiologic response. Physiologic predisposing factors thus occur because of the interplay of the sympathetic and autonomic nervous systems and the vasocenters controlling the contractile and chemical adjustment of the capillaries and their endothelia. These phenomena influence and regulate the nutrition of the capillary walls and adjacent structures and pathologic changes that occur are the result of nutritional imbalances within the tissues. Contrary to popular opinion, the primary developmental period of periodontal pathology probably also begins early in life. The really important periods may actually be from the prenatal period to adolescence with emphasis on prenatal to 6 years of age, even though the clinical manifestations do not generally arise before adolescence, and the more severe clinical manifestations may not appear until after 30 years of age. If this hypothesis of the early development of periodontal disease should prove to be true, this would accord well with the formulation given earlier of predisposing factors occurring early in development.

Predisposing Social Determinants. The mother-child relationships, the family and finally the peers and the school situation each play an important role in the child's attitudes, conflicts and physiological responses. It is interesting in this regard that oral dependency associated with inadequate parental attention has been found to be present in a large percentage of patients with periodontal disease. Another form of inadequate parental attention is that in which there is inconsistent parenting; that is, the mother is responsive to the child at times and is unavailable or unresponsive at other times. It should be remembered that in infancy and early childhood the predominant fear is that of being abandoned by the parent. Therefore, this inconsistency on the part of the mother can be the factor that provides the necessary early trauma that later in life leads to oral dependency and fear of abandonment. However, before this can occur, the child must have reached a period of awareness of the presence of and responsiveness to the mother. Weaning is another important period. Infants may react to weaning as a punishment, a rejection or a withdrawal on the part of the gratifying mother.[2] As a result, during this period the child may experience pain, anger and hurt feelings that are very intimately associated with the mouth. In cases where breast feeding lasts into the biting stage, there is a social dilemma added to a physical one in that the child must now learn how to continue sucking without biting so that the mother will not withdraw the nipple in pain or anger. One can see, therefore, how the mouth can take on the qualities of aggression and active acquisition and at the same time can become a site of potential deprivation, hurt and suffering.

There are also aggressive fantasies occurring during childhood that involve the teeth, such as the common childhood threat, "I'm going to eat you up." In this expression there is an obvious close relationship between feeding and feeling.

Feeding attitudes also have obvious dynamic inferences depending on the relationship of the feeding to the mothering at any given time. For instance, a clenching of the teeth can represent either a conscious aggressive refusal to be fed, or a negative reaction to being forced to accept food into the mouth.

Fortunately, most of the predisposing social determinants are of such a nature that the child is able to handle them through reliving them in play, shutting them out from perception at the time of their onset, or by absorbing only pieces of the experience. Perhaps, as an alternative solution, some feelings and ideas are added to an unconscious conflict around fears of abandonment and feelings of deprivation.

Predisposing Psychological Determinants. In periodontal disease the predisposing psychological determinant could be a conflict between the primitive extreme dependency the child has toward mother and an attitude of extreme anger with mother because of early disturbances in the child-mother relationship. The disturbance in the relationship implies a failure of mother and child to mesh successfully during the very early years of development. This could be due to an interplay of factors mentioned earlier, that is, the child's genetic endowment could, through an unusual sensitivity or insensitivity, require more or less contact from mother in order to satisfy the needs. It is well known that physiologic states in children vary from exquisite sensitivity to relative insensitivity with a resulting lack of harmony depending on the mother's temperament and sensitivity. In other words, a child very sensitive to separation would require more time from mother and perhaps suffer more trauma if mother were unusually absent for one reason or another.

Inconsistency in parenting could be responded to with a combination of emotional and physiological responses mentioned earlier and then later go on to feelings of oral deprivation and fear of abandonment. The deprivation resulting from episodes of inconsistency, where mother was expected but did not appear, or when arriving did so with a change in feeling tone that the infant sensed as rejection, could lead to oral dependency or a continuing need for gratification of early unmet needs around feeding and fear of separation from mother or abandonment.

The role that each small trauma plays in the eventual clinical symptoms of the various periodontal diseases might possibly be considered as the final insult that resulted in the clinical signs and symptoms of the disease. Traumatic experiences can readily result if a child is subjected to stimuli which come in such abundance and concentration or intensity that he cannot assimilate, digest and master them. It should be remembered that the child has not developed the protective shell that adults have built from repeated experiences. Anna Freud speaks of trauma of this nature as so overwhelming the ego that the child is unable to perform the usual ego functions of perception, integration and the executive function of acting on the incoming stimuli.[7] She sees this as a destructive experience which the child must relive perhaps many times in his play in an attempt to gain mastery and resolution. Traumatic experiences of this nature have very little learning value and none at all when the ego is overwhelmed. Perhaps pieces of the bad experience are taken in and the child in his attempt to form a meaningful pattern forms his own very distorted one. His distortion of what occurred may at times be considerable but fortunately, it diminishes as the child grows and becomes capable of operational thinking. This happens at about a year and a half to six years of age.

In view of the physiological, psychological and social predisposing factors, we must look carefully at the developmental phases early as well as later in adolescence when the precipitating factors may bring about the overt disease process.

If in truth, periodontal disease goes through a latent process first, it may be unrecognizable with our current method of study. In order to exert proper preventive measures they would have to be undertaken with an understanding of the early predisposing factors—physiological, psychological and social—that would be influential in the later development of the disease process. First there would have to be an awareness of the genetic disposition of the periodontal tissues. Then there would have to be an understanding of the neurologic mediation and physiologic changes occurring in the salivary, vascular and endocrine processes in conjunction with stimulation in response to the normal social and psychological experiences of early development. These experiences at times are imprinted by certain traumatic situations that could later, under stressful circumstances, evolve into the pathologic changes characteristic of the various periodontal diseases.

Precipitating Physiological Determinants. Little is known about the role of physiologic determinants for either periodontitis or periodontosis. Studies however, have shown that the physiological precipitating determinants for acute necrotizing ulcerative gingivitis may be preexisting gingivitis, recent extractions or other trauma about the mouth, as well as hospitalization for other illnesses or operations not connected directly with the mouth.[10,12,18] Social experiences accompanied by considerable drinking which result in fatigue, and psychological situations which cause feelings of guilt and which can also produce fatigue may, through the fact that they do produce fatigue, act as physiological determinants. Fatigue, tension and strain can cause a decrease in circulating antibodies. It is also a well-known fact that salivary factors and the endocrine glands are affected by emotional stimuli that may also play a role as precipitating physiological determinants.

Precipitating Psychological Determinants. The precipitating psychological determinants are states of anxiety or alarm set off by a threat, an actual rejection or abandonment. This could be associated with a collision between the patient and the assumed standards or value system of the parent or parent substitute. The patient feels morbidly dependent on this person and the dependency is resented. When the relationship is disturbed the patient reacts with intense hostility and bitter resentment. The hostility dilutes the anxiety about the possible separation, since, if the person is bad, unworthy or cruel, he is no great loss to the patient. In psychotherapy these reactions can be traced back to feelings of fear of abandonment early in life and frequently have been substantiated by actual or emotional separation from significant figures during early childhood development.

Investigators using a word association test and an interview evaluated a group of patients with gingivitis and acute necrotizing ulcerative gingivitis and noted that the acute necrotizing ulcerative gingivitis group was more seriously disturbed than the gingivitis group and the amount of recent stress experience differed considerably between the groups.[11] Members of the acute necrotizing ulcerative gingivitis group showed either a moderate degree of tension, had a serious problem giving the individuals a good deal of worry but not incapaciting them, or felt overwhelmed with the tension spilling over into other areas of their life. Sexual, family, vocational, and educational maladjustment were present in a preponderance of these patients. The ANUG group was almost four years younger than the other and 41 percent of them had undergone either severe or moderate stress just prior to their illness, while only 15 percent of the gingivitis group had suffered any type of difficulty. The ANUG group were people who generally were more unstable and tended to lead unhappier lives. The acute anxiety present as a precipitating psychologic determinant was associated with separation from loved ones and was exaggerated by predisposing psychologic determinants of ambivalence and conflict around oral dependency needs. In fact, oral dependency was the outstanding character pattern of patients with necrotizing ulcerative gingivitis.[16] When there is a conflict between the need to be dependent and the wish to be independent, ambivalence can result; that is, feelings of an unconscious need and love for the person the patient depends upon and an unconscious hatred of that person for permitting the dependent relationship can occur simultaneously. These feelings have their source in childhood and the person these feelings are invested in is usually a parent or a parent substitute.

Inadequate parental attention is a characteristic of early deprivation or overprotection. Overprotective mothers may cause their children to be either immature and overdependent, or may cause them to attempt to rebel and break the independency. This concept agrees with the findings that there is a very high correlation between dominance-nonsubmissive ratings on the Edward personal preference profile and a broader representation of ANUG patients than would be anticiapted.

Precipitating Social Determinants. In a study that compared 41 preflight students who had acute necrotizing ulcerative gingivitis with 41 normal control students, it was found that the personality profile of the students with ANUG was significantly higher in their dominance-nonsubmissive scores than was the control group.[6] It was felt that such a dominant individual would not be able to argue for his point of view and would be unable to exert leadership in the indoctrination phase of his military training. Also, this type of individual would lack the ability to humble himself when required as a trainee. Therefore, he would find it difficult to adjust to the military situation. In this way, the social determinant could become a precipitating factor in the onset of the acute necrotizing ulcerative gingivitis. As can be seen, the social predisposing determinants can shade into the social precipitating determinants.

In other studies involving military personnel it was found that the time of entering the army was particularly significant in the onset of acute necrotizing ulcerative gingivitis.[12] Visits home could stir up feelings concerning a coming separation as well as feelings concerning the entrance into the service.

Episodes of sexual searching which occur in a very dependent oral individual can be interpreted as an extension of fear of further separation from the person on whom he depends, whether it be mother or spouse, with the production of guilt and anxiety. If the individual followed through with a new sexual alliance, there was always the fear of separation from the earlier dependency bond, as well as concern over the reliability of the new dependency bond that was formed. In this way, the ambivalent conflict around the dependency and the unhappiness over the need to be dependent and the wish for independence can be understood in terms of the sexual searching behavior. This, in turn, leads to the psychological precipitating determinants which were discussed earlier.

Patient Management

Patient management will also be discussed from the standpoint of predisposing and precipitating determinants; however, here the physiological, social and psychological factors blend. Though separating them for examination and increased understanding is a very difficult task, it is helpful in exploring methods of management.

After the age of 2 years at which time the child has his full complement of primary teeth, there is a lag of approximately 4 or 5 years before his first permanent teeth appear. By that time he may have had traumatic oral experiences, such as a tonsillectomy, pain from a traumatic tooth or from a restorative procedure, or premature loss of some of his teeth.[2] At the age of 6 years with the eruption of the permanent teeth and loss of primary teeth, there is again a renewed and more active focus on the teeth with a variety of associated feelings that depend upon fateful circumstances for their management. From the point of view of teeth as possessions, the child may experience shameful embarrassment and humiliation about the loss of teeth and he may be constantly bombarded with warnings about neglecting his teeth. The adolescent, however, runs the gamut of vacillating between being very concerned about his teeth to appearing to be very nonchalant about his teeth, his appearance and care of himself, all depending on the role the teeth and the mouth play in his current peer relationship.

The dentist himself is a predisposing social determinant in his handling of the child and adolescent. It is, therefore, important for the dentist to engender a feeling of safety in the child patient so that he does not feel abandoned by those to whom he looks for protection and security.[5] The dentist can positive-condition the child by treating him with respect and according him a certain dignity, personal pleasantness and cordiality and letting the child know that the dentist likes him. The dentist should also give the child a period of familiarization with the office through early painless experiences so that the child can cope successfully initially and strengthen his inner resources for handling such situations in the future. Permitting the child to see the parents in a dental situation and helping the child to relax during his sessions are other positive ways of conditioning the child. Once the dental work is started, thought processes go on continuously and vividly. The dental patient is continuously stimulated by thoughts of the dental tray, the lighting, the condition of the equipment, the view, interruptions, the dentist's manner and fingers and his slight clumsiness, the sound of air jets, nozzles, self-awareness of tensions, the condition of the headrest, the elevating and lowering of the dental chair, the peculiar positions of the dentist as he works in various parts of the mouth, the white gown, and the patient's own localized sensations such as salivation and his taste.[8] It is almost impossible for the patient not to have heightened self-awareness once dental work is going on. Some patients keep their eyes closed with marked sensation of inner tension and pressure; some open their eyes at times when there is any change of procedure, but all patients are in a position to manifest as much outward control as possible in order to be cooperative as continual thoughts of harm, hurt and pain are being born. Feelings of inner shame, comparison with other patients and reflections on what the dentist will think of them are very close to awareness in many people. As the dentist repeats many procedures, is interested in the techniques and mechanical procedures, he should never be unmindful of the psychic phenomena that are continually going on and which are as important as the more impersonal scientific aspects of the procedure.

The dentist's awareness of the psychological predisposing determinant as it operates in the children he sees should be directed first toward the recognition of any emotional disturbance between mother and child, and later between child and family. Most dentists can sense the inconsistent parenting or the smothering parent. If such a situation is suspected, the next step is for the dentist to refer these troubled parents for help for the psychological management of their child. The tendency in the past has been for dentists to be somewhat hesitant to make a psychiatric referral. However, once the parent knows the dentist, the most seemingly unapproachable parent may actually be quite grateful for a referral to an agency or person skilled in dealing with emotional problems. It is important to help the parent view the problem as one necessary for the eventual welfare of their child and as a preventive measure rather than one directed primarily toward their own difficulties. The dentist himself can help in his procedure by his consistency in keeping appointments, his warmth and understanding as well as his nonjudgmental attitude toward the parent and the child. This should in no way interfere with the firmness necessary in dealing with both parent and child.

In those instances where the patient is extremely apprehensive about the dental procedure, a careful discussion of what will be done is important in the treatment. In some patients it is better to discuss the problem before any treatment is started, while in others it might be wiser to withhold this information until some exploratory examination and preparations have been completed. In general, it is important not to press the patient in these areas, but to wait until he is able to discuss them openly.

The physiologic predisposing determinant is associated with local stress situations, such as mechanical trauma to the gingival or periodontal tissues, the gnashing or grinding of the teeth or some other destructive dental habit. Many times if the dentist discusses the destructive habit with the child-patient and the family it can be very effective in preventing the development of certain types of periodontal or oral diseases.

The physiologic precipitating determinant, in contrast to the predisposing physiologic determinant, is a general systemic stress factor induced by anxiety related to the fear of abandonment, that is, rejection activating an old underlying fear of abandonment. This factor would come to the dentist's attention by the history of social trauma in the nature of a separation or rejection and would, therefore, in addition to the local dental management, require the handling of the social precipitating determinant.

In addition to the physiologic, psychologic and social determinants predisposing or precipitating a periodontal disorder, there are certain other facts that should be known in dealing with adolescent patients. First, the dentist should be aware that there are certain developmental tasks the adolescent must struggle with and overcome before he is able to see himself as an individual who is competent to perform in an adult way, making choices regarding his life's activities and his relationships with people. The adolescent patient behaves differently depending on the particular stage he is going through, the intensity of the relationships with his parents and the struggle around separation from parents and parent figures. Age is no criterion of the maturational level and many adolescents well into puberty are still interacting at the maturational level of the latency age child (i.e., 7 to 11 years of age).

One of the most important procedures in dealing with the adolescent is to discuss honestly and clearly what is coming next in terms he can understand. The problem as the dentist sees it and the necessary steps that must be undertaken in correcting the problem have to be very carefully and clearly communicated to the patient. Since one of the greatest fears for the patient undergoing dental care is fear of the unknown, it is necessary in dealing with adolescents to be absolutely honest and not to permit prejudices to interfere with the routine of the treatment. Adolescents are very sensitive to prejudices and feelings of impatience and disapproval even though they themselves may be very prejudiced, impatient and disapproving. It is a mistake to try to go from the position of expert and in a sense parent substitute to one of equality and camaraderie. In the long run it has been shown over and over again that the adolescent does not want a pal when he goes to see an expert. When a dentist is confronted by aggressive or defiant behavior, he must clearly understand that this may not be toward him as a person but toward adults or parent figures. If he can view it in this way, impersonally, he is in a much better position to be patient with the adolescent's anger and defiance. Following a treatment session, adolescents may show resentment and hostility for having been put in a defenseless, dependent position; or there may be a reaction formation to this, that is, after finding themselves at the mercy of the dentist in the dental situation, they may repress these feelings and instead show submission and acceptance.

A further consideration in dealing with adolescents is their sensitivity to defect and perhaps tooth extraction. It is necessary, therefore, to clearly define not only any procedure that might have a cosmetic effect but also the time necessary to institute such procedures.

A number of other important considerations have to do with the fact that the more patients do open up about themselves the more frequently they are likely to have feelings of discomfort and perhaps distrust. As a result, resistance may develop so that in subsequent sessions there may be a period when these patients will wish not to talk about themselves. The dentist must be aware of such behavior so that he will not take it as a personal disapproval on the part of the patient toward him, but will recognize it as a sign of their initial trust and the strength of the impulse to uncover their inner conflict.

REFERENCES

1. Alexander, F., and French, T. P., Psychosomatic Specificity. vol. I., University of Chicago Press, 1968.
2. Belmont, H. S., The development of the oral cavity as related to the development of the total personality. J.D.Med. *19*:86, 1964.
3. Belting, C., and Gupta, O. P.: The influence of psychiatric disturbances of the severity of periodontal disease. J. Periodont., 1961.
4. Dunbar, H. F.: Emotions and Bodily Changes. New York, Columbia University Press, 1935.
5. Fisher, G. C.: Management of fear in the child patient. J. Amer. Den. Assoc. *57*:792, 1958.
6. Formicola, A. J., Witte, E. T., and Curran, P. M.: Ulcerative gingivitis. J. Periodont. *41*:36, 1970.
7. Freud, A.: Normality and Pathology in Childhood. New York, International University Press, 1965.
8. Friend, M. R.: Everyday psychiatric problems of dentistry. N. Y. J. Dent., Vol. 23, 1954.
9. Gerard, M.: Genesis of Psychosomatic Symptoms in Infancy—The Psychosomatic Concept in Psychoanalysis. New York, International University Press, 1953.
10. Giddon, D. B., Zackin, S. K., and Goldhaber, P.: Acute necrotizing ulcerative gingivitis in college students. J.A.D.A., *68*:381, 1964.
11. Goldberg, H., Ambinder, W. J., Cooper, A. L., and Abrams, A. L.: Emotional status of patients with acute gingivitis. N.Y. State Dent. J., *22*:308, 1956.

12. Goldhaber, P., and Giddon, D. B.: Present concepts concerning the etiology and treatment of acute necrotizing ulcerative gingivitis. Int. Dent. J., *14*:468, 1963.
13. Grinker, R. R.: The physiology of emotions. *In* Simon, A., Herbert, C. C., and Strauss, R. (eds.): The Physiology of Emotions. Springfield, Ill., Charles C Thomas, 1961.
14. McLean, P. D.: The limbic system (visceral brain) in relation to central gray and reticulum of the brain stem. Psychosom. Med., *17*:355, 1955.
15. Mirsky, I. A.: Physiologic, psychologic and social determinants in the etiology of duodenal ulcer. Am. J. Dig. Dis. *3*:247, 1958.
16. Moulton, R., Ewen, S., and Thieman, W.: Emotional factors in periodontal disease. Oral Surg., *5*:833, 1952.
17. Reusch, J.: The infantile personality: the core problem of psychosomatic medicine. Psychosom. Med., *10*:134, 1938.
18. Schluger, S.: Necrotizing ulcerative gingivitis in the army: incidence, communicability and treatment. J.A.D.A., *38*:174, 1949.
19. Spitz, R. A.: Hospitalism: an inquiry into the genesis of psychiatric conditions in early childhood. Psychoanal. Study Child, *1*:53, 1945.
20. Spitz, R. A.: Relevancy of direct infant observations. Psychoanal. Study Child, *5*:66, 1950.
21. Weisman, E.: Diagnosis and treatment of gingival and periodontal disorders in children with cerebral palsy. J. Dent. Child., *23*:73, 1956.
22. Wolff, H. G.: Life stress and bodily disease; formulation. A. Res. Nerv. Ment. Dis. Proc., *29*:1659, 1950.

20

Retained Primary Tooth Fragments and Periodontal Lesions

Primary tooth fragments can cause isolated periodontal lesions about teeth in the permanent dentition as seen in Figure 20-1, and Figure 20-2. (See also Fig. 10-2 and Fig. 10-20 and the discussion of primary teeth and periodontosis in Chap. 10.) Recently a method of classifying these tooth fragments, based upon the roentgenographic location of the fragment to the alveolar crest, was devised. (See Table 20-1.)[2]

TABLE 20-1. CLASSIFICATION OF RETAINED TOOTH FRAGMENTS

Class 1 – Fragment apical to alveolar crest
Class 2 – Fragment partially apical to alveolar crest
Class 3 – Fragment coronal to alveolar crest.

Etiology. There are apparently two basic processes by which this phenomena occurs.[1,2] First, there may be irregularities in the resorption and shedding processes, such as those shown in Figure 20-3, and Figure 20-4, whereby the erupting permanent tooth slips past the apical portion of the primary tooth and results in resorption coronal to the root apex.

The second basic situation relates to the fracture of a primary root which occurs during extraction and which may be deliberately left in place. If this fractured root is not left in place the underlying permanent tooth may be damaged with the efforts made to remove it.

Treatment of Periodontal Lesion. Removal of tooth fragment is usually sufficient therapy. In those instances where the fragment is located apical to the alveolar crest, the fragment should be removed and the infrabony defect should be treated separately. (See Chap. 10, Fig. 10-2.)

REFERENCES

1. Gleckner, J. F., and Hurt, W. C.: Retained deciduous root tips and intrabony pocket formation. Armed Forces Med. J. *11*:1049, 1960.
2. Mahan, C. J., and Hurt, W. C.: Retained deciduous tooth fragments and periodontal lesions: Radiographic, Clinical and histologic observations. Oral Surg. *35*:708, 1973.

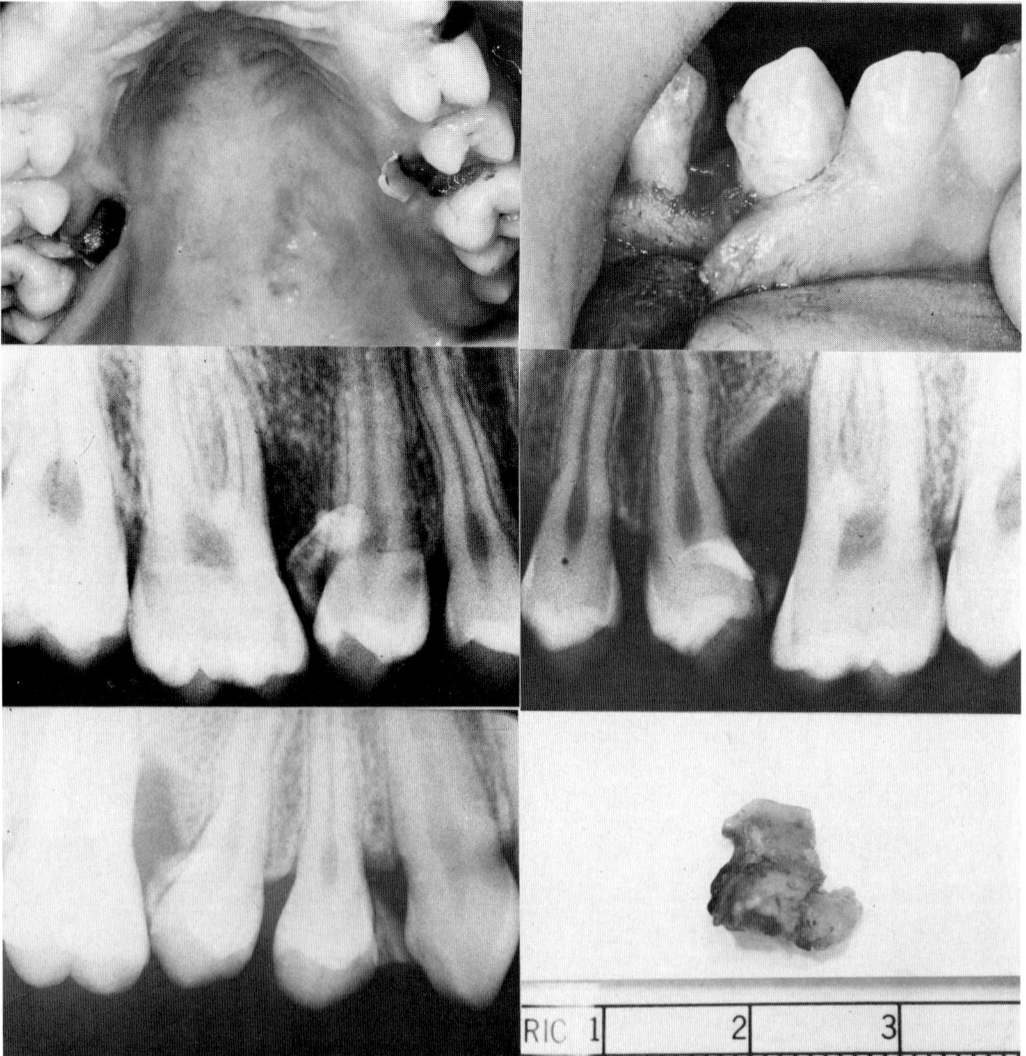

Fig. 20-1. A 15-year-old female. *Top left.* This clinical photograph shows retained primary tooth fragments between the first molar and the second bicuspids on the palatal surface, and the buccal surface between the cuspid and the first bicuspid. *Top right.* A clinical view of the 11-12 area, revealing bone loss not apparent on the roentgenogram. *Center left.* A roentgenograph of the 13-14 area, showing the retained fragment and the adjacent radiolucent area. *Center right.* The retained fragment and adjacent radiolucency in the 3-4 area. *Bottom left.* A retained fragment in the 11-12 area and another in the 13-14 area. *Bottom right.* A specimen of the 3-4 area of biopsy. (Courtesy of C. J. Mahan and W. C. Hurt.)[2]

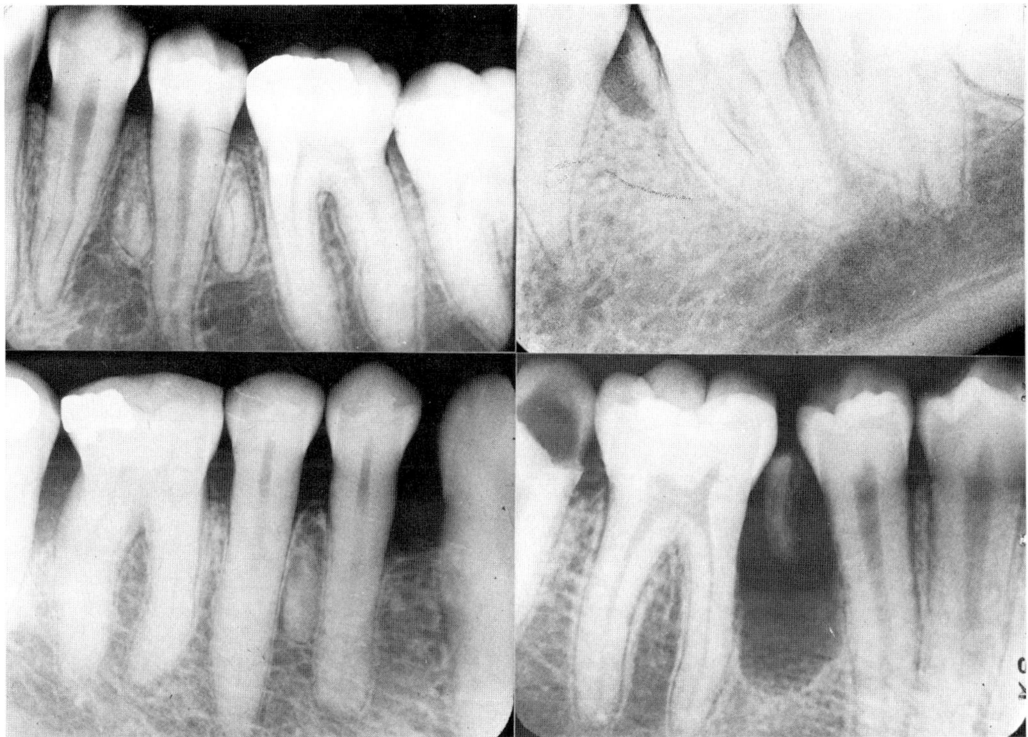

Fig. 20-2. A 16-year-old female. *Top left.* Class 1 retained primary tooth fragments. *Top right.* A Class 1 retained primary tooth fragment with some evidence of resorption of the alveolar crest. *Bottom left.* A Class 2 retained primary tooth fragment between the roots of the permanent bicuspids. *Bottom right.* A Class 3 retained primary tooth fragment showing evidence of an extensive periodontal lesion in a 15-year-old boy. (Courtesy of C. J. Mahan and W. C. Hurt.)[2]

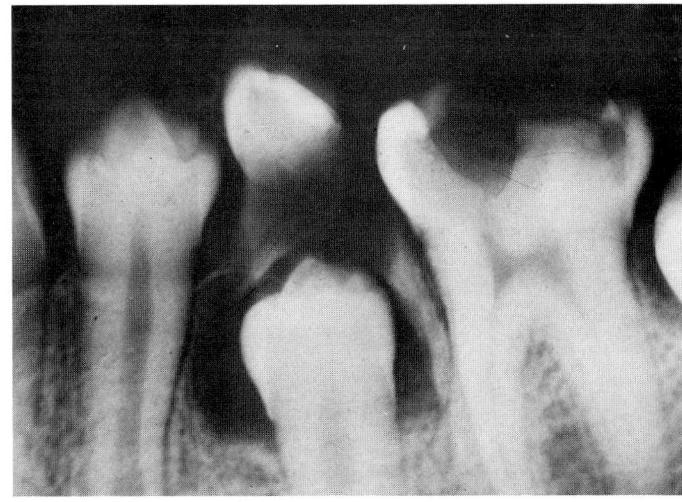

Fig. 20-3. Evidence of lateral root resorption of a primary second molar in a 10-year-old boy. The crown of the erupting second premolar has moved past the widely divergent root apices of its predecessor. (Courtesy of Dr. Richard E. Jennings.)

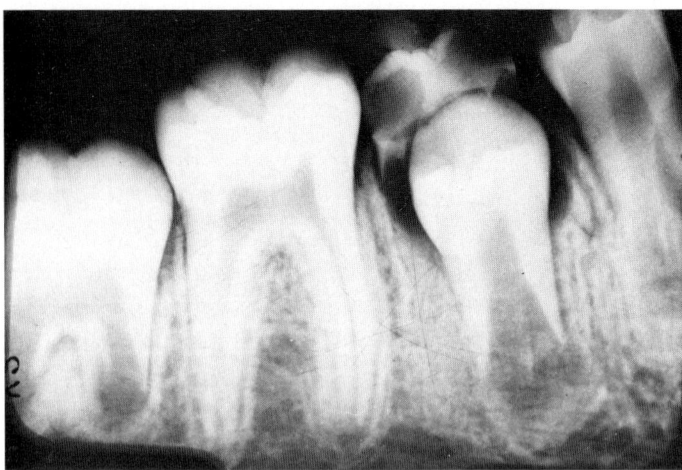

Fig. 20-4. A variation in the eruptive and resorptive events that could lead to a Class 2 or Class 3 retained primary root fragment. (Courtesy of C. J. Mahan and W. C. Hurt.)[2]

Index

Numerals in italics indicate a figure, "t" following a page number indicates a table.

B

C

H

N

O

P

R

S